Portland Community College

WITHDRAWN

Pain

PAIN
DYNAMICS AND
COMPLEXITIES

Daniel M. Doleys, PhD

Director, The Doleys Clinic and Pain and Rehabilitation Institute

Birmingham, Alabama

OXFORD
UNIVERSITY PRESS

OXFORD
UNIVERSITY PRESS

Oxford University Press is a department of the University of Oxford.
It furthers the University's objective of excellence in research, scholarship,
and education by publishing worldwide.

Oxford   New York
Auckland   Cape Town   Dar es Salaam   Hong Kong   Karachi
Kuala Lumpur   Madrid   Melbourne   Mexico City   Nairobi
New Delhi   Shanghai   Taipei   Toronto

With offices in
Argentina   Austria   Brazil   Chile   Czech Republic   France   Greece
Guatemala   Hungary   Italy   Japan   Poland   Portugal   Singapore
South Korea   Switzerland   Thailand   Turkey   Ukraine   Vietnam

Oxford is a registered trademark of Oxford University Press
in the UK and certain other countries.

Published in the United States of America by
Oxford University Press
198 Madison Avenue, New York, NY 10016

Library of Congress Cataloging-in-Publication Data
Doleys, Daniel M., author.
Pain: dynamics and complexities / by Daniel M. Doleys.
   p.; cm.
Includes bibliographical references and index.
ISBN 978–0–19–933153–6 (alk. paper)
I. Title.
[DNLM: 1. Chronic Pain. WL 704]
RB127
616'.0472—dc23
2013034353

9 8 7 6 5 4 3 2 1
Printed in the United States of America
on acid-free paper

To my parents, Julia and John, to my father-in-law, Rev. H. T. Henderson, and to my children, Thomas, Dannette, Nicholas, and Brad.

To the thousands of patients with chronic pain who entrusted our clinic with their story and care.

And most especially to my wife, Sue, for her patience endurance and support during the long days and weeks in the office and all those working "vacations." She cannot imagine the influence her love, intellect, and insight have had on this project.

Contents

Preface

This book is a mixture of neuroscience, psychology, and philosophy of science. It is designed to present the evolving concept and complex nature of pain, especially chronic pain. It does so by reviewing the history of pain and outlining the current concepts and theories regarding the mechanisms involved in the experience of pain. The experimental and clinical research in a broad number of areas, including infant pain, empathy and pain, psychogenic pain (medically unexplained symptoms), and genetics and pain is summarized. The notion of pain as a disease process rather than a symptom is also highlighted.

Although there is continued interest in activation of the peripheral nociceptive system as a determining factor in the experience of pain, there is a growing appreciation for the brain as the ultimate pain-generator, this is noted here. The definition of consciousness and conscious awareness and a theory as to how it relates to nociceptive processing is also outlined. In addition to putting the study of pain in an historical perspective and summarizing current research and theories, the manner in which concepts from systems theory to quantum theory can be applied is illustrated. A rationale for considering pain as an emergent phenomenon and hypothetical construct is also outlined. In part, the intent of *Pain: Dynamics and Complexities* is to encourage and promote a broadening of the existing paradigm within which pain is viewed and understood.

The book is designed primarily for health care professionals, paraprofessionals, academicians, and students interested in pain. This book is not a clinician or patient manual. There are, however, illustrations of how experimental and clinical research can be being translated into treatment options and provide implications of a broader view of pain for future therapies. Although many of the chapters contain a summary of the relevant research, no attempt was made to conduct an exhaustive review of the literature. Commentary, clinical anecdote, and observation are used to provide real-life illustrations, when appropriate.

Daniel M. Doleys

Acknowledgments

I owe a debt of gratitude to Andrea Miller, Carolyn Holmes, and Erin Thrift for their invaluable assistance in obtaining the many references needed for this book. I appreciate Doctor Roger Fillingim's thoughtful review and comments on Genetics and Pain (Chapter 12), and those of Doctor Michael Ferrante on Pain Mechanisms and Types (Chapter 3) and Pain and the Brain (Chapter 4). My interest in and understanding of pain were greatly influenced by my interactions with Doctors Richard North, Peter Staats, Sam Hassenbusch, Hugh Rosomoff, and Jaimie Henderson. Special thanks are owed to Doctor Thomas Kraus. His passion for his work and his insistence that his patients participate in their care is a model for all pain clinicians. Finally, I thank Doctor Kenneth Follett, clearly one of the most thoughtful and systematic persons I have encountered. In my many conversations with Ken, I learned to think beyond the facts. In one way or another, each of these individuals, knowingly or unknowingly, stimulated critical thinking and expanded my conceptual horizons in the area of pain.

Acknowledgment

1 Introduction

For all the happiness mankind can gain is not in pleasure, but in rest from pain.

–John Dryden, *17th century English poet and playwright*

SCOPE OF THE PROBLEM

Pain is perhaps the most fundamental, complex, and common of all human experiences. Chronic pain results in limitations in daily function and physical activities, compromised emotional health, impaired quality of life, and a significant increase in health care utilization. Pain knows no gender, age, ethnic, or socioeconomic boundaries. People with chronic pain represent the largest group of individuals with a long-term disability. About 90% of the U.S. population will experience pain, and 30–50% (some 100 million adults) will go on to have chronic pain. The estimated health care cost (in 2010 dollars) ranges from $261 to $300 billion, and the loss of work productivity from $299 to $335 billion. In 1996 the total cost of chronic non-cancer pain was $150 billion and the average cost of treatment per patient approximately $35,000.00 per year. The health care costs for patients in moderate pain are some $4,200.00 more per year than a person in no pain and about $7,700 more for those in severe pain (Gaskin and Richard, 2012). The overall emotional impact of chronic pain is reflected in the lifetime prevalence among patients expressing their wish to die: it is 1.47 times higher than that for non-patients. Patients in pain report an "active" suicidal ideation or plan up to six times more than non-pain controls, and suicidal attempts occur 14% more often (Fishbain, 1999; Fishbain et al, 2008).

The American Pain Society (APS) estimates that some 50 million Americans live with some type of chronic pain (Quinlan-Colwell, 2008). The origin of pain varies widely and includes those with a genetic basis, such as sickle cell anemia or osteogenesis imperfecta, pain intrinsic to another disorder, such as rheumatoid arthritis (RA) or fibromyalgia, or pain as a consequence of injury, illness, surgery, cancer, or aging. Cancer-related pain and headache (HA) each account for about 10%, and neck/back and musculoskeletal/joint pain make up 30% of chronic pain. The 2008 U.S. Census report on persons over the age of 18 years complaining of pain in the low back, neck, face, or jaw or with HA indicated that of those reporting persistent pain, 51% were 18 to 44 years of age, and 33% were 44 to 64 years old. Approximately 57% of those reporting a disability were 16 to 64 years of age. Some 52% were women; 83.8% were white and 11.5% were African American (Quinlan-Colwell, 2008).

DEFINITIONS OF PAIN

Pain appears to be one of those events in life that nearly everyone experiences. Yet, it seems to defy description. The concept of pain seems clear enough but remains elusive and continually evolving. Attempting to define it has been a like trying to capture smoke in a net. Below are some of the many definitions of *pain*, beginning with the one offered by the International Association for the Study of Pain (IASP), which is the most frequently quoted and adhered to among pain-oriented societies, clinicians, and researchers.

Pain is an unpleasant sensory and emotional experience associated with actual or potential tissue damage, or described in terms of such damage. (Merskey and Bogduk, 1994, p. 210)

Pain is that sensory experience evoked by stimuli that injure or threaten to destroy tissue, defined introspectively by every man as that which hurts. Pain is composed of a separate and distinct sensation and the individual's reaction to pain. The adequate stimulus for pain is the rate of destruction of tissues innervated by pain fibers. (Mountcastle, 1974, p. 349)

Pain is an enigma. It differs from the classical senses (vision, hearing, touch, taste, and smell) because it is both a discriminative sensation and a graded motivation (or behavioral drive). It is a leading clinical complaint that can present mystifying symptoms, such as allodynia (sensitization to normally innocuous stimuli), referral from deep tissue to skin, radiation over wide regions, temporal summation (windup), persistent after-sensations, emotional variability, and hyperpathia (hysterical responses). It can attain intolerable intensity, but it can disappear in the heat of battle. It is a universal human experience that is commonly generalized to psychic suffering of any sort. (Craig, 2003, p. 1)

Pain is a multidimensional sensory experience that is intrinsically unpleasant and associated with hurting and soreness. It may vary in intensity (mild, moderate, or severe), quality (sharp, burning or dull), duration (transient, intermittent, or persistent) and referral (superficial or deep, localized or diffuse). Although essentially a sensation, pain has strong cognitive and emotional components; it is linked to, or described in terms of, suffering. It is also associated with avoidance motor reflexes and alterations in autonomic output. All of these traits are inextricably linked in the experience of pain. (Woolf, 2004, p. 441)

Pain, like all subjective experiences, has no contents. It is about something and that something is the process and neural representation of nociception, but it has no substance, nothing to measure or to observe- no contents. Pain is an experience, not an emotion. Surprise, fear, grief or anger that are evoked by pain are emotion, pain is not. Pain therefore, is a state of consciousness, a subjective experience. (Moskovitz, 2011, p. 13)

[Pain is a] homeostatic emotion.... [I]t is represented by the forebrain integration of both specific labeled lines and convergent somatic activity in a well-organized hierarchical system that subserves homeostasis.... [I]t is one aspect of the representation of the physiological condition of the body (interoception). (Craig, 2003, p. 4)

In 2009, the American Academy of Pain Medicine (AAPM) recommended separating pain into two broad categories: eudynia and maldynia. *Eudynia*

is *physiological pain* that describes a nociceptive process beginning with a noxious stimulus and then ascending from the point of tissue stimulation to the brain through the peripheral and central nervous systems. Eudynia refers to pain as a symptom of an underlying pathological disorder, either an illness or an injury. (Dubois et al, 2009, p. 983)

Maldynia denotes

pathological pain... [or] a neuropathological disorder or disease process that occurs due to changes at the cellular and molecular levels. Maldynia is usually the result of an injury to the nervous system; however, maldynia can result from a persistent and intractable eudynia, and can persist due to neuropathological changes in the nervous system even when the initial tissue pathology is no longer present. It serves no useful purpose and is destructive to the organism. It can shorten lifespan, inhibit function and ability to work, frequently causes psychiatric disorders, and is associated with suicidal ideation and suicide. (Dubois et al, 2009, p. 983)

Maldynia is viewed as a failure of the organism's homeostatic pain modulatory system.

One's perspective on pain tends to guide the structure of the definition. Most often pain is interpreted as a consequence of an injury, tissue or nerve damage, or an accompanying symptom to a disorder or disease state. Considerable effort has been put into discovering the neurophysiological and neurochemical aspects of nociception. However, this pain-transmission system appears to function in a nonlinear fashion. That is, the pain experienced is not proportional to the degree of physical damage. Furthermore, pain processing can be quite different for acute, chronic, and cancer-related pain, and for neonates and infants compared to pain processing in adults. Using a fractal dimension analysis, Foss et al (2006) demonstrated that nociceptive and neuropathic pain possessed unique characteristics. In addition, the peripheral nociceptive system does not explain phenomena such as socially mediated analgesia and hyperalgesia found in both animals and humans. Melzack's observations regarding the disconnect between the degree of physical pathology and pain, as well as the occurrence of pain in the absence of any activation of the peripheral nociceptive system, led to the development of his neuromatrix theory (see Chapter 5). This and other similar theories attempt to explain how the experience of pain can be generated by the brain itself.

The notion of pain as a sensation with an emotional or affective component appears common among many definitions. The idea of a "hierarchical system that subserves homeostasis" (Craig, 2003) is unique and may well represent a paradigm shift in the way pain is understood. It implies that pain encompasses and emerges from a complex interplay among many aspects of the system (organism) and not just the peripheral or central nervous system. Furthermore, the term *homeostasis* suggests that this interaction is an ongoing and dynamic one. If this is true, then this has implications for the manner in which we evaluate and treat pain. It is noteworthy that Darwin spoke of pain as a "homeostatic emotion" as early as 1872.

COMPLEXITIES OF PAIN

As difficult as it may be to define pain, pain also seems to defy satisfactory measurement. Consider the following descriptions of pain: "pain (chronic) fills the space of our conscious experience, demands our attention, and diverts attention and motivational resources away from other agenda" (Price, 1999, p. 207), and "pain degrades and impoverishes the human spirit, brings us back to our physicality, and raises the possibility of our annihilation" (Buytendyck, 1961; from Price, 1999, p. 208). How does one begin to capture the totality of this type of physical and emotional experience by asking a patient to rate their pain using a 0 to 10 numerical pain rating scale? Some have suggested a less quantitative approach, such as patient narratives. Numerous questionnaires have been developed in an effort to measure the quantitative and qualitative aspects of pain. Most are left wanting. Deyo et al (1998) recommended a comprehensive approach to assessment that would include the patient's pain, functioning, mood, and personality. Although more comprehensive, even this approach seems, at times, to be inadequate.

The problem of measurement is compounded when considering different species and stages of development. Infants, toddlers, young and old adults, as well as many species of animals appear to "feel" pain; but is it felt in the same way? Is the emotional pain felt in the face of social rejection comparable to the more physical pain that is associated with an injury or disease? Recent decades have witnessed an increased interest in the unpleasant or affective components of pain from its intensity. The Heisenberg principle of uncertainty, however, questions whether one can, in fact, measure two related features, such as pain intensity and unpleasantness, at the same time with equal accuracy.

The devastating effects of pain are becoming more evident. Suppression of the immune system, morphological changes in the spinal cord dorsal horn, reduction in cortical gray matter volume, altered activity in the endocrine system, and the release of proinflammatory substance resulting in heightened pain sensitivity have all been well documented. It seems obvious that a fuller understanding of the concept of pain may require a consideration of the entire system. It has been in this context that pain is gradually being appreciated as a disease entity rather than a symptom. Chronic pain has even been described by some as a neurodegenerative disease. Recognizing pain as a disease entity would have significant implications for the manner in which patients with pain, especially chronic pain, are viewed and treated. For example, maintaining an adaptive system and avoiding decomplexification become important ingredients in therapy.

The role of genetics in pain sensitivity and effectiveness of treatment is complex and complicated. The premature and often tragic death of those unfortunate individuals with congenital insensitivity to pain highlights the survival value of pain. The availability of genetic screening to differentiate those most likely to respond to a particular pharmacological agent is already at hand. Epigenetics has emerged as a potential means of accounting for what is often referred to as functional or "medically unexplained" symptoms (MUS). The inherited sensitivity to pain acquired by offspring from its mother may well render the organism vulnerable to pain throughout its life. Gene therapy as a therapeutic approach is under exploration, but the downstream effects on the system are almost too numerous to contemplate.

At first glance, consciousness or conscious awareness would seem to be a necessary ingredient to the experience of pain. Nevertheless, there is some evidence that individuals in a minimally conscious state show activation of many aspects of the brain's pain matrix in response to experimentally induced pain, just as fully conscious individuals do. The relationship between the brain and what we ordinarily think of as the mind and consciousness has always been of some philosophical interest. Efforts to locate anatomical and physiological correlates have met with varying degrees of success. At least one approach has emphasized the role of the insular cortex in creating re-representations of what goes on in the body and how one feels (interoception). Other proposals have borrowed concepts from quantum theory, such as wave coherence and entanglement.

It would seem obvious that any condition as devastating as pain appears to be would demand early and aggressive treatment. However, there is a lack of consensus on this issue. In his book, *The Truth About Chronic Pain*, Arthur Rosenfeld interviewed several persons whom he felt to be key thinkers in the area of pain. One interviewee, Marilyn Vos Savant, was described as an author, thinker, and commentator. In response to the question, "Do you think that to live as pain-free as possible is a right?" she responded, "No, I don't. I think it is in conflict with nature" (p. 201). There are those that feel that a little pain (suffering) is "good for the soul" or will reiterate the chant of "no pain, no gain." Indeed, several religions view pain as a sign from their deity or even an opportunity for spiritual growth.

The emphasis on the importance of access to treatment has been accompanied by an unprecedented increase in the use of pharmaceuticals, especially opioids (McCabe et al, 2008; Simoni-Wastila, 2008). Unfortunately, this has been associated with an increased incidence of drug abuse (Turk et al, 2008; Webster, 2008). For example, among 12-year-olds, the abuse of prescription drugs is second only to that of marijuana, and since 2002 the number of persons using pain relievers for nonmedical purposes has exceeded the number of new marijuana users. In 2006, 5.2 million individuals age 12 years or older in the United States reported nonmedical use of opioids in the previous month (Office of Statistical Analysis, 2006). In 2005, 12.4% (4 million) of 18- to 25-year-olds reported nonmedical use of prescribed opioids in the previous year. The cost of managing and controlling opioid abuse is up to $300 billion a year. Beyond the issue of opioid abuse is the uncovering of the detrimental effects of opioids on the immune and endocrine systems. Some analgesics have even been linked to an increased risk of renal cell carcinoma (Gago-Dominguez et al, 1999). The need for safer and more effective treatments is clear.

No one would argue that pain is a part of life; but what about suffering? Might there be ways of altering the impact of pain on the individual such that, although present, its disabling impact on one's quality of life and emotions could be minimized? Patients often bemoan the fact that we can send a man to the moon and a probe to Mars, yet they are told they must "live with their pain." It is almost as though they believed that an available remedy was being withheld from them. It is out of this sense of desperation that so many patients succumb to the temptation of unproven, untested, and sometimes potentially harmful remedies. They readily submit to recommended treatments with irreversible consequences, in the hope of relief.

Assisting the patient to become an active participant in their treatment rather than a passive recipient of it could yield big dividends. It has been shown that when properly educated and well informed, patients submit to spine surgery up to 30% less often. In addition, there are a large number of proven psychological and functionally based therapies that can be used as adjuncts to or in place of more invasive and medically oriented approaches. For example, there is evidence to support the impact of cognitive behavioral therapies (CBT) on reorganizing the brain's response to pain and potentially reversing the loss of cortical gray matter seen in patients with chronic pain.

The brain (mind) has an enormous capacity to influence our perceptions and experiences, including pain. But it can be fooled. This has been highlighted by research involving placebos. The idea that an otherwise inert or nontherapeutic substance (placebo) can have a positive treatment effect is well known. Usually the placebo is administered under the guise of being beneficial. Thus, the positive effect is attributable, at least in part, to the patient's expectation or brain response. In a 2010 study, Kaptchuk and his colleagues deviated from the standard protocol. The participants were actually told that they were, in fact, getting a placebo, but also that they should appreciate the potential for a beneficial effect through the mind–body connection. Despite this lack of deception, the participants demonstrated a statistically and clinically significant response.

So, what in their brain (mind) produced this outcome? Was there some type of unconscious mechanism that overrode the "logical" brain? Was the effect tied to a desire to get better or to having had a previous positive experience with pills? Recent technological advances have finally allowed for a more detailed investigation of the brain's response in such situations. Real-time biofeedback using functional magnetic resonance imagining (fMRI) technology and heart rate variability (HRV) training may provide a means of harnessing the mind–brain connection and its potential for neuroplasticity. The effect of such treatments may be one of self-directed neuroplasticity that could bypass the negative consequences of more invasive therapies.

In the midst of pain and suffering, many people gravitate to their religious or spiritual foundations. What is it about desperation that drives one to unseen forces? The impact of religion and religious philosophies on our understanding of pain and the types of treatments employed can be traced back thousands of years. The ancient religious ways are often seen as naive and lacking any scientific validity. Yet, most do believe in miracles. Even modern medicine encourages faith, hope, and prayer, and in the absence of any objective evidence to explain a cure, accepts the notion of a miracle. Our tendency to scrutinize outcomes on the basis of sample size, reproducibility, and level of statistical significance often discounts the rare or unusual observation. Moreover, the scientific legitimacy of an event is frequently linked to an explanation that fits our contemporary scientific methodology, dismissing the alternative as lacking scientific merit.

PHILOSOPHY OF SCIENCE

Modern science had its beginnings in the late 16th century with Galileo. It was Galileo who introduced the notion of taking measurements. Late in the 17th century Isaac Newton created the foundational model for science. Newton maintained that systems could be precisely predicted through the laws and associated equations of motion. Newton was able to explain planetary motion by application of his scientific methods and calculus. He also formulated the three laws of motion that became the foundation of physics. According to Goerner (1994), Newton's mathematical approach to systems can be represented by the following: (a) any system that can be integrated can be represented as a set of independent elements, all changing in isolation from one another; (b) all integrable systems exhibit smooth continuous change; (c) all integrable systems can be broken down and approximated by simpler curves; and (d) once their equations of motion are known, precise prediction and control are, in principle, possible.

The 20th century brought with it a commitment to scientific endeavor. Eradication of disease, putting a man on the moon, and establishing a leadership position in the world was thought most achievable though science. Much of what is known about the neurobiology of pain has come from the rigorous application of scientific methodology handed down by Newton (Newtonian physics). The embracing of the scientific endeavor has produced some marvelous discoveries and treatments. It has also established and reinforced reductionism and materialism as the cornerstones of scientific philosophy.

Philosophical materialism made its appearance in the 16th century during the Age of Reason, in part to discredit the religious dogma of the day. It asserts that the universe is a material, three-dimensional phenomenon. The only thing that exists is matter, and all that is real can be measured. Furthermore, all things are composed of material matter, and all phenomena are the result of the material interactions of its physical components. As such, the universe operates in accordance with natural physical laws rendering it deterministic and causal in nature. Philosophical materialism would reject the notion of an essential wholeness or interconnectedness found in quantum theory. Religion and spirituality are relegated to the status of superstitions. Consciousness is seen as an outcome of the activity of the physical brain. Physical death marks the end of existence; nothing exists beyond death.

A companion concept is that of philosophical reductionism. Reductionism embraces the notion that any complex system is a product of the sum of its parts. Thus, the most appropriate and complete means of understanding a complex system is to reduce it to its most basic constituent components. It is the interaction of these most simple and fundamental components that make up the system or phenomenon. For example, boiling water is best understood by examining it at the level of the atom, which enables one to explain why liquid boils at a given temperature. In this sense, reductionism is wholly deterministic and causal. Determinism, especially causal determinism, states that events are causally bound together such that any particular event is determined by, or is the consequence of, previous events. Causality specifies the relationship of two events, A and B, such that A predetermines B, or that if B, then it was preceded by A. The deterministic universe, therefore, is a chain of events governed by the law of cause and effect, allowing for the existence of only one state at a particular point in time.

Phenomena that cannot be objectively measured or described in terms of some set of fundamental elements and whose total is not equal to the sum of its parts (nonlinear) are relegated to the vestiges of pseudo- or epiphenomena to be pursued by those lacking in true scientific training and methodology. Indeed, Aristotle forewarned us of this possibility, noting that the whole *was* greater than the sum of its parts.

Only in recent decades have pursuits in cognitive sciences gained in stature in the traditional scientific community, as witnessed by publications in such prestigious journals as *Science*. This acceptance has been propelled, at least in part, by the neurocognitive scientist's ability to demonstrate some physiological correlates, such as metabolic or blood flow variations, in the brain that are associated with a specific cognitive or mental activity. These observations have been made possible by the advent of sophisticated neuroimaging technology, such as fMRI, positron emission tomography (PET), and single-photon emission computerized tomography (SPECT) scans. Thus, in a sense, the rigorous application of traditional scientific methodology has opened the door to the understanding of otherwise unacceptable areas of inquiry, such as consciousness and the mind.

In so far as our everyday experience is concerned, Newtonian physics provides a meaningful way of comprehending our world. However, it does not seem to apply at the atomic and subatomic level. Understanding the behavior within and between biological systems at this level may enhance our comprehension of the experience of pain.

SYSTEMS THEORY

It may be useful to extend the paradigm through which we study pain to include some aspects of systems theory and quantum mechanics. This could provide a means of expanding our understanding of the totality of the experience of pain and all of its nuances. Systems theory is an interdisciplinary field of study whose goal is to identity principles that can be applied to all types of systems. In this context the word *systems* refers to self-regulating systems (self-correcting through feedback). Nature is made up of many such self-regulating systems, including the physiological systems of the human body, and human learning processes.

Nested within systems theory are chaos and complexity theories. Their goal is to explain complex systems. These complex systems are made up of a large number of mutually interacting and interrelated parts. In this instance, *chaos* has been defined as unforeseen behavior in a deterministic system (Elbert et al, 1994; Gleck, 2008). What appears to be random behavior in fact is not, but represents part of a nonlinear-dynamic system. The presence of chaotic behavior, however, can introduce an element of unpredictability. In fact, Skarda and Freeman (1987) see chaos as that which underlies the brain's ability to respond in a flexible manner to demands imposed by the external and internal world, producing novel brain patterns.

Complex-adaptive systems (CAS) represent a particular type of a complex system. They are *complex* in that they are diverse and made up of multiple interconnected elements and *adaptive* in that they have the capacity to change and learn from experience. Some of the common attributes of complex systems or phenomena include the following:

(a) The whole is made up of parts and is greater than the sum of its parts.
(b) There is a reciprocal and causal relationship between parts and the whole.

(c) Interesting wholes can arise simply from interacting parts and/or from apparent chaos or randomness (which is a property of physiologically normal as well as abnormal systems).

(d) Elements that appear resistant to change in the parts or their properties may suddenly and mysteriously change.

(e) Change does not necessarily indicate the presence of an outside force or agent.

(f) The relationship between parts and wholes may change for a given whole.

Pain, especially chronic pain, appears to manifest many of these attributes and thus could be considered a complex emergent phenomenon. This may be especially true when considering the interaction between the emotional/affective and sensory/discriminative systems involved in the processing of nociceptive information. Indeed, Martinez-Lavin and Vargas (2009) and Newell (2003) have provided examples of the application of the concepts of CAS to an analysis of fibromyalgia and low back pain, respectively.

QUANTUM THEORY AND MECHANICS

Quantum mechanics (QM) is essential to understanding the behavior of systems at atomic and subatomic levels. Quantum theory has revealed that matter exhibits a wave-like and particle-like behavior simultaneously; in other words, matter is not as solid as we thought. QM deals with scientifically demonstrable facts that seem to contradict everything we see around us. It has been successful in explaining the behavior of subatomic particles that make up all forms of matter (electrons, protons, neutrons, photons, etc.). It is important for understanding how individual atoms combine to form chemicals and molecules, as well as for understanding the function of different biological systems. QM has found practical application in the development of the laser, transistor, electron microscope, and MRI.

There are a number of QM principles that may well be applicable to the study of pain, for example, the observer effect. The *observer effect* refers to changes that the act of observation will make on the phenomenon observed. This effect is frequently a consequence of the measuring instrument used; the instrument itself may alter that which is being measured. A corollary of the observer effect is the Heisenberg uncertainty principle, which addresses the actual process of measurement. The uncertainty principle states that when measuring certain pairs of physical properties, referred to as *conjugate variables*, their properties cannot be known with absolute precision. In physics, *quantum entanglement* refers to a state in which two or more constituent objects (particles, atoms, molecules, etc.) become linked in such a fashion that one object can no longer be adequately described without full mention of its counterpart. In essence, when these particles become entangled, the behavior of one is simultaneously reflected in the behavior of the other, even though they are spatially separated. Although mostly studied at the anatomic or micro level, this phenomenon may well exist at the the more macro level. For example, quantum biologists are begining to examine how quantum entanglements can affect our body, sensory experiences, and conscious processes. Déjà vu, sympathy pains (Couvade syndrome), premonitions, shared experiences and pain between indentical twins, and Hebbian-cell assemblies are possible examples. The well-documented relationship between attention/cognitive activity and pain, shown by the work of both Eccleston (1995; Eccleston and Crombez, 1999) and Seminowicz (Seminowicz et al, 2004; Seminowicz and Davis, 2007), may serve as an example in the area of pain. The principles of nonlocality and coherence may also be relevant and will be discussed in Chapters 4 and 13.

CONCLUSION

The absence of data supporting any substantial change in the statistics regarding the incidence, development, and persistence of chronic pain, despite the proliferation of pain clinics and various pain-oriented therapies over the past 50 years, is both surprising and disappointing. Perhaps it is too early in the process. Alternatively, there may be a need for a fundamental shift in the way we view pain. Insanity has jokingly been defined as doing the same thing over and over yet expecting a different result. There appears to be an effort to find new reasons for recapitulating the past rather than learning from it. Sequestering our imagination to the confines of the present methodologies and knowledge is a one way of all but ensuring theoretical and therapeutic stagnation.

An understanding of, and appreciation for, the complexities of pain requires more than anecdotal reports of the heroic day-to-day battle waged by those afflicted. Outlining the past failures of pain therapies and anticipated future innovations adds perspective. A review of the research relating to the suspected mechanisms and causes of pain is fundamental, but it has to be placed in context. There is also a need to go beyond the data and probe the many pain-related issues, ranging from genetics to theories of pain to consciousness.

Fortunately, pain research and treatment appear to be on the precipice of change. At the very least there is a need to broaden the current paradigm used to understand the experience of pain. Pain may emerge as something very different from the way it is currently conceptualized. The use of concepts from systems and quantum theory may prove beneficial. The appreciation of pain as a disease entity, the role of homeostasis, and the consideration of the entire system (organism) represent a significant paradigm shift. In the present context, homeodynamics might be a more descriptive term than homeostasis, as *homeostasis* refers a system seeking some neutral state, whereas *homeodynamics* suggests an ongoing adaptation and adjustment of the system to changing external and internal environments (Lloyd et al, 2001). Hopefully, this book will provide a glimpse of these changes in the context of where pain theory, research, and therapy have come from, where they are currently, and where they might be headed.

REFERENCES

Buytendyck FJJ. *Pain*. London: Hutchinson Press; 1961.

Craig, AD. Pain mechanisms: Labeled lines versus convergence in central processing. *Annu Rev Neurosci*. 2003;26:1–30.

Darwin C. *The Expression of Emotions in Man and Animals*. London: John Murray; 1872.

Deyo RA, Battie M, Beurskens AJ, et al. Outcome measures for low back pain research: a proposal for standardized use. *Spine*. 1998;23(18):2003–2013.

Dubois MY, Gallagher RM, Lippe PM. Pain medicine position paper. *Pain Med*. 2009;10(6):972–1000.

Eccleston C. Chronic pain and distraction: an experimental investigation into the role of sustained and shifting attention in the processing of chronic persistent pain. *Behav Res Ther.* 1995;33(4):391–405.

Eccleston C, Crombez G. Pain demands attention: a cognitive-affective model of the interruptive function of pain. *Psychol Bull.* 1999;125(3):356–366.

Elbert T, Ray WJ, Kowlik ZJ, Skinner J, Graf KE, Birbaumer N. Chaos and physiology: deterministic chaos in excitable cell assemblies. *Physiol Rev.* 1994;74(1):1–40.

Fishbain DA. The association of chronic pain and suicide. *Semin Clin Neuropsychiatry.* 1999;4:221–227.

Fishbain DA, Cole, B, Lewis JE, Rosomoff RS, Rosomoff HL. What percentage of chronic non-malignant pain patients exposed to chronic opioid analgesic therapy develop abuse/addiction and/or aberrant drug-related behavior? A structured, evidence-based review. *Pain Med.* 2008;9(4):444–459.

Foss JM, Apkarian AV, Chialvo DR. Dynamics of pain: fractal dimension of temporal variability of spontaneous pain differentiates between pain states. *J Neurophysiol.* 2006;95:730–736.

Gago-Dominguez M, Yuan JM, Castelao JE, Ross RK, Yu MC. Regular use of analgesics is a risk factor for renal cell carcinoma. *Br J Cancer.* 1999;81(3):542–546.

Gaskin DJ, Richard P. The economic cost of pain in the United States. *J Pain.* 2012;13(8):715–724.

Gleck J. *Chaos: Making a New Science.* New York: Penguin Books; 2008.

Goerner SJ. *Chaos and the Evolving Ecological Universe.* Luxembourg: Gordon and Breach; 1994.

Kaptchuk, TJ, Friedlander E, Kelley JM, et al. Placebos without deception: a randomized controlled trial in irritable bowel syndrome. *PLoS ONE.* 2010;5(12):e15591, 1–7.

Lloyd D, Aon MA, Cortassa S. Why homeodynamics, not homeostasis? *Scientific World Journal.* 2001;1:133–145.

Martinez-Lavin M, Vargas A. Complex adaptive systems allostasis in fibromyalgia. *Rheum Dis Clin North Am.* 2009;35(2):285–298.

McCabe SE, Cranford JA, West BT. Trends in prescription drug abuse and dependence, co-occurrence with other substance use disorders, and treatment utilization: results from two national surveys. *Addict Behav.* 2008;33(10):1297–1305.

Merskey H, Bogduk N, eds. *Classification of Chronic Pain.* Seattle: IASP Press; 1994.

Moskovitz P. Giving severe and chronic pain a name: maldynia. *Practical Pain Management.* 2011;11(5):12–20.

Mountcastle VB. Pain and temperature sensibilities. In Mountcastle VB, ed. *Medical Physiology*, 13th ed. St. Louis: Mosby; 1974.

Newell D. Concepts in the study of complexity and their possible relationship to chiropractic health care: a scientific rationale for a holistic approach. *Clin Chiropr.* 2003;6:15–33.

Office of Statistical Analysis, Substance Abuse and Mental Health Services Administration. How young adults obtain prescription pain relievers for nonmedical use. The NSDUH Report. Issue 39, 2006. www.samhsa.gov/data/2k6/getPain/getPain.pdf. Accessed October 3, 2013.

Price DD. *Psychological Mechanisms of Pain and Analgesia.* Seattle: IASP Press; 1999.

Quinlan-Colwell, A. People living with chronic pain: who are they? *SPS Newsletter*, 2008; June: 4–5.

Rosenfield A. *The Truth About Chronic Pain.* New York: Basic Books; 2003.

Seminowicz, DA, Davis KD. Interactions of pain intensity and cognitive load: the brain stays on task. *Cereb Cortex.* 2007;17:1412–1422.

Seminowicz DA, Mikulis DJ, Davis KD. Cognitive modulation of pain-related brain responses depends on behavioral strategy. *Pain.* 2004;112:48–58.

Simoni-Wastila L. Increases in opioid medication use: balancing the good with the bad. *Pain*. 2008;138:245–246.

Skarda CA, Freeman WJ. How brains make chaos in order to make sense of the world. *Behav Brain Sci*. 1987;10:161–173.

Turk DC, Swanson KS, Gatchel RJ. Predicting opioid misuse by chronic pain patients: a systematic review and literature synthesis. *Clin J Pain*. 2008;24:497–508.

Webster L. *Determining the Risk of Opioid Abuse. Emerging Solutions in Pain Monograph*. Morrisville, PA: MedCom Worldwide; 2008.

Woolf CJ. Pain: moving from symptom control toward mechanism-specific pharmacologic management. *Ann Intern Med*. 2004;140:441–451.

2   The History of Pain

Pain is at once one of life's great tragedies and greatest triumphs;
[p]ain on occasion becomes the site of encounters we can do nothing except witness in respect.
–Jody Lynee Madier *(2006, p. 43)*

INTRODUCTION

In a sense, the history of pain is the history of humankind (see reviews by Todd, 1985; Parris, 2000). Pain is an essential feature of the sentient human. The inability to experience it is more of a curse than a blessing. Although animals are relied on in research, pain, at least as currently defined, and its associated suffering can only be fully realized and understood in the human context. The manner in which the infliction of pain or its management is regarded is a reflection of perceived value of a person or group of people. Philosophers, religions, and scientists have struggled to define its source and its meaning, if indeed one exists. Pain of some type is a common theme in literature and seems capable of eliciting fascination and horror. Only recently has the concept of pain begun to be considered in the context modern-day systems and quantum theory. As always, knowing the past may help to prevent committing the mistakes of the past.

ANCIENT VIEWS

Ancient civilizations, including early Egyptians and Babylonians, tended to view pain as a result of the influx of demons or mysterious and magical fluids. Indeed, the Egyptians considered the left nostril to be the pathway through which diseases and demons entered the body. Babylonians believed that well-localized pain represented the demon consuming that specific portion of the body. Pain resulting from being impaled by a spear made sense; pain from what we now know as a disease was more confusing, given the absence of any external injury, and reinforced the invocation of unseen mystical forces.

Logically, at least to these ancients, the cure was providing a means of allowing the fluids or demons to escape. Vomiting, sweating, urinating, and sneezing were some of the means of expelling pain-causing fluids or demons. Trepanning (scrapping of the skull or drilling of a hole into the skull), used to expose the dura as a means to release pressure and evil spirits, appeared during the Neolithic Period beginning about 9500 BCE. The use of polished stones or rocks as the trepanning tool was replaced with metal objects by 2000 BCE. Marks resembling a tattoo have been found on the spine and joints of mummies dating back to 3000 BCE, suggesting a type of trepanning. Trepanning was still practiced in the 1800s.

The shaman emerged as another means of treating pain and illness. The shaman created wounds of a specific type and location, releasing the fluids or demons. In some cases, the intrusive pain-causing substances were sucked out and neutralized by applying special potions to the open wound. These treatments set the stage for matching the magical powers of the shaman with those of the evil spirits.

Egyptians viewed the heart as the center of all sensations. An array of vessels, they thought, carried the breath of life and various perceptions to the heart. Anything that might disrupt this flow to the heart could alter one's perceptions. The use of "electric fish" from the Nile to spread over some areas of pain or wounds as a means of interrupting this flow dates back as far as 2700 BCE. Sometime later, the Greeks made use of the electrogenic torpedo fish (*Scribonius largus*) to treat the pain of arthritis and headache. These experiences seemed to have foretold the development of modern-day transcutaneous electrical nerve stimulation (TENS). By the first century CE, Romans had discovered the analgesic value of a seawater bath and an ointment made of poppy and wild cucumber. As early as 1200 CE sponges soaked in opium and herbs were used during surgery.

Judaism introduced the notion of a single omnipotent God instead of the prevailing polytheistic beliefs. Sin occurred when the laws handed down by God were violated. Sin resulted in some type of punishment, often in the form of pain. This view of pain carried over into Christian doctrine. Indeed, the term *pain* derives from the Latin word *poena*, meaning "punishment," and *patient* from *patior*, "to endure suffering or pain." Illness and disease became synonymous with wickedness and a sinful nature while good physical health was reflective of moral purity. In Genesis, God destined women to endure pain during childbirth in response to Eve's disobedience when she ate of the forbidden fruit. Prayer, rituals, ceremonies, and sacrifices were used in an effort to gain forgiveness and thus relief from the pain. Exorcism emerged as a means of "casting out" evil forces thought to have invaded the unsuspecting individual and causing the infirmity and associated pain.

The Greeks began to distinguish sensation and sensory perception as occurring in the brain, not the soul or the heart. Pythagoras (580–497 BCE) believed pain and suffering were necessary to the development of the self-control and self-discipline needed to demonstrate the cardinal virtues of courage, temperance, justice, and wisdom. By adhering to these virtues one could determine the future of one's soul. For example, enduring severe pain demonstrated nobility and courage, guaranteeing the soul's returning to the gods upon death, instead of being punished by having to return to earth.

Philosophical debates as to the nature of the human body and soul can be found in the third century. Aristotle (384–322 BCE) believed the heart and not the brain to be center of all sensory experiences, as well as all feelings, including pain. Thus, pain resulted from increased sensitivity of the senses—touch, sight, smell, taste, and hearing. The heart functioned to modify this increased sensitivity, the outcome of which was felt as pain. Plato (423–347 BCE) thought pain was a product of the interaction of the earth, fire, air, and water with the soul (believed to reside in the body), which somehow intruded on the body. These interactions were considered to be particularly violent at the beginning of life, implying that for the infant all feelings were essentially painful. The experiences of pain and pleasure had a negative effect on the soul, as they tended to distract the soul from knowing what was real. Sensations were assimilated in the heart and the liver and ultimately transmitted to the brain. The brain's function was to expand upon the information acquired from sensory perceptions.

Anatomical dissections carried out in the second and third centuries BCE revealed the brain to be connected to a system of nerves traveling from the periphery through the spinal cord. One set of nerves was thought to be involved in movement, another with feelings. This evidence seemed to re-establish the brain as the center of sensation and not the soul, heart, or liver as proposed by Plato and Aristotle. Some 400 years later, Galen (130–201 CE) confirmed these anatomical findings through dissections of the nerves and spinal cord of the pig. He described three types of nerves: (a) "hard nerves" associated with movement, (b) "soft nerves" associated with sensation, and (c) those of least sensitivity to be associated with pain. Nevertheless, Aristotle's notion of the five senses (touch, smell, sight, taste, and hearing) and pain as a "passion of the soul" originating in the heart held sway for many centuries thereafter.

During this period in history and extending into the Middles Ages, infant and pediatric pain was readily recognized and acknowledged to be equal to or more severe than adult pain (Unruh, 1992). Several accounts were given for this. First, it was believed that the lack of life experiences contributed to pain sensitivity. Second, infants and children were thought to be particularly susceptible to demonic influence or possession. And third, pain sensitivity was linked to developmental and physiological immaturity. In general, it was thought that experience with pain diminished one's sensitivity to it. The absence of the ability on the part of the infant or child to accurately describe their experience was a noted problem. However, Galen highlighted the role of crying as an indicator of distress and pain, and suggested holding and rocking the child and singing lullabies. In the second century CE, Soranus reiterated the potential importance of crying as well as other behavioral and physiological changes as indicators of distress and pain. In fact, he observed different reactions in the infant to bruising, being bitten, and constipation. Aurelianus (fifth century CE) described groaning while asleep, gnashing of teeth, sudden crying, outstretched hands, pale color, and perspiration as indicators of pain.

Ancient physicians were surprisingly concerned over the prevention of injury and the treatment of pain in infants and children. Treatment of infant pain varied. Egyptian records indicate the use of opium in the 1500s BCE. Egyptians also made frequent use of amulets hung about the neck. Others provided various agents to the wet-nurse, believing that beneficial effects would be passed on to the infant via the breast milk. Some favored administering remedies directly to the infant. Rubbing the gum with chicken fat or a hare's brain was used for teething. Soranus recommended suppositories created from boiled honey.

MIDDLE AGES AND RENAISSANCE

As the Roman Empire started to decline in the fifth century, the Christian church began to exert its considerable influence in the areas of philosophy and medicine. Beginning with the first century, many Christians believed that the pain and suffering associated with martyrdom identified them more closely with Christ. St. Augustine declared that all of the diseases of Christians, even those of innocent babies, was the work of evil demons. Many of the Greek teachings were labeled as pagan and were banned. Therefore, Greek scholars fled to Persia. Several of the classical Greek works were translated into Arabic and other local languages, thus influencing the thinking of the region. Avicenna, a well-known tenth century Arabic physician and philosopher, theorized the body to be composed of four temperaments: heat, cold, dryness, and moistness. Each organ and limb had its own unique and ideal mixture. Pain was viewed as an independent sensation that occurred when there was a disturbance or perturbation in this ideal mixture. Indeed, 15 different types of pain were identified, including pricking, boring, heavy, corrosive, compressing, incisive, dull, fatigue, irritant itching, relaxing throbbing, stabbing, tearing, and tension. It is noteworthy that many of these pain types (descriptors) are part of the McGill Pain Questionnaire, developed in 1971. Each type of pain was associated with a specific type of change in the four temperaments. Pain and the other senses were thought to be felt or experienced in the ventricles of the brain.

In the Middle Ages, the interpretation and meaning of pain were dictated predominately by the Christian church. St. Thomas Aquinas was perhaps the most influential medieval theologian and philosopher. The human condition with all of its pain and suffering was seen as a direct result of Adam's original sin in the Garden of Eden. Life's purpose was to gain salvation for one's soul. Emphasis was placed on moral and spiritual responsibilities and not on the alleviation of pain and suffering. Indeed, attempts to relieve pain and suffering could be construed as an offense against God, as the very condition one tried to improve may have been imposed by God. Thus, the disease that punished, also cleansed. This is perhaps best exemplified by Job's response in the Old Testament to the apparently unwarranted infliction of painful diseases and personal loss. His patient endurance, even in the face of the inexplicable, was seemingly rewarded by the restoration of his family and wealth. Recall Paul's letter bemoaning the "thorn in his side" thought to be put there by the devil. Upon asking God to remove it, Paul noted God's response: "My grace is sufficient" (2 Corinthians, 12:7–10).

During the 15th century, with the beginning of the Renaissance, concepts of pain and of the body moved away from theologically dominated thinking and toward scientific methodology. Leonardo de Vinci, among others, proposed that nerves were tubular in nature and that the purpose of the spinal cord was to convey information to the brain, the center of sensation. The "sense of pain" was linked to the sense of touch. The notion of pain and suffering as a consequence of original sin gave way to the concept that humans are born "pure," only to be corrupted once exposed to the evils of life, including poverty, injustice, and disease. Thomas Hobbes reasoned that the existence of natural laws was ordained by God and therefore moral. The study of the laws of nature, that is, God, was considered a form of religious worship. By coming to understand how to manipulate destructive social and natural phenomena, such as disease, humans could affect their future. The proper methodology for conducting experiments designed to discover these laws of nature was fashioned by Francis Bacon. Rationalism was thus adopted as the preferred philosophy. Rationalists maintained that the acquisition of knowledge was essentially an intellectual and valued enterprise.

The use of reason and analytical deduction became a trademark of Renaissance philosophers and scientists. One of the most notable was René Descartes (1596–1650), a French mathematician and philosopher. He considered all physical things, including the human body, to function according to the laws of mechanics. Nerves were once again seen as hollow tubes within which fibrils (fibers or tiny threads), originating in the brain, meandered through the body, terminating in the skin and organs. These tubules carried both sensory and motor information to the brain. Descartes theorized the existence of a gate between the brain and these tubules. A tug on the fibril was created by a sensory cue. This opened the gate between the brain and tubules, allowing "animal spirits" to flow throughout. This sensory input "opened" pores thought to line the ventricles of the brain, allowing these animal spirits to elicit a motor response. Pain was considered a perception felt in the brain in response to a sufficiently intense "tug." A weaker tug was associated with a tingling sensation. He also thought the pattern and intensity of stimulation were important, but he appeared to reject the notion of a dedicated "pain pathway" (Moayedi and Davis, 2013).

Thus, sensory stimulation of the skin was transmitted to the brain via activation of these tubules, similar to ringing a bell by pulling on the end of an attached rope. Descartes illustrated this by his now-famous drawing of a boy with his foot near a fire (see Figure 2.1). Minute particles from the fire were thought to activate a spot on the skin, which in turn resulted in a pulling motion of the thread(s). Incoming sensations interacted with the mind or soul, which was considered to be distinct from the body and thus immune to the influence of external and mechanical forces. However, the mind and the body were integrated, as it were, within the pineal gland. Therefore, pain was the product of enhanced sensory awareness modulated by the mind.

Descartes' theory was quite disparate from that of William Harvey (1578–1657 AD). Harvey's discovery of circulation prompted him to theorize the heart as the center of pain sensation. Thus, the Aristotelian notion of the existence of five senses and the heart being the center of sensation continued to dominate well into the 18th century. It was the work of Isaac Newton (1642–1727) and physician David Hartley (1705–1757) that shifted the view of pain and other sensations from being dependent on some agent outside the body that transported them to the heart or brain, to being sensations that are a consequence of these external agents, causing a vibratory motion of minute particles inside the nerves themselves.

MODERN ERA

The 19th century witnessed unprecedented concern over social injustices and an increased effort toward reducing human suffering. Also, empiricism emerged, introduced by John Locke in the 1600s. Contrary to the rationalists, empiricists believed that knowledge was acquired rather than existing in an a priori fashion. Knowledge was gained through experience, and learning and was not God-given. Likewise, pain

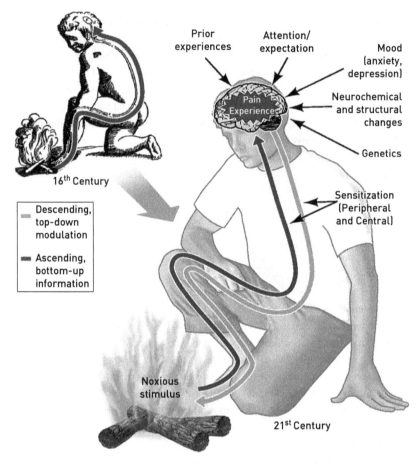

Prior experiences

Attention/ expectation

Mood (anxiety, depression)

Neurochemical and structural changes

Genetics

Pain Experience

16th Century

Descending, top-down modulation

Ascending, bottom-up information

Sensitization (Peripheral and Central)

Noxious stimulus

21st Century

FIGURE 2.1

Note the difference in conceptualization of pain between Descartes' original cartoon (upper right) from the 16th century and a more contemporary, 21st-century model, from Bingel and Tracey (2008). Image on the right from Bingel U, Tracey I. Imaging CNS modulation of pain in humans. *Physiology*. 2008;23:372. Reprinted with permission.

was considered one aspect of learning instead of being interpreted in a religious or spiritual context. These events launched an age of scientific study using systematic investigations into physiology and anatomy that were based on sound experimental methodology. An era of materialism and reductionism as the dominating philosophies was ushered in. Pain nonetheless continued to be seen as an indicator the patient's vitality, life's power and energy, and treatment effectiveness. This view of pain, however, gave way to the utilitarian philosophy of the early 1800s. The emergence of individual rights and the importance of the individual's experience paved the way for embracing pain relief as a beneficial enterprise.

In addition to this transitional phase in the scientific and medical view of pain, there was what Morris (1998) describes as "the invisible history of pain." He has chronicled the impact of the 19th-century Romantic poets in Britain and American, including Coleridge, Emerson, Bryon, Shelley, and Keats, on the modern understanding of pain. Indeed, anesthesiologist E.M. Papper (1990) credits the change in public attitudes toward pain brought about by the British Romantic poets' concept of self and subjectivity as a driving force in the development of surgical anesthesia.

At the time, science and medicine were struggling with the concept of pain. The lack of coordination among experimental studies, therapeutic research, and clinical activity, along with a stubborn adherence to and fruitless investigation of unsubstantiated theories, slowed progress. The search shifted from "What is wrong with you?" to "Where does it hurt?". The focus was moving toward the visible and objectifiable, or "lesion-illuminated," approach, the legacy of which was to transform pain "into a visible object of clinical medicine" (Morris, 1998, p. 192). The unfortunate subtext was permission, even implicit encouragement, to overlook if not ignore anything beyond the lesion. The distinction between emotional and physical pain was endorsed in the medical textbooks of the early 19th century, which declared that pain either had an objective, physical, visible cause or was emotional, imaginary, and all in one's head. This approach was further strengthened as the clinician's ability to "observe" was enhanced by the subsequent development of imaging technology. Ironically, despite a tacit acceptance of pain being "subjective," somehow science of the day was convinced its origin and ongoing foundation could be objectified.

Morris notes that England and early colonial America shared a propensity toward public inflictions of pain and the execution of criminals. These public spectacles took on the quality of a spectator sport. However, he states,

in the 19th century the judicial system began to substitute incarceration for the public infliction of pain. Incarceration transformed punishment into a private act at the exact moment when the clinical gaze redefined pain as something visible only to the physicians as they peer, with the objectifying light of science, inside the human body. Indeed, pain in the early 19th century had clearly begun its long retreat from public spaces. (Morris, 1998, p. 193)

The Romantic writers' emphasis on reconstruction of the self through suffering, pain, and affliction became influential. Morris highlights Prometheus' comment in Shelley's "Prometheus Unbound": after being exposed to the daily ravages of vultures, Prometheus withdraws his curse on Jupiter, declaring, "I wish no living thing to suffer pain." In writing about the New England reformers Emerson said, "We crave a sense of reality, though it comes in strokes of pain." Likewise, Byron wrote, "The great object of life is sensation to feel that we exist-even though in pain." His work seems to draw inescapable attention to "lesion-less" pain, which had been generally displaced by the scientific appeal to the visible and objectifiable.

It was also the Romantic poets' attention to the human condition—the plight of the downtrodden, the disenfranchised, and marginalized—that helped to revolutionize the concept of pain and suffering, particularly in relation to women. Although seen as fragile, unstable, hysterical, and not worthy of participating in the higher educational system, women were nonetheless given the duty of attending to those in pain. Indeed, so complete was the impact of Romantic literature on this role for women that in 1835 Princess Victoria's name appeared on a list supporting the newly formed Society for the Prevention of Cruelty to Animals (SPCA).

It was about this period of time that the use of opium began to flourish. European physicians had some familiarity with opium. Although Thomas Sydenham introduced "laudanum," a mixture of opium and sherry, in the 1680s, blood-letting as a means of eliminating the evil humors and amputation of diseased limbs continued as part of mainstream medicine. Opium, however, came into common use during the American Civil War and the Napoleonic wars, to treat pain from all types of wounds. It emerged as a treatment for other ailments as well, including dysentery, the common headache, diarrhea, and gastrointestinal discomfort. Unregulated, its use soon extended outside the medical arena. In "Confessions of an English Opium Eater" (1821), Thomas De Quincey records his addiction to opium, describing it as "divine poppy-juice, as indispensable as breathing." He claimed that the English chemist shops displayed 1- to 3-gram pills on the counter awaiting the usual weekend patrons.

Morphine, as a product of crude opium, was discovered and produced industrially in Germany in the 1820s. In 1855, Alexander Wood introduced the first syringe. As early as the 1870s, concern was expressed about the "morphine habit" or "narcomania." It was about 1895 when druggist John Pemberton was wounded while serving in the Confederate Army. Like many other solders, he became addicted to morphine. He began experimenting with coca (the source of cocaine) and coca wines in search for a cure for his addiction. He created Pemberton French Wine Coca—a combination of kola nut and damiana (a small plant that has an aromatic flower and produces a fruit similar to a fig; it has aphrodisiac properties and can be found in Mexican liqueurs). In the late 1930s a variety of opioid-type preparations were introduced, including meperidine, oxycodone, methadone, and pentazocine, under the auspices of the National Institutes of Health in the United States. Nonopioid drugs such as acetaminophen (Tylenol(R)) and ibuprofen (Motrin(R)) began to appear in the mid-1900s.

In addition to the development and refinement of opioid therapy, surgeons began to take greater pride in minimizing the pain of surgery by becoming more efficient. On October 16, 1846, William T.G. Morton introduced anesthesia. Chloroform was used during childbirth with Queen Victoria in 1847, and by 1850 its use was commonplace during childbirth and surgery. This modern marvel of medicine was not without its critics. Some argued that the relief of pain might well retard the healing process. Others found anesthesia an abomination and a violation of God's law. They believed pain to be divinely imparted as a means of strengthening one's faith. For the birthing mother, pain was seen as an opportunity to learn self-sacrifice for her children. Ironically, it was only a few decades earlier, about 1774, that a German physician, Franz Mesmer, had used magnetics and hypnosis as nonpharmacological approaches to reducing the pain of childbirth. It would be some 200 years later, in the mid-1900s, when the French obstetrician Fernand Lamaze took note of the use of "psychoprophylaxis," a type of relaxation therapy, during childbirth in the Soviet Union. He developed the Lamaze method as a non-drug alternative to alleviating the pain of childbirth.

Crawford Long (1815–1876), a rural physician in Georgia, removed a cyst from the neck of James Venable using an ether-soaked towel in March of 1842. Much to the amazement of the medical students and other onlookers, the ether anesthesia resulted in a relatively painless procedure for which Venable was changed the tidy sum of two dollars. As word spread of this new and painless surgery, Long was suspected by some of practicing witchcraft, while others simply thought it to be unnatural. The religious traditionalists objected, declaring that pain was God's way of cleansing the soul. So impassioned were the outcry and threats against Long and this unnatural surgery that he was reportedly compelled to abandon his home and relocate. However, there were some religious groups that began to accept reduced pain during childbirth and surgery as nonheretical. Late in the 19th century, Pope Pius XII stemmed the tide of resistance by declaring that the use of scientifically discovered preparations to reduce pain during surgical procedures was not immoral. Surgeons saw anesthesia, rather than pain, as the "divine blessing," allowing for procedures previously unimaginable to be undertaken.

Anatomical and histological investigations in the early and mid-1800s along with new-found methods of experimentation regarding the transmission of information from the spinal cord to the brain revealed that sensory pathways tended to be segregated in the dorsal aspect of the spinal cord and motor pathways in the ventral portion. The identification of these two separate pathways led some to posit the presence of a straight-through system of specific nerve energies. Indeed, The doctrine of specific nerve energies was published by Johannes Müller in 1826 (Müller, 1940). He declared that each of the five senses (vision, auditory, touch, smell, and taste) had its own sensory nerve which carried information to the brain. Individual sensory nerves served a specific function, and each somatic sensation was associated with separate and distinct nerve fibers. Pain, therefore, was a result of the stimulation of a specific sensory receptor (nerve fiber).

Specificity theory grew out of this view. It was outlined by Schiff in 1858 and refined by von Frey and colleagues in the 1890s (von Frey, 1894). Specificity theory, not unlike Descartes' notion of pain, postulated that pain was a specific modality, independent of touch and similar to vision and hearing, with its own particular central and peripheral mechanism(s). In specificity theory, emphasis was placed on the presences of separate and distinct receptors for the modalities of pain, touch, warmth, and cold. Free nerve endings in the skin were thought to function as "pain receptors." When stimulated, these particular nerve endings generated "pain impulses," which were transmitted by A-delta and C-fibers through the spinothalamic tract to the "pain center" in the thalamus.

In 1874, Erb outlined the intensive (explicit) theory of pain, suggesting that any stimulus could evoke pain. He proposed that it was the intensity of the stimulus which produced a type of "sensory overload" that was crucial, rather than the activation of a specific receptor. Therefore, any stimulus of sufficient intensity, including cold and light, was capable of producing pain. Goldscheider (1884) expanded the intensive theory of pain to include both stimulus intensity and central summation of stimulation. Goldscheider proposed that each tactile nerve fiber could evoke three distinct qualities of sensation depending on the intensity of the stimulation: tickle, touch, and pain. He also suggested that, over time, input from peripheral fibers could accumulate (summate) in the dorsal horn of the spinal cord, and once a given threshold of activity had been achieved, a pain-signaling fiber in the spinal cord would be activated.

The notion of central summation of stimulation, expressed in the summation theory, was expanded upon by Sherrington. In 1906, Sherrington described the existence of injury sensitive nerve endings and referred to them as "nocicipent," later renamed as nociceptive nerves or nociceptors. He noted that these nociceptive nerves could be activated by mechanical, thermal, or chemical stimuli. He characterized the nociceptive reaction as consisting of a reflex withdrawal, autonomic responses, and pain, and the initiating event as a noxious stimulus. He also proposed the existence of pools of nerves in the spinal cord that functioned to separate out the incoming signals form the periphery. The ability of incoming impulses to activate or create excitatory or inhibitory states in the central nervous system, which could be summated, was used to explain how sensory experiences could outlast the duration of the stimulus.

Despite rigorous investigation, the search for a modality-specific pain fiber (nerve) failed. A verifiable relationship between the makeup (morphology) of a sensory receptor and its function could not be established. Thus, in the 1950s, Lele, Waddell, and Sinclair (see Sinclair, 1958), among others, also argued against the existence of a specific cutaneous pain receptor and, incorporating some of the features of summation theory, proposed the pattern theory of pain as an alternative to the specificity theory. These researchers reasoned that it was the spatial and temporal patterns of nerve impulses and their summation that was important. These spatiotemporal patterns were transmitted to the brain, where they were summated and translated into various sensations. Spatial summation was demonstrated when previous subthreshold stimulation applied to a small area of the skin provoked a pain response upon being applied to a larger area of the body. Likewise, a stimulus of sufficient intensity to evoke a response when applied to small area resulted in a more intense response when applied to a larger area. Temporal summation, by contrast, was observed when stimulation at a given frequency did not produce a pain sensation, but did at another frequency. Some of the pattern theories emphasized the importance of the summation of cutaneous (peripheral) spatiotemporal patterns, while others, such as that by Livingston, highlighted the role of "central summation." In fact, Livingston (1943) and Hebb (1949) proposed a type of reverberating circuit in the spinal cord that was established in response to pathological stimulation. These circuits, or central summation mechanisms, could then be activated by ordinarily nonpainful stimulation, thus generating abnormal impulses that would be interpreted by the brain as pain.

On the more clinical side, observations of patients in severe pain without an apparent lesion or injury were being recorded. Furthermore, such pain seemed recalcitrant to opioid therapy. Two theories emerged to explain this phenomenon. In 1826, Francois Broussais (1826) proposed the concept of a "functional" lesion, and Benjamin Brodie the notion of spinal irritation and "cenesthesia" (the inability to correctly perceive one's internal sensations). In 1872, Silas Weir Mitchell, an American neurologist, published his now famous *Injuries of Nerves and Their Consequences*. In this book he chronicled his observations during the Civil War of what is now know to be phantom limb pain and causalgia (neuropathic pain). In both instances, the complaints of the injured soldiers seemed fantastic and inexplicable. Severe pain was felt not only in response to merely touching the injured limb but often in anticipation of it being touched. The fact that these pains lasted for decades seemed to strain credulity. In the absence of any definitive diagnostic test or medical explanation, the suffering victim was thought to manifest symptoms of some psychiatric or emotional disorder or, worse yet, to be malingering. In a similar vein, William K. Livingston (1943) maintained the existence of an organic basis for similar complaints of soldiers from World War I and II. The eventual advent and demonstrated effectiveness of local anesthetic nerve blocks ultimately validated the reality of these pain complaints.

Ironically, Henry Beecher, a Harvard anesthesiologist working at Anzio during World War II, noted a striking contrast between the complaints of pain in seriously wounded soldiers and those of his civilian patients with similar or less remarkable injuries. Indeed, those of the soldiers were significantly muted (Beecher, 1946). He reasoned that this was associated with the competing positive emotions of the soldier realizing that the injury would result in his returning home to his family. Beecher thus brought to light the potential contribution of cognitive and emotional factors in the experience of pain. This notion led to the exploration of the placebo effect, through which administration of a relatively inert substance produced an unexpected analgesic response. The efforts to dissect out those nuances of the human brain ("mind") that make it capable of creating something (pain relief) out of nothing (a placebo) continue and are spearheaded by researchers such as Antonio Benedetti (Benedetti et al, 2005).

In the 1960s and 1970s, Edward Perl and his colleagues (Mason, 2007; Perl, 2007) introduced the notion of pain occurring in response to activation of specialized high-threshold nociceptors. They described primary afferents responsible for the detection of noxious stimulation of the skin. Several types of afferents were discovered via meticulous recordings involving some 513 lightly myelinated and 131 unmyelinated primary afferents and 110 dorsal horn cells. These included (a) a group of lightly myelinated primary afferents that only responded to noxious mechanical stimulation; (b) two populations of unmyelinated primary afferents that respond to noxious stimulation: polymodal nociceptors and high-threshold mechanoreceptors; and (c) a group of about 10% of the cutaneous afferents that were unresponsive to all forms of stimulation. This latter group may have represented those afferents that have come to be known as "silent nociceptors," as they are only activated by severe cutaneous damage or inflammation The polymodal nociceptors were so named because they could be activated by a variety of noxious stimuli, including mechanical, thermal, and chemical stimuli.

Two of the most recognized names in the history of pain are Ronald Melzack and Patrick Wall. In 1959, psychologist Ronald Melzack, a student of D.O. Hebb, was exploring the effects of early sensory deprivation on pain perception and had already suggested that the brain exerted descending inhibitory influence on pain. Patrick Wall was chairman of the Department of Biology at the Massachusetts Institute of Technology and interested in spinal cord physiology. The two men initially met in response to Melzack's search for research space. Wall was able to free up space in his building, which was occupied by members of MIT's Department of Food Technology who had received funds from the U.S. Space Agency to study the effects of a hard landing on the moon on cans of food in the space vehicle. They accomplished this by using a catapult-like apparatus to sling cans of food against a cement surface. Reportedly, Wall was able to convince them that they could do this in more limited space. Thus the long-standing relationship between Melzack and Wall began.

Stimulated by visits from W.K. Livingston and by W. Noordenboos' 1959 book *Pain*, Melzack and Wall were convinced of the inadequacy of the existing theories of pain. First, they felt that the anatomical and physiological specificity described by many of the existing theories of pain did not account for the vast array of discrepancies noted between the degree and type of peripheral stimulation or injury and the experience of pain. Second, they believed brain processes, which had been relatively ignored, were crucial to an integrated theory of pain, and that this theory had to include consideration of feedforward and feedback transmission. And third, they felt that a new hypothetical spinal cord mechanism with sufficient power to explain existing data was needed. In 1965, Melzack and Wall coauthored "Pain Mechanisms: A New Theory." In this article they posited the existence of a gate control system that modulated sensory input before evoking the perception of pain and accompanying response(s). Their gate control theory (GCT) forever altered the manner in which pain and its treatment was conceptualized.

The GCT of pain emphasized the importance of central processing. Melzack and Wall noted that pain was related to the rate of firing of certain spinal neurons, which they called the first central transmission (T) cell. The rate of firing of these spinal neurons was in turn determined by the degree of large- and small-fiber input. Furthermore, small-fiber input into a hypothetical spinal gate was modulated by descending activity from the brain. Shortly after this, Melzack and Casey (1968) expanded on the role of the central control processes in the brain that interacted with a motivational-affective and sensory-discriminative system activating an action system. The GCT essentially rejected the notion of a specific pain receptor or dedicated pain pathway to the brain. These researchers effectively proclaimed psychological factors to be as important as sensory factors in the experience of pain. The GCT stimulated a paradigm shift in the understanding and treatment of pain, from surgical and pharmacological approaches designed to alter the sensory input to one that also considered motivational, affective, and cognitive factors (Meldrun, 2003).

In the 1950s, John Bonica, a noted anesthesiologist in Seattle, Washington, convened a group of pain experts from around the world and initiated the International Association for the Study of Pain (IASP), with emphasis on the multidisciplinary approach to the study and treatment of pain. Seattle became the site of one of the first truly multidisciplinary treatment clinics in America, headed by John Loeser, a neurosurgeon, and Wilbert Fordyce, a psychologist. Another well-known neurosurgeon on the other side of the country, in Miami, Florida, Hubert Rosomoff, began a pain clinic also founded on this multidisciplinary model. Fordyce's 1976 book, *Behavioral Methods for Chronic Pain and Illness*, heralded the onset of extensive investigations and experimental studies into the role of behavioral and conditioning procedures and theory in pain. Some two decades later, Donald Price wrote *Psychological Aspects of Pain and Analgesia* (1999), in which he provided a detailed account of the impact of psychological variables. His work was facilitated and greatly expanded by the advent of functional neuroimaging techniques which, for the first time in history, allowed one to capture an image of the functioning brain rather than its mere anatomical structure.

Scientific knowledge of the sensory processing system expanded as well (Carli, 2011; Perl, 2007). Free nerve endings in the skin were identified that responded to thermal, chemical, or mechanical stimulation. Noxious levels of stimulation sufficient to cause tissue injury or damage were discovered to result in the release of chemicals producing a local inflammatory response, which in turn was associated with the experience of pain. A-delta and C afferent fibers were found to be responsible for transmitting sensory input to the spinal cord. Once these primary afferents entered the spinal cord gray matter, they synapsed with second-order neurons, eventually ascending to the brain within the spinothalamic tracts. All pain, however, was not the same. Clifford J. Woolf (2004, 2007) outlined the general properties of four types of pain: nociceptive, neuropathic, inflammatory, and functional pain. He enumerated the different mechanisms involved in each and promoted a mechanism-based approach to pain diagnosis and treatment.

Over time, it became apparent that pain, especially chronic pain, was more than just a symptom or a product of poor coping. Quite the contrary, the 21st century has witnessed the most remarkable change in the history of pain. Michael Cousins of Australia and other pain experts around the world have begun to view pain as a "disease process" (Cousins, 1999; Siddall and Cousins, 2004). Consistent with the accepted criteria for a condition to be considered a disease entity, pain has be found

(a) to manifest its own pathology (physiological and chemical), (b) to be independent and self-perpetuating, (c) to have a constellation of signs and symptoms, and (d) to impair or modify vital functions. The basis for considering pain as a disease process will be discussed in detail in Chapter 8.

CONCLUSION

Pain has been viewed as a symptom for the better part of its history. The cause has varied from evil spirits and demons to the activation of specialized nerve endings. An organized scientific exploration of pain is but 150 years old; an awareness of the existence of modulatory influences is about 50 years old; and formal investigation of cortical and subcortical involvement is less than 20 years old. The emergence of pain as a disease unto itself represents a quantum shift in how pain is understood.

Despite having come a long way from interpreting pain as a result of demon intrusion, much remains to be done. The theories outlined above, some of which will be discussed in greater detail in upcoming chapters, have illuminated the way for new and novel approaches to pain. To date, however, the incidence and prevalence of various types of pain remain relatively unchecked. Although the therapeutic approaches are more scientifically based and, in many respects, more humane, the outcomes, especially when viewed worldwide, are woefully inadequate.

The next step in the evolution of the concept of pain may profit from extending beyond the scientific principles of materialism and reductionism that have guided most of the research efforts up to this point. There may be advantages to reframing and expanding the paradigm in which pain is viewed. In doing so, there is no need to abandon the current theories and clinical practices. However, it is important not to be held hostage by these theories and modes of thinking. The willingness to explore and embrace a broader view of pain will prove to either strengthen the existing notions or reveal complementary and perhaps alternative conceptualizations. Either way, as shown by history, the understanding of pain and the patients experiencing it will be advanced. In much the same fashion that ancient approaches to pain seem crude when examined in light of current scientific principles and knowledge, expanding beyond the present-day notion of pain may provide new and valuable insights. Chaos theory, quantum physics, decomplexification, and the notion of nonlinearity offer unique opportunities to go to the next level. The remaining chapters in this book will explore these arenas and their potential contribution to the understanding of pain.

REFERENCES

Beecher HK. Pain in men wounded in battle. *Ann Surg.* 1946;123:96–105.

Benedetti F, Mayberg HS, Wager TD, Stohler CS, Zubieta JK. Neurobiological mechanisms of the placebo effect. *J Neurosci.* 2005;25:10390–10402.

Bingel U, Tracey I. Imaging CNS modulation of pain in humans. *Physiology.* 2008;23:371–380.

Broussais F. *Traité de physiologie appliquée à la pathologie* (2 vols). Paris: Mile Delauney; 1822–23. [*A Treatise on Physiology Applied to Pathology.* Bell J, LaRoche R, trans. Philadelphia: H.C. Carey and I. Lea; 1826.]

Carli G. Historical perspective and modern views on pain physiology: from psychogenic pain to hyperalgesia priming. *Arch Ital Biol.* 2011;149(Suppl):175–186.

Cousins MJ. Pain: the past, present, and future of anesthesiology. *Anesthesiology*. 1999;91:538–551.

De Quincey T. *Confessions of an English Opium Eater*. New York: Dover; (1821) 1995.

Erb W. *Handbuch der Krankheiten des Nervensystems. II*. Leipzig: F.C.W. Vogel; 1874.

Fordyce W. *Behavioral Methods for Chronic Pain and Illness*. St. Louis: Mosby; 1976.

Goldscheider A. Die spezifische Energie der Gefühlsnerven der Haut. *Mh Prakt Derm*. 1884;3:283.

Hebb DO. *Organization of Behavior: A Neurophysiological Theory*. New York: John Wiley and Sons; 1949.

Livingston WK. *Pain Mechanism: A Physiological Explanation of Causalgia and Its Related States*. New York: Macmillan; 1943.

Madier JL. Recognizing Odysseus' scar: reconceptualizing pain and its empathic role in civil adjudication. *Fla State Univ Law Rev*. 2006;34:43.

Mason P. Placing pain on the sensory map: classic papers by Ed Perl and colleagues. *J Neurophysiol*. 2007;97:1871–1873.

Meldrum ML. A capsule history of pain management. *JAMA*. 2003;290(18):2470–2475.

Melzack R, Casey K. Sensory, motivational and central control determinants of pain: a new conceptual model. In Kenshalo D, ed. *The Skin Senses*. Springfield, IL: Thomas; 1968:23–42.

Melzack R, Wall P. Pain mechanisms: a new theory. *Science*. 1965;150:971–979.

Mitchell SW. *Injuries of Nerves and Their Consequences*. Philadelphia: J.P. Lippincott; 1872.

Moayedi M, Davis KD. Theories of pain: from specificity to gate control. *J Neurophysiol*. 2013;109:5–12.

Morris DB. An invisible history of pain: early 19th-century Britain and America. *Clin J Pain*. 1998;14(3):191–196.

Muller J. *Handbuch der Physiologie des Menschen für Vorlesungen*. Koblenz, Germany: Verlag von J. Holscher; 1840.

Noordenboos W. *Pain*. Amsterdam: Elsevier; 1959.

Papper EM. The discovery of anesthesia: its relationship to the literature of the Romantic Era. *Anesthesia History Association Newsletter*. 1990;8(1):10–13, 16.

Parris WCV. The history of pain medicine. In Raj PR, ed. *Practical Pain Management*, 3rd ed. St. Louis: Mosby; 2000:3–9.

Perl ER. Ideas about pain, a historical view. *Nat Rev Neurosci*. 2007;8:1–80.

Price DD. *Psychological Aspects of Pain and Analgesia*. Seattle: IASP Press; 1999.

Schiff JM. *Lehrbuch der Physiologie des Menschen. I. Muskel- und Nervenphysiologie*. Lahr, Germany: M. Schauenburg; 1858.

Sherrington CS. Observations on the scratch-reflex in the spinal dog. *J Physiol*. 1906;43:1–50.

Siddall PJ, Cousins MJ. Persistent pain as a disease entity: implication for clinical management. *Anesth Analg*. 2004;99:510–520.

Sinclair DC. The anatomy of pain. *Aust J Physiother*. 1958;4:150–156.

Todd EM. Pain: historical perspectives. In Aronoff GM, ed. *Evaluation and Treatment of Chronic Pain*. Baltimore: Urban & Schwarzenberg; 1985:1–16.

Unruh AM. Voices from the past: ancient views of pain in childhood. *Clin J Pain*. 1992;8:247–254.

Woolf CJ. Pain: moving from symptom control toward mechanism-specific pharmacologic management. *Ann Intern Med*. 2004;140:441–451.

Woolf CJ, Ma Q. Nociceptors—noxious stimulus detectors. *Neuron*. 2007;55:353–364.

von Frey M. Beiträge zur Physiologie des Schmerzsinns. *Berichte der Königlichen Sächsische Akademie der Wissenschaften zu Leipzig Math. Phys. Classe*. 1894;46:185–196.

3 Pain Mechanisms and Types

The labeling of nociceptors as pain-fibers was not an admirable simplification but an unfortunate trivialization.
–P.D. Wall and S.B. McMahon (1986, p. 255)

INTRODUCTION

The term *nociception* is derived from *noci*, which in Latin means "to injure, to hurt; injury, harm, or harmful." The term *nociception* is used in place of *pain* to convey an important notion—that is, the nociceptive system involves the activation of specialized sensory nerves (axons) referred to as *nociceptors*, so named because they tend to be activated by events that are damaging or potentially damaging to the individual, such as getting burned from touching the stove. The term *nociception* has at times referred to the transmitting of sensory information, at other times as the entire process encoding and processing of sensory information (Loeser and Treede, 2008). The nociceptive system "signals" the individual of the need to make a response, for example, withdraw the hand from the hot stove. This nociceptive reflex may occur with little thought and exists in organisms with limited brain capacity, such as rodents.

The experience of pain, however, is much more complex and complicated, arguably requiring more sophisticated processing, such as that found in the human brain. Tracey and Mantyh (2007) described pain as "a conscious experience, an interpretation of the nociceptive input influenced by memories, emotional, pathological, genetic, and cognitive factors. Resultant pain is not necessarily related linearly to the nociceptive drive or input; neither is it solely for vital protective functions" (p. 377). Therefore, the creation of an electrical signal or impulse and the manner in which it makes its way to the brain will be referred to as *nociception* rather than *pain*. This distinction will aid in understanding how two individuals can be subjected to the same external stimulus activating their respective nociceptive systems, yet only one describes the experience as "painful." One of the more time-honored approaches to the study and understanding of the phenomenon of nociception has been to dismantle it into its four components: transduction, transmission, modulation, and perception.

NOCICEPTIVE PATHWAYS

Peripheral System

The periphery (peripheral nervous system [PNS], consisting of spinal and cranial nerves) contains many sensory nerve fiber endings (Johnson, 2000). Each nerve is made up of several axons, including somatic and visceral, whose cell body (nucleus) is found in the dorsal root ganglion. One end of the axon terminates in the skin and serves a specific area (receptor field), and the other end terminates in the dorsal horn of the spinal cord. A particular axon is only influenced by stimuli occurring within its receptor field. This configuration results in the ability to precisely locate the origin of a stimulus. Afferent axons conduct information into the central nervous system (CNS—spinal cord and brain), and efferents convey information from the CNS. The term *primary afferent* is given to the nerve activated by a peripheral stimulus, making it the initial "link" in the nociceptive chain. Depending on their anatomical structure, these axons respond to different types of stimulation, such as thermal, mechanical, or chemical. Some axons require only a small amount of stimulation (low threshold); others require more intense stimulation (high threshold). In addition, some axons respond to a single stimulus, and others, called *polymodal*, respond to a variety of stimuli.

Visceral nociceptors do not respond to cutting or burning injury like their counterparts in the peripheral cutaneous tissue. Instead, they are activated in response to pathological change. A hollow viscus needs to identify and transduce distention, stretch, and isometric contraction. A solid organ needs to signal distention of the capsule that contains it, as well as inflammation. Gebhart and Ness (1991) identified the following as naturally occurring visceral stimuli: distention of hollow organs, ischemia, inflammation, muscle spasm, and traction.

The skin and deep tissues also contain so-called silent nociceptors. These nociceptors are normally unresponsive to noxious mechanical stimulation. However, they become "awakened" (responsive) to stimulation in the presence of inflammation and after tissue injury. It is thought that continuous stimulation from inflammation or damaged tissue reduces the threshold of these nociceptors, causing them to be responsive to stimulation. Activation of these silent nociceptors may contribute to the development of hyperalgesia, central sensitization, and allodynia.

The peripheral end of the axon contains encapsulated proteins called *transduction proteins* (TRP), which can be activated by a specific stimulus. Once released by an effective stimulus, these proteins faithfully initiate a chemical reaction, or *depolarization,* generally involving sodium (Na) or calcium (Ca). Depolarization of the terminal results in "opening" of a sodium or calcium gate, allowing for the creation of an electrical impulse, or action potential, to be conducted along the axon. This process, *transduction*, results in an external stimulus trigging an internal reaction. The nature of the transduction protein defines the response properties of the nerve fiber. For example, certain proteins only react to a thermal stimulus over 43°C, others to one greater than 53°C, and still others only to temperatures between 34 and 38°C.

A variety of neurotransmitters are sequestered in the vesicles at the other end of the axon awaiting release by an effective electrical impulse. Activation of these voltage-sensitive Ca channels culminates in the mobilization and release of a neurotransmitter or neurotransmitters. Genetically linked dysfunction in these ion channels (channelopathy; Raouf et al, 2010) has been associated with a variety of abnormal pain conditions (see Chapter 12). While there are numerous neurotransmitters, the three most common participating in nociceptive transmission are peptides, purines, and excitatory amino acids (EAA). Some primary axon terminals co-contain and co-release both peptides and EAA. These proteins and neurotransmitters are synthesized in the axon's cell body and transported to their respective terminals. Once released, these substances transverse a gap (synapse) between two axons. Upon engaging the second order axon's receptor, the process of depolarization repeats itself, and the impulse is propagated along the chain of axons. The EAA, particularly glutamate, produce the initial excitatory response on the postsynaptic, second-order, neuron, followed by the release of peptides, including substance P, causing a more prolonged depolarization and sustained nociceptive transmission. The electrical-chemical properties of this nociceptive system have been and continue to be the object of much investigation (Heavner and Willis, 2000).

Sensory nerves in the PNS are made up of many smaller nerves. These smaller nerves are classified by their structure and response properties. The *A-beta* nerves, for example, tend to be relatively large and very specialized, and are covered by an insulating myelin sheath that allows for the rapid conduction of an impulse in the range of 40 to 50 meters per second (approximately 110 mph). These fibers are activated by low-threshold mechanical stimulation such as light touch, brushing, or positioning of a joint. *A-delta* myelinated nerve fibers are also specialized but are somewhat smaller and conduct at slower speeds of between 10 and 40 meters per second. Depending on the specific characteristics of a particular fiber, it will be activated by a low or high, mechanical or thermal stimulus (room temperature). The A-delta fibers are generally responsible for the initial sudden, sharp sensation that immediately follows an injury, sometimes referred to as *first pain.*

C-unmyelinated fibers are the smallest and slowest conducting fibers, at less than 2 meters per second. Unlike the A-beta and A-delta fibers, C-fibers are free nerve endings responding to thermal, mechanical, and chemical stimuli alike, but only at high enough thresholds to be potentially damaging or aversive (noxious) to the organism. Thus, they are referred to as *C-polymodal* nociceptors. C-fibers tend to transmit what is often referred to as *second pain.* This is felt as an aching, dull, or burning sensation and lasts long after the noxious event has ended. One example is the prolonged burning sensation felt after removing one's hand from a hot stove. Because of their propensity to respond only to high-threshold stimuli, some A-delta fibers are also considered to be nociceptors.

Primary sensory afferents enter the spinal cord through Lissauer's tract and terminate in the dorsal horn of the spinal cord (see Figure 3.1). They send spinal projections into various areas, or *laminae,* of the spinal cord, which collectively has the appearance of a butterfly. These laminae, or layers, of which there 10, were first described by the neurophysiologist Rexed (1954) and are thus referred to as the "Rexed laminae." They

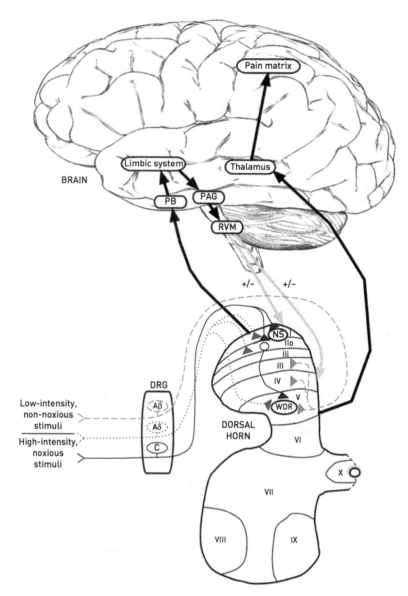

FIGURE 3.1

Pain pathways from periphery to the brain. Primary afferent fibers (A-beta, A-delta, and C-fibers) transmit impulses from the periphery, through the dorsal root ganglion (DRG), and into the dorsal horn of the spinal cord. Nociceptive specific (NS) cells are mainly found in the superficial dorsal horn (laminae I–II), whereas most wide dynamic ranges (WDRs) are located deeper (lamina V). Projection neurons from lamina I innervate areas such as the parabrachial area (PB) and periaqueductal gray matter (PAG) and such pathways are affected by limbic areas. From here, descending pathways (yellow arrows) from brainstem nuclei such as the rostral ventromedial medulla (RVM) are activated and modulate spinal processing. Lamina V neurons mainly project to the thalamus (spinothalamic tract), and from here the various cortical regions forming the "pain matrix" (primary and secondary somatosensory, insular, anterior cingulate, and prefrontal cortices) are activated. From D'Mello R, Dickenson AH. Spinal cord mechanisms of pain. *Br J Anesth*, 2008;101(1):8–16. Reprinted with permission.

are designated by Roman numerals I to X. Different fibers send spinal projections into different laminae (lam). For example, A-delta and C-fibers terminate in lam I, II, and V and, to a lesser extent, lam X; A-beta and A-delta fibers terminate in in lam III–VI; and A-beta fibers in lam VII–IX.

Lam I–V are most prominently featured in nociceptive transmission. Lam I is the outermost layer of the dorsal horn and referred to as the *marginal zone*; lam II is referred to as the *substantia gelatinosa*; and lam III–V as the nucleus proprius. Careful examination has failed to reveal any overlapping of fiber types. That is, high-threshold fibers are found in lam I–II, and low-threshold axons in lam III–VI. A-beta fibers tended to go into deeper laminae and then make a type of U-turn, with some terminating in the deep aspects of lam II. Both A- and C-fibers send collaterals rostrally (cephalad; toward the head) and caudally (toward the base of the spine) along Lissauer's tract up to as many as four to six segments, creating a three-dimensional pattern—that is, superficial and deep, up and down. Therefore, activation of primary afferents in the lumbar spine at the fourth lumbar area (L4) will also create some excitation to L5 and as high as T12 (in the human), with progressively lesser penetration by the dendrites of the axon at the more remote sites. The A fibers also tend to travel along the dorsal column, and the C-fibers in Lissauer's tract. Clinically, this may account for why an injury at a specific lumbar spinal level can be associated with complaints of pain beyond that particular level.

Once in the dorsal horn of the spinal cord, primary afferents synapse with two main classes of second-order neurons, marginal cells or wide dynamic range (WDR) neurons. The marginal cells have their position in the marginal zone or lam I and receive input from high-threshold A-delta and C-fibers. WDR neurons have their cell body in lam V, where they synapse with A-beta fibers but also send dendrites to lam I and II, thus activated by A-delta and C-fibers as well. The process of receiving input from many types of primary afferents in called *fiber convergence*. Therefore, a primary C-fiber, its second-order neuron or marginal cell, will respond only to intense, high-threshold, potentially damaging stimuli. WDR neurons by contrast respond to (encode for) a wide array of stimuli—brushing, pressing, pinching, and squeezing (noxious). Their discharge frequency tends to be proportional to the stimulus intensity, suggesting a linear relationship.

There are two types of convergence: (a) different fiber types converging on a WDR neuron, discussed above, and (b) convergence of different types of afferents. For example, patients with ischemic heart disease often report pain in their left arm as well as their chest. This phenomenon is called *referred pain*. It is accounted for by the fact that primary afferents that innervate visceral organs (heart, colon, liver, esophagus, etc.) travel along sympathetic nerve pathways, but, in fact, tend to have their cell bodies in the same dorsal root ganglion as somatic afferents and synapse with the same WDR neuron as the somatic or peripheral primary afferents described above. Therefore, superficial tenderness can be created by noxious input from a deep structure.

Ascending–Descending System

Transmission pathways extend from the dorsal horn of the spinal cord to higher centers (brain) where perception is said to occur. The brain receives information from both spinal and trigeminal (face and mouth) sensory neurons. Although several tracts are involved, only the three most commonly cited nociceptive spinal transmission tracts will be reviewed here: spinoreticular, spinothalamic, and spinomesencephalic. The postsynaptic dorsal column tract (PSDCT) has been receiving a good deal of research attention as well, possibly because of its involvement in conveying visceral pain information from the pelvic organs to the ventroposterior lateral nucleus (VPL) of the thalamus.

The names of the three primary tracts denote the origin and termination of the signal. The *spinoreticular tract* carries information from the dorsal horn of the spinal cord to the reticular system in the brainstem. This is particularly important, as it services the "reflexive" response to nociception by virtue of its direct contact with the reticular arousal centers. Some projections also go to the thalamus (*spinoreticulothalamic tract*). These pathways tend to run ventrally and laterally from the cord (ventrolateral spinoreticulothalamic tract).

The *spinothalamic tract (STT)* has two trajectories, the lateral, or *neospinothalamic tract*, and the medial, or *paleo* (old) *spinothalamic tract*. These tracts are made up of second-order neurons that cross over to the opposite (contralateral) side of the cord and ascend to higher centers. The *lateral STT* is the primary somatosensory project system and goes directly to the thalamus, perhaps sending off the occasional collateral. This somatosensory projection system allows for precise mapping of the physical characteristics of the sensory stimulus. Second-order WDR neurons from lam V cross over to the contralateral side and ascend up the ventrolateral tract (VLT) to the lateral aspect of the ventral basal complex (VBL) of the primary sensory thalamus.

The primary thalamus is somatotopically organized, in that it provides specific mapping of body sites. The ventroposterior medial nucleus (VPM) tends to encode for the face and receives its input from the trigeminothalamus tract, and the ventroposterior lateral nucleus (VPL) encodes for the body. From here, third-order neurons project to the primary and secondary somatosensory (S1 and S2, respectively) cortex. S1 and S2 cells are organized into somatotopically separated regions, with their small, receptive fields being contralateral. S1 and S2 cells encode for the specific modality, intensity, and location of stimulation. It is this somatosensory system that allows a person, after stubbing his or her toe, to declare that the right great toe is throbbing at an intensity of 7 out of 10 on a numerical rating scale. Indeed, damage to S1 and S2 cells, such as from a focal infarction (an area of dead or dying tissues as a result of obstructed blood flow) results in significantly impaired ability of the individual to discriminate the spatial, temporal, and intensity component of innocuous and noxious peripheral stimuli. In the schema introduced by Melzack and Casey (1968), this function is referred to as the *sensory-discriminative* aspect of nociception. The lateral STT seems to act to arouse the organism to potential tissue damage, instigating neuroendocrine, autonomic, reflexive, and emotional responses to "pain" (see Figure 3.2).

The *medial STT* contains neurons from lam I that cross over and ascend to the more medial aspects of the thalamus. The medial and medial–dorsal aspects of the thalamus do not contain the precise somatotopic organization like that of the lateral thalamus. They appear to process information in a more general fashion and send their third-order neurons to the anterior cingulate cortex (ACC). The ACC is part of the limbic system, which is well known for its involvement in processing emotional states including depression and anxiety. Insula cortex, prefrontal cortex, the amygdala, and the hippocampus are also part of this limbic system and provide input to the hypothalamus. The periaqueductal gray matter (PAG) of the midbrain receives afferent input from limbic structures and in turn sends projections to the medial thalamus

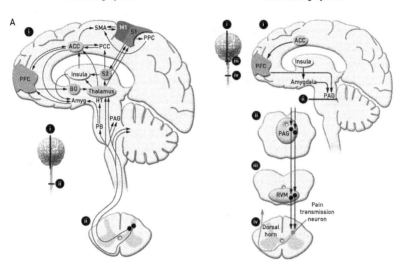

Ascending Sytem

Descending System

FIGURE 3.2

Schematic representation of ascending and descending pain pathways and brain regions involved in pain processing. The highlighted regions superimposed on an anatomical MRI (coronal slice) are S1, S2, anterior cingulate cortex (ACC), insula, thalamus, prefrontal cortex (PFC), and primary motor cortex (M1). SMA, supplemental motor area; PCC, posterior cingulate cortex; BG, basal ganglia; HT, hypothalamus; Amyg, amygdala, PB, parabrachial nuclei. Descending pain modulatory pathways that might be involved in psychological modulation of pain are also shown. One pathway involves descending input from the ACC to the PFC and then to the periaqueductal gray matter (PAG). Another descending pathway arrives at the PAG from the insula via the amygdala. A descending pathway from the PAG through the rostral ventromedial medulla (RVM) to the dorsal horn of the spinal cord influences nociceptive afferent transmission. From Schweinhardt P, Bushnell MC. Pain imaging in health and disease—how far have we come? *J Clin Invest.* 2010;120(11):3788–3797. Reprinted with permission.

and hypothalamus. Therefore, it is this more medial system that encodes for the emotional response to stubbing our toe as that it feels horrible and we fear that the toe is broken. Melzack and Casey (1968) described this as the *motivational-affective,* or *suffering* component. Patients with lesions in this system demonstrate pain asymbolia: they can discriminate the qualitative aspects of noxious input but lack the usual emotional or affective response.

Sophisticated brain imaging techniques have confirmed altered activity in the somatosensory cortex associated with different modalities and intensities of stimulation. The activity correlates very highly with intensity ratings of nociceptive input. Activity in the ACC, however, appears more related to the noxious quality or aversiveness of the stimulation–what Price (1999, 2000) calls pain "unpleasantness." Experimental studies have documented altered activity in the ACC when, as a result of posthypnotic suggestion, subjects noted the same intensity of stimulation to be less upsetting or bothersome despite little or no change in their rating of its intensity.

A third tract is the *spinomesencephalic tract.* Its second-order neurons originate in lam I, IV–VI and appear to be nociceptive specific. They ascend in the dorsal lateral funiculus, particularly those from lam III and IV. It travels via the ventral horn to the mesencephalic reticular formation, PAG, and parabrachial (PB) nuclei. Third-order projects go to the amygdala. It is thought that the dorsal column system functions to alert and prepare the cerebral cortex for incoming nociceptive information. The cortex, in turn, can activate appropriate descending modulatory systems, which can serve to alter the incoming nociception at the level of the dorsal horn.

In addition to this ascending nociceptive system, there is a descending modulatory system that is inhibitory in nature and travels down the dorsal longitudinal funiculus. This descending pathway extends from the cortex to the periventricular gray matter, periaqueductal gray matter (PAG), dorsolateral pontine tegmentum, and on to lam I, II, and V of the dorsal horn. In general, descending modulation involves the cortex and midbrain structures including the PAG and rostral ventromedial medulla (RVM). The primary neurotransmitters include opiates, serotonin (5-HT), and norepinephrine (NE). Activation of this system inhibits nociceptive transmission at the level of the dorsal horn.

In summary, A-delta and C nociceptive afferent fibers extend from the skin to lam I and II of dorsal horn of the spinal cord. Second-order neurons comprise the STTs conducting information to the brain. The lateral tract makes up the sensory discriminative component of nociception and involves the thalamus, basal ganglia, and primary and secondary somatosensory cortex. The more medial nociceptive system involves the motivational-affective components. Cortical structures participating in the processing of this information include the amygdala, hippocampus, brainstem, PAG, insula, ACC, and prefrontal cortex. The descending inhibitory system involves the cortex, amygdala, PAG, hypothalamus, RVM, and parabrachial nucleus. Neurotransmitters involved in the ascending systems include substance P, cholecystokinin (CCK), glutamate, calcitonin gene–related proteins (CGRP), and nerve growth factor (NGF). Opioids, NE, 5-HT, and perhaps gamma-aminobutyric acid (GABA) are involved in the descending system.

NEUROCHEMISTRY OF NOCICEPTION

Sensory fibers carry nociceptive and non-nociceptive information to the central nervous system. The thinly myelinated A-delta and unmyelinated C-fibers primarily transmit nociceptive information. Polymodal C-fibers respond to mechanical, thermal, and chemical stimulation. One group of C-fibers expresses the P2X3 purine receptor, a binding site and receptor for glial cell–derived neurotrophic factor (GDNE). Another group of C-fibers synthesizes substance P and CGRP and expresses the high-affinity NGF receptor TrkA. New molecules are expressed by sensory neurons following damage or inflammation. Damage to sensory neurons also unveils a group of silent nociceptors. These silent nociceptors may be involved in helping to create peripheral sensitization or a heightened response in the peripheral system to otherwise non-noxious or tissue-damaging stimulation.

The physiological and biochemical status of sensory nerves is maintained by growth factors such as NGF, brain-derived neurotrophic factor (BDNF), neruotrphin-3 (NT-3), and GDNF from innervated tissues. Injury to a peripheral nerve results in predictable changes in the chemical milieu, which can be reversed by peripheral or intrathecal delivery of NGF or GDNF. The architectural changes that occur in the superficial layer of the spinal cord as a result of sprouting of A-fiber terminals into the more superficial area of the spinal cord and the retracting of C-fibers from this area can also be prevented by intrathecal NGF.

In general, then, there are two subpopulations of C-fibers: those that are sensitive to NGF and those sensitive to GDNF. GDNF has been implicated in the development of chronic-pain states and are associated with C-fibers that do not express peptides. Tissue inflammation increases NGF, resulting in the sensitization of the primary afferents and the release of substance P and other peptides in sensory neurons and the central nervous system. NGF has been found to be related to pain sensitivity. Blocking the increase of NGF can forestall the development of peripheral sensitivity or hyperalgesia (Treede, 2006).

There are approximately six molecules that signal nociception and are expressed by nociceptive-sensitive neurons. However, the vanilloid receptor 1 (VR1; also known as the transient receptor potential cation channel subfamily V member 1, or TRPV1) and the sensory nerve–specific (SNS) sodium channel have garnered the most interest. TRPV1 receptors are activated by thermal and chemical stimuli including capsaicin and are sometimes referred to as the capsaicin receptor. They appear to play a role in inflammatory pain and hyperalgesia. Alteration of VR1-related genes reduces the emergence of inflammatory related hyperalgesia without affecting the organism's response to noxious thermal or mechanical stimulation. However, TRPV1 receptors have also been found in several brain regions, including the thalamic and hypothalamic nuclei, locus coeruleus, PAG, cerebellum, and cortical and limbic structures, including the hippocampus, and they may play a significant role in learning and memory (Gibson et al, 2008). The SNS sodium channels are classified according to their sensitivity to tetrodotoxin (TTX), a toxin found in the puffer fish. The increased expression TTX-resistant channels tend to be associated with delayed development of hyperalgesia.

In the spinal cord dorsal horn, neurons in lamina 1 expressing the NK1 receptor appear to signal only the presence and intensity of noxious stimulation. However, neurons in the parabrachial area receiving input from NK1-positive spinal neurons send projections that terminate in the ventromedial hypothalamus and amygdala, an area known to be related to the affective-emotional component of pain. Other neurons that do not express the NK1 receptor seem to project information regarding the quality and type of pain. This arrangement reinforces the notion of two separate but interrelated mechanisms involving the sensory and affective components of pain.

The activity of the descending modulatory system should not be ignored and is thought to be part of the process involved in "resetting" nociceptive thresholds. As such, the descending modulatory system, along with the local circuits in the spinal cord, may be as responsible for the hyperalgesia and allodynia that is observed following an injury. Knocking out or deactivating the NK1 system reduces a good deal of the stress-related, anxiety-related, and aggressive behavior usually associated with an injury. NK1 receptor antagonists, therefore, are not likely to reduce the sensory components of pain perception but may impact the affective or unpleasant components.

Morphine and related compounds act at the mu-opioid receptor, which is expressed in nociceptive sensory fibers, spinal cord neurons, forebrain, and brainstem neurons. Morphine efficacy is compromised by drug tolerance, side effects, and fear of abuse and addiction. Evidence suggests that morphine tolerance may be related to cholecystokinin-B (CCK-B) receptor and NK1-receptor activity.

Tolerance can be divided into associative (learned) and nonassociative (pharmacological) (Grisel et al, 1996). Associative tolerance is demonstrated when an organism shows tolerance to the effect of a drug in one particular setting but this tolerance to the drug does not generalize to another setting or is functionally reversed when the drug is administered in a novel environment. This associative tolerance can also be reversed by administering a CCK-B antagonist into the amygdala. The psychologically rewarding effects of morphine contribute to the development of drug abuse and addiction, but can be separated from its analgesic effects. NK1-receptor antagonists have been shown to reduce the rewarding effects of morphine, such as euphoria, without interfering with its analgesic effects.

LONG-TERM POTENTIATION

Long-term potentiation (LTP) has been defined as a long-lasting increase of synaptic strength that can be mediated by either pre- or postsynaptic mechanisms, or both. Sandkuhler (2007) describes synaptic strength as the magnitude of a monosynaptically evoked postsynaptic current or potential in response to a single presynaptic action potential. LTP is generally induced experimentally by the application of a high-frequency (HF; although low-frequency stimulation and pharmacological agents have also been used) conditioning stimulus to primary afferent C-nociceptive fibers and consists of at least two phases: early phase and late phase. The early phase can last up to 3 hours. The late phase, which appears to be dependent on protein synthesis, can last for the duration of the organisms' existence and may involve structural changes (plasticity) at C-fiber synapses.

LTP occurring at the first synapse in the superficial dorsal horn appears to contribute to the hyperalgesia seen is response to inflammation, trauma, or neuropathy. Furthermore, LTP of synaptic strength in the hippocampus forms an excellent model for learning and memory formation (Gibson et al, 2008; Goosens and Maren, 2002). In the brain, LTP requires synchronization of high levels of presynaptic activity or the pairing of a low level of presynaptic activity with a strong postsynaptic depolarization.

LTP in the spinal cord is known to last for a matter of hours or perhaps a few days. In cortical structures it can persist for the lifetime of the organism in accordance with the conditioning stimulus, its repetition, and the experimental conditions.

The evidence indicates that LTP induction occurs in spinal cord lamina-1 neurons, which send projections to the PB area but not those with projections to the PAG. In addition, LTP requires coactivation of NK1 and NK2 receptors and the opening of NMDA-type glutamate and T-type voltage-gated calcium channels. Postsynaptic calcium (Ca^{2+}) appears essential for LTP induction and is linearly related to the magnitude of the LTP (Reyes and Stanton, 1996). LTP can spread to neighboring synapses (heterosynaptic) that are not directly affected by the conditioning stimulus. This accounts for the experience of pain outside the receptive field of the stimulated C-fiber (secondary hyperalgesia). LTP at synapses of nociceptive C-fibers is also been shown to be related to the hyperalgesic response seen with acute opioid withdrawal and is a shared mechanism with opioid-induced hyperalgesia (OIH).

The LTP concept is based in part on the Hebbian notion of cell assemblies (Hebb, 1949). Hebb noted, "When one cell repeatedly assists in firing another, the axon of the first cell develops synaptic knobs (or enlarges them if they already exist) in contact with the soma of the second cell" (p. 63). He also noted that "any two cells or systems of cells that are repeatedly active at the same time will tend to become 'associated,' so that activity in one facilitates activity in the other" (p. 70). Hebb speculated that this coordinated activity between a presynaptic terminal and post-synaptic neuron would strengthen their connection. These combinations of cells would form a processing unit, or "cell assembly...a diffuse structure comprised of cells in the cortex and diencephalon capable of acting briefly as a closed system delivering information to other such systems" (p. xix). Synaptic terminals strength-ened by this coordinated activity would persist or sprout new branches, while those with uncoordinated activity would be weakened. Over time, complex behaviors are formed from sets of cell assemblies called *phase sequences*. Hebb reasoned that indi-vidual neurons do not work in isolation and thus cannot themselves account for any perception or ability. Originally he postulated that this type of behavior of synapses in neural networks enabled the process of learning and allowed for the networks to store memories. However, Hebb's notions have now been applied to the under-standing of long-term alterations in synaptic strength (plasticity). The phrase "neu-rons that fire together wire together" is commonly referred to as Hebb's law. In later chapters it will become clear how Hebb's notions fit well with contemporary systems theory approach to brain functioning and the development of systems neuroscience (Nicolelis et al, 1997).

LTP can be prevented or reversed. Using the animal model of low-frequency induced LTP, Drdla-Schutting et al (2012) demonstrated what they referred to as the "erasure of a spinal memory trace of pain." Brief administration of a high dose of remifentanil, an ultra-short-acting opioid, was given at 1 or 4 hours after the con-ditioning stimulus. The remifentanil effectively reversed LTP and prevented synap-tic plasticity (opioid-induced depotentiation, OID) at both time periods. The effect was observed in a variety of LTP models, including capsaicin-induced hyperalgesia, but only with high- and not low-dose remifentanil. They suggested that this calcium (Ca^{2+})-dependent depotentiation at the nociceptive C-fiber synapses in the superficial lumbar dorsal horn may erase a "memory trace" of pain. By extension, there would be suppression of activity in the ascending nociceptive pathways, virtually preventing the experience of acute, and therefore chronic, pain. These and other findings suggest that the use of a mu-opioid analgesic along with general anesthesia is more likely to shield the cord from noxious input, the result being less postoperative acute pain and, perhaps, less emergence of chronic pain.

A companion concept to LTP and OID, and an associated form of synaptic plas-ticity, is long-term depression (LTD) of synaptic strength. LTD is characterized by a decrease in synaptic strength (pain perception) following the administration of a conditioning stimulus—usually low-frequency (LF) vs. high-frequency stimulation, depending on the degree of depolarization. The "weaker" depolarization created by the LF stimulation only partially displaces the Mg^{2+} ions, resulting in a lower amount of Ca^{2+} entering the postsynaptic neuron and thus a lower concentration of intracel-lular Ca^{2+} at the postsynaptic neuron. LTD can also be instigated at inactive synapses if (a) the Ca^{2+} concentration is increased to the minimum level required by heterosyn-aptic activation or (b) the extracellular concentration is increased. There also seems to be a narrow time period in which the pairing of a postsynaptic potential with synaptic input will occasion LTD. Thus, in general, it is the level and timing of the rise in Ca^{2+} which determine whether LTD or LTP will emerge.

From a system's perspective there is the possibility of a bifurcated outcome (LTD or LTP), based on the frequency of the conditioning stimulus (high vs. low), amount of pre- and postsynaptic Ca^{2+}, and timing of the conditioning stimulus. Once created, LTP can be short-lived (few hours) or indefinite, depending on subsequent stimulation. Furthermore, this neural network represents only a fraction of the overall pain perception network. LTP and LTD are examples of how relatively small perturbation may be associated with strong and long-standing consequences, exemplifying a non-linear system.

PAIN TYPES

There are many ways to categorize pain. These include by intensity (mild, moderate, sever), location (low back, pelvis, joint, headache), quality (sharp, burning, throbbing, nauseating), duration (transient, persistent, intermittent), or referral pattern (superficial, deep, generalized, localized). Traditionally, pain has been described as acute, chronic, or cancer related. *Acute pain* is generally seen as adaptive, in that it warns the person of potential damage or harm. *Chronic pain* is considered maladaptive and void of any survival value to the organism. *Cancer pain* has been reserved for those cases in which the presence of cancer is the cause of the pain. Although arguably a form of chronic pain, by virtue of its association with a frequently fatal disease and often indicative of tissues or organ destruction, cancer pain is classified separately.

Headache or *head pain* is another unique category containing *recurrent-acute* types of pain, such as that from migraine. Yet the acute episodes, though very painful, are not brought on by tissue damage.

Another means of categorizing pain is according to the suspected underlying mechanism, as outlined by Woolf (2004, 2010). *Nociceptive pain* is brought on by activation of neural or peripheral nociceptive pathways in response to a tissue-damaging or potentially damaging stimulus. Postoperative pain, mechanical low back pain, and pain from sports and exercise injuries are some examples. *Neuropathic pain* by contrast is caused by damage, injury, or dysfunction involving the central or peripheral nervous system. Postherpetic neuralgia, diabetic neuropathic pain, trigeminal neuralgia, and post-stroke pain are examples. *Inflammatory pain* is defined by spontaneous pain and hypersensitivity to pain in response to tissue damage and inflammation, such as that in rheumatoid arthritis.

Finally, *functional pain* is highlighted by hypersensitivity to pain stemming from abnormal central processing of normal input. In the case of functional pain, there is an apparent lack of an identifiable neurological deficit or peripheral abnormality. Conditions commonly found in this category are irritable bowel syndrome, fibromyalgia, and noncardiac chest pain, commonly referred to as medically unexplained symptoms (MUS; see Chapter 7).

There is evidence that all types of pains are not alike. For example, Honore and colleagues (2000) examined neurochemical changes found in animal models of inflammatory, neuropathic, and cancer pain. Inflammatory pain was created in a group of mice by injecting an inflammatory substance (Freund's adjuvant) under the skin of the subject's hind paw. Within days there is evidence of swelling and tenderness. Neuropathic pain was generated by two different approaches. One used a suture that was tightly tied (ligating) around the L5 nerve in the spine of the animal. The other approach involved cutting (transecting) the sciatic nerve. Finally, cancer pain was created by injecting osteolytic sarcoma cells in to the leg bone (femur).

After these procedures were carried out, an extensive and detailed immuno-histochemical analysis was conducted on various markers in the primary afferent fiber, spinal cord neurons, motor neurons, and astrocytes. The results showed unique changes in the cellular markers for each type of pain. There was significant up-regulation of SP and CGRP in the dorsal horn of the mice exhibiting inflammatory pain. However, these same neurotransmitters were down-regulated in the primary afferents of the mice with neuropathic pain, and no change was observed in those with cancer pain. Furthermore, galanin (GAL) and neuropeptide Y (NPY) were dramatically up-regulated in the DRG neurons in animals with neuropathic pain but were unchanged in the cancer pain model. Differential changes were also noted in the spinal cord. The most significant one was an up-regulation of GFAP for cancer pain. Lesser and more localized increases in GFAP were found in neuropathic pain. It was concluded that cancer pain is not simply some variant or combination of inflammatory and neuropathic pain, but a distinct pain entity unto itself.

NEUROPATHIC PAIN

Neuropathic pain merits a more detailed discussion, as it tends to have some unique features that make it especially damaging to the organism and recalcitrant to treatment (Woolf and Mannion, 1999). About 3% of the U.S. population suffers from neuropathic pain. The cost in terms of treatment and loss productivity is estimated at some 40 billion dollars a year. It can be associated with "positive" signs, such increased response to provocative stimuli, or "negative" signs (loss of feeling or sensation, or decreased responsiveness). Causes of neuropathic pain are many and varied and include trauma, inflammation, transaction of a nerve, nerve compression, ischemic or metabolic injury to cell bodies, cancer, diabetes, multiple sclerosis (MS), Parkinson's disease, an infections agent (HIV), and toxic side effects of drugs.

In general, peripheral sensory or nociceptive neurons are damaged by diseases, injuries, or drugs. This damage results in hyperexcitability in the primary afferent nociceptor referred to as *peripheral sensitization*. If the nerve is able to repair itself, such as with a sunburn, the sensitization resolves. However, in the case of a chronic disease like diabetes, the damage is ongoing as a result of hyperglycemia. Ultimately, the damage alters the processing mechanism of nociceptors, leading to further sensitization characterized by a lower threshold for activation, increased response, and/or abnormal spontaneous activity (*spontaneous discharge*), commonly seen in diabetic neuropathic pain.

Chronic peripheral nerve damage can result in abnormal electrical connections being formed among damaged and undamaged nerves. These abnormal connections cause "cross-talk" or ephaptic transmission associated with amplification of the pain impulses. Ephaptic transmission can occur between sensory and sympathetic fibers contributing to sympathetically mediated pain (SMP). Therefore, any event that activates the sympathetic nervous system, including stress, can increase the experience of pain. Neurotransmitters such as norepinephrine mediate the increased pain and become therapeutic targets. Impaired sympathetic activity can lead to other conditions, such as vasoconstriction, which results in decreased regional blood flow, further complicating the clinical problem. Damage to the peripheral nerve axon can also cause the accumulation of sodium channels at the injury site and along the axon, promoting ectopic discharges or increased bursts of pain impulses. The increased discharge to the dorsal horn of the spinal cord affects the gating mechanism and increases expression and release of substance P, a primary neurotransmitter in the pain system.

Several changes can occur in the dorsal horn. For example, sympathetic and afferent nerve fibers are linked or coupled together. Sympathetic nerve fibers sprout basket-like terminals around the primary afferent. There is abnormal release of substance P, normally found only in C-fibers, from A-fibers as well. These various structural and functional changes lead to hyperexcitability of CNS neurons, or central sensitization. This central sensitization is thought to result from increased neuronal expression and activation of ion channels, such as voltage-gated sodium channels, and the receptors that initiate and mediate abnormal generation of action potential and synaptic transmission in pain pathways. Sprouting of the central terminal of low-threshold (A-beta) fibers into the superficial layer of the dorsal horn, usually occupied exclusively by nociceptive terminal, occurs within weeks of the nerve injury. Similarly, nerve injury leads to the selective death of GABAergic inhibitory interneurons, resulting in the loss of inhibition (disinhibition), thus contributing to hypersensitivity. One week after nerve injury produces hypersensitivity neurons begin to undergo *apoptosis*, which may become excitotoxic due to excessive glutamate release or failure of glutamate uptake or can result from cell death–inducing signals.

This peripheral and central hyperexcitability activates the N-methyl-D-aspartate (NMDA) receptor, located postsynaptically in the dorsal horn. Glutamate, an excitatory neurotransmitter, is released, causing neuronal membrane depolarization that allows stimuli to produce a much larger postsynaptic potential than would otherwise be the case. This is referred to as *synaptic potentiation*. This LTP is found in many chronic neuropathic pain states and may account for the enhanced intensity and duration of the pain.

CONCLUSION

Pain has been viewed as a sensation and a perception. As a sensory phenomenon, pain is interpreted as being akin to the auditory and visual system—that is, directly explainable by the functional properties of receptors, afferent nerve fibers, and the central sensory system. This version of pain is depicted by the now-famous and classic cartoon drawing of Descartes showing a boy with his toe by a fire (see Figure 2.1 in Chapter 2). It was thought that particles from the fire stimulated molecules of some type, activating a nerve pathway that transmitted a pain signal directly to the brain. There was little indication of the pain signal being altered. This linear approach to pain held sway for many centuries. Pain as a perception, by contrast, embodies the total psychological experience. Contemporary theories recognize pain as the result of a complex set of sensory and perceptual processes. In this regard, pain is somewhat unique among human experiences.

There appear to be several types of pain, differentiated, at least in part, by the inciting event; these include inflammatory, nociceptive, and neuropathic pain. More often than not, these types are not mutually exclusive in the clinical setting. Furthermore, this classification system does not take into account the differences between acute, chronic, cancer-related, and experimentally induced pain. In the case of phantom pain, the sensation seems to be generated from within the system. What meaning should be attached to the fact that different types of chronic pain exist is unclear. Should a mechanistic approach to treatment be taken? Or, given that the brain appears to be the vital organ, should it be the therapeutic target? Merely suppressing nociception is clearly not the answer but cannot be overlooked.

There may be some advantage to considering the notion of "persistent" pain vs. "chronic" pain. *Persistent pain* would represent the ongoing awareness of the patient regarding the presence of an uncomfortable sensation or feeling involving the processing of nociceptive information. Persistent pain might be characterized by patients with such conditions as inflammatory arthritis, diabetic neuropathy, or postoperative epidural scarring. In these cases the patient is well aware of the sense of discomfort; however, by virtue of the degree of pathological damage, genetic background, pain acceptance (activity engagement), and motivation, the impact is minimal. These patients maintain a relatively active, productive, and meaningful life. Their utilization of the medical system may surpass that of an individual with no pain but is far less than that of the patient with the disease of chronic pain. The term *chronic pain* would be reserved for those patients exhibiting all the various psychological, functional, and behavioral abnormalities generally associated with any disabling disease process.

The understanding of the neurochemical and physiological aspects of the nociceptive process has expanded exponentially in recent decades. What was once seen as a static and fixed system needs to be understood as very dynamic and made up of a variety of components and networks interacting in a very complex fashion (Koch and Laurent, 1999). The pain processing system has proven to be susceptible to external and internal forces and demonstrates enormous plasticity. Because it shares many of the characteristics of complex adaptive systems, it should be viewed as such. The capacity for the PNS and CNS to adjust and accommodate can be seen in conditions such as sensitization and wind-up, which appear to be characteristic of many chronic pain conditions. The ability of the system to reorganize itself (plasticity) has been effectively demonstrated. The nonlinear aspects are attested to by the vast discrepancies between the magnitude of the inciting event and consequent experience of pain.

REFERENCES

Berthier M, Starkstein S, Leigyards R. Asymbolia for pain: a sensory-limbic disconnection syndrome. *Ann Neurol.* 1988;24:42–49.

Drdla-Schutting R, Benrath J, Wunderbaldinger G, Sandkühler J. Erasure of a spinal memory trace of pain by a brief, high-dose opioid administration. *Science.* 2012;335:235–238.

Gebhart GF, Ness TJ. Central mechanisms of visceral pain. *Can J Physiol Pharmacol.* 1991;68(5):627–634.

Gibson HE, Edwards JG, Page RS, Van Hook MJ, Kauer JA. TRPV1 channels mediate long-term depression at synapses on hippocampal interneurons. *Neuron.* 2008;57:746–759.

Goosens KA, Maren S. Long-term potentiation as a substrate for memory: evidence from studies of amygdaloid plasticity and pavlovian fear conditioning. *Hippocampus.* 2002;12:592–599.

Grisel JE, Watkins LR, Maier SF. Associative and non-associative mechanisms of morphine analgesic tolerance are neurochemically distinct in the rat spinal cord. *Psychopharmacology.* 1996;128:248–255.

Heavner JE, Willis WD. Pain pathways: anatomy and physiology. In Raj PP, ed. *Practical Management of Pain*, 3rd ed. St. Louis: Mosby; 2000:107–116.

Hebb DO. *The Organization of Behavior*. New York: John Wiley and Sons; 1949.

Honore P, Rogers SD, Schwei MJ, et al. Murine models of inflammatory, neuropathic and cancer pain each generates a unique set of neurochemical changes in the spinal cord and sensory neurons. *Neuroscience*. 2000;98:585–598.

Johnson BW. Pain mechanisms: anatomy, physiology, and neurochemistry. In Raj PP, ed. *Practical Management of Pain*, 3rd ed. St Louis: Mosby; 2000:117–143.

Koch C, Laurent G. Complexity and the nervous system. *Science*. 1999;284:96–98.

Loeser JD, Treede RD. The Kyoto protocol of IASP basic pain terminology. *Pain*. 2008;137:473–477.

Melzack R, Casey K. Sensory, motivational, and central control determinants of pain: a new conceptual model. In Kenshalo D, ed. *The Skin Senses*. Springfield, IL: Thomas; 1968:23–42.

Nicolelis MAL, Fanselow EE, Ghazanfar AA. Hebb's dream: the resurgence of cell assemblies. *Neuron*. 1997;19:219–221.

Price DD. *Psychological Mechanisms of Pain and Analgesia*. Seattle: IASP Press; 1999.

Price DD. Psychological and neural mechanisms of the affective dimension of pain. *Science*. 2000;288(5472):1769–1772.

Raouf R, Quick K, Wood JN. Pain as channelopathy. *J Clin Invest*. 2010;120(11):3745–3752.

Reyes M, Stanton PK. Induction of hippocampal long-term depression requires release of Ca^{2+} from separate presynaptic and postsynaptic intracellular stores. *J Neurosci*. 1996;16(19):5951–5960.

Rexed B. A cytoarchitectonic atlas of the spinal cord of the cat. *J Comp Neurol*. 1954;100:297–379

Sandkuhler J. Understanding LTP in pain pathways. *Mol Pain*. 2007;3:3–9.

Tracey I, Mantyh PW. The cerebral signature for pain perception and its modulation. *Neuron*. 2007;55:377–391.

Treede RD. Pain and hyeralgesia: definitions and theories. In Cervero F, Jensen TS, eds. *Handbook of Clinical Neurology*, New York: Elsevier; 2006: Vol 81, 3–10.

Wall PD, McMahon SB. The relationship of perceived pain to afferent nerve impulses. *Trends Neurosci*. 1986; 254–255.

Woolf CJ. Pain: moving from symptom control toward mechanism-specific pharmacologic management. *Ann Intern Med*. 2004;140:441–451.

Woolf CJ. What is this thing called pain? *J Clin Invest*. 2010;120(11):3742–3744.

Woolf CJ, Mannion RJ. Neuropathic pain: aetiolgy, symptoms, mechanisms, and management. *Lancet*. 1999;353:1959–1964.

Yaksh TL. Basic lectures in the biology of pain processing. Handout, Dannemiller Review Course, Chicago IL; August 2009:1–65.

4 Pain and the Brain

Although the data are not conclusive regarding causality, [they] clearly show that the brains of patients suffering chronic pain are fundamentally disturbed in ways neither considered nor appreciated before.
–I. Tracey and P.W. Mantyh (2007, p. 386)

INTRODUCTION

Koch and Laurent (1999) describe the brain as "1.5 kilograms of flaccid matter, convoluted folds, about 100 billion neuronal components, hundreds of trillions of interconnections, many thousand kilometers of cabling" (p. 96). The billions of neurons in the brain are highly interconnected, forming intricate and complicated networks of communication and cell assemblies of various sizes. The complexity of these networks is far more advanced than the Internet, with synapses numbering in the trillions. These connections are highly individualized and very dynamic, changing over the course of a lifetime, depending on the individual's experiences. The activation of any of these many circuits, which may take only tens of milliseconds, can be occasioned by local events, such as the activity of the adjacent neurons and circuits, or more remote factors, including substances released elsewhere and transported via the circulatory system. The brain produces millions of such impulses across a variety of regions every second. The chemical signaling agents and electrical currents found in these networks organize one's personality, thoughts, consciousness, and memories. Perhaps one of the great anatomical ironies is that the very organ most responsible for the experience of pain does not contain any pain receptors.

The brain represents about 2% of one's total body weight, yet it uses about 20% of the metabolic energy (oxygen) created. Gray matter (unmyelinated cell bodies) makes up about 40% of the brain but utilizes approximately 90% of the cerebral oxygen. White matter (myelinated bundles of axons) makes up some 60% of the brain but only uses an estimated 6% of the oxygen. In general, gray matter is associated with processing and cognition, while white matter coordinates the communication among various brain regions. Using a computer network as a model, white matter represents the array of cables connecting the computers together and gray matter the computers themselves. The amount of oxygen extracted from the blood varies in accordance with the rate of blood flow. Changes in blood oxygen content correlate with increased brain activity and can be detected with functional magnetic resonance imaging (fMRI), generally referred to as blood oxygen level-dependent (BOLD) contrast imaging. Positron emission tomographic (PET) scans can provide a quantitative measure of the amount of available oxygen utilized (oxygen extraction fraction, OER).

Developmentally, the brain achieves about 90% of its adult weight by early childhood. However, changes in the brain's architecture occur throughout the life of the organism. Primary motor and sensory areas mature earliest. Gray matter shows a nonlinear growth pattern with increasing density during childhood; decreased density occurs during adolescence and young adulthood. White mater increases linearly throughout this period.

As sophisticated and complex as the brain is, it can be deceived. "Somatic delusions," such as the sensation of something crawling on one's skin, are not uncommon. Sudden contact with ice can produce a burning sensation. As early as 1896, Thunberg reported on the "thermal grill illusion" (Craig and Bushnell, 1994). This experiment employed a device whose surface contained 15 one-cm wide sterling silver bars set 3 mm apart. Thunberg noted that simultaneously applying innocuous warm and cool stimuli through the use of these interlocking spiral tubes elicited a sensation of painful heat not unlike the burning sensation that accompanies cold pain. Another example of the difference between perception and reality is provided by the "cutaneous rabbit illusion" (Blankenberg et al, 2006; Geldard and Sherrick, 1972). Stimulating electrodes are placed along the arm—P1 at the wrist, P2 at mid-forearm, and P3 just below the elbow. Repeated rapid stimulation at the wrist (P1) and then at the elbow (P3) gives the sensation of a rabbit hopping from P1 to P2 to P3, even though P2 is never stimulated.

One final example of deceiving the brain is provided by Raij et al (2005). They selected 14 "suggestion-prone" subjects. The brain activity of each subject was monitored during "suggestion-induced" pain and compared with activity from laser stimulation–induced pain. Both suggestion-induced and laser-induced pain states were associated with activation of the brain's pain matrix. Very similar changes were noted in the somatosensory (SS) cortex, anterior cingulate cortex (ACC), and insula cortex. The ACC tended to be more highly active in the suggestion condition. The researchers concluded that events often tend to feel as though they are real, rather than known to be such. This sentiment was echoed by Gallagher and Firth (2003): "Even when it conflicts with reality, it is belief and not reality that determines behavior" (p. 77). These phenomena may also be examples of a type of synesthesia (union of the senses) or ideasthesia (sensing of concepts or ideas; Simner, 2012) in which the brain mixes up senses or concepts, for example, hears color and sees words.

The breadth and depth of neuroscientists' knowledge has grown exponentially with the advent of highly sophisticated and sensitive neuroimaging techniques (see reviews by Casey, 2000; Casey and Bushnell, 2000). Imaging technology such as X-ray, MRI, computed tomographic (CT) scanning, and ultrasound and magnetic resonance angiography (MRA) have been available for decades. These technologies allowed for a detailed assessment of anatomical structures, including the integrity of the arterial and venous structures. Electroencephalographic (EEG) readings provided a measure of brain function but lacked the specificity needed to reveal unique stimulus–response relationships and the dynamic interaction among various brain structures. It has only been in the last 15 years or so that the technology has evolved to the point of being able to assess brain function and structure.

Structural anomalies sometimes referred to as "incidental findings" do not always correlate with alterations in function. Likewise, the fact that a structure appears normal says little about how well it works.

Technologies used for the study of the brain can be divided in to three main types: hemodynamic, neuroelectrical, and neurochemical. In 1890, Roy and Sherrington reported that changes in the functional activity of the brain were accompanied by local variations in blood supply that resulted in chemical by-products as a function of increased cerebral metabolism. This relationship between metabolic demand and neuronal activity formed the basis for modern imaging technology. Hemodynamic studies take advantage of the fact that synaptic activity, which can be generated by sensory, motor, or cognitive events, requires increased energy. This demand for increased energy is met by the delivery of glucose and oxygen through increased local blood supply. There is a close spatial and temporal relationship between this energy demand and increased regional cerebral blood flow (rCBF). Indeed, changes in rCBF have been detected within 2 to 3 seconds of presenting a stimulus. Studies using this technology date back to the 1970s.

PET and SPECT

Positron emission tomography (PET) and single-photon emission computed tomography (SPECT) measure various physiological and neurochemical aspects of brain functioning. These tests are based on the assumption that neuronal activity, rCBF, and the regional metabolic rate of glucose utilization (CMRglu) are linked. That is, changes in brain activity are reflected in alterations in CMRglu. The use of tomographic imaging provides a three-dimensional (3D) representation of this altered activity. PET was initially used along with ^{18}F-fluorodeoxyglucose (FDG). However, the radioisotope ^{18}FDG has a long half-life approximating 110 minutes, which makes it difficult to perform repeated scanning in the same subject within a short time interval. In addition, the stimulation or task has to persist and remain constant for some 10 minutes, the length of time it takes for fixation of the radiotracer uptake in the brain. These limitations were overcome by the use of ^{15}O with a labeled water or gas, with a half-life of only 124 seconds. Thus images can be repeated after only a few minutes.

In practice, radiolabeled substances and tracers are introduced intravenously while the subject is performing a task or undergoing some type of stimulation. Shorter duration radiotracers allow for repeated scans. Therefore, several control or stimulation conditions could be carried out in the same subject within the same experimental session. With newer generation PET scanners, data can be transformed to a common coordinated system, making it possible to average information from several subjects. These scanners can detect the product of compounds such as radiolabeled FDG metabolism, which is held in the presynaptic terminal the nerve. The magnitude of these changes tends to correlate with measures of reported pain intensity and unpleasantness, as well as motor and cognitive functioning.

Although fMRI assumed prominence in brain imaging studies after its introduction in 1992, Minoshima et al (2000) believe that PET continues to have several advantages. These include that it (a) is noninvasive, (b) has a known relationship between signals and physiological mechanisms, (c) has uniform sensitivity throughout the brain, and (d) is an established methodology.

MRI and fMRI

As synaptic activity increases there is enhanced utilization of oxygen, and oxyhemoglobin is transformed to deoxyhemoglobin. About 2 seconds later there is a marked microvascular response raising the oxyhemoglobin levels, thus altering the oxyhemoglobin/deoxyhemoglobin ratio. These two forms of hemoglobin manifest different magnetic resonance signals. The shifting from one type of signal to the other is referred to as the *magnetic blood-oxygenation-level dependent (BOLD)* signal. The magnitude of the signal correlates with rCBF and is a functional measure of neuronal activity and forms the basis for fMRI. Thus, the application of MRI technology to the study of pain assumes "that the nociceptive or pain signal is manifested as an increase in metabolic activity evoking an increase in blood flow, increased cerebral blood volume, decreased deoxyhemoglobin, and thereby an increased magnetic resonance imaging (MRI) signal" (Stephenson and Arneric, 2008, p. 570).

Functional MRI is similar to MRI except the degree of brain activation is measured by examining the change in magnetization between oxygen-rich and oxygen-poor blood. Statistical procedures eliminate the noise. The resulting degree of activation across the brain or in specific regions is identified through color-coding. deCharms et al. (2004, 2005) demonstrated the application of real-time fMRI (rtfMRI) as a means of training individuals to alter activity in specific parts of the brain in the classic biofeedback fashion. Using rtfMRI, subjects are able to get real-time feedback regarding the effectiveness of particular mental strategies. For example, by learning to reduce the level of activity in the ACC, subjects reported less pain in response to a noxious stimulus. In some cases different pharmacological agents can be used and their effects on brain functioning studied using pharmacological magnetic resonance imaging (phfMRI). phfMRI can be used to study drug-induced changes in brain activity as well as pharmacological modulation of task-induced activities.

The absence of radiation and high spatial resolution make fMRI preferable to PET and SPECT. The disadvantages of fMRI include (a) the inability to bring magnetic materials, as might be used to present various stimuli, into the scanner, (b) less well-established imaging and statistical analysis of whole-brain responses, (c) the inability to obtain resting or baseline rCBF, and (d) the lack of fMRI suitable for animal studies. However, studies by Thompson and Bushnell (2012) and Seminowicz et al (2012) suggest that the difficulties encountered with using fMRI for animals may have been overcome. Apkarian et al (2005) have expressed concern over fMRI's rather slow temporal resolution, suggesting that the rapid events that underlie the activity of dynamic networks could go undetected. They recommended EEG as a means of detecting the synchronization or desynchronization of pain-related events.

Generally, however, fMRI, PET, and SPECT are considered complementary rather than competing technologies in the study of pain-related brain activity.

DTI

Diffusion tensor imaging (DTI) is an MRI technique that is sensitive to the diffuson of free water and is the only technique for tracing white matter pathways in the living organism (Johansen-Berg and Behrens, 2006). Difffusion is orientation dependent and essentially shows the path of less resistance—there is greater resistrance across the white matter fibers than along them. Tractography involves the use of diffusion data to trace brain pathways. White matter tract integrity can be assessed by examining microstructural changes in directional water diffusion in the brain. With DTI, images of neural tracts (tractography) revealing complicated 3D networks formed by connections among different cortical and subcortical regions can be generated. MRI sequences are used to examine the symmetry of brain water diffusion. Bundles of fiber tracts make the water diffuse asymmetrically in what is referred to as a *tensor*. Tensors can be used to describe the properties of the system.

Color-coding (anisotropic map) makes it possible to describe how the fibers are oriented in a 3D-coordinate system. For example, red can indicate directions in the X axis (right to left or left to right), green the directions in the Y axis (posterior to anterior or anterior to posterior), and blue the direction in the Z axis (foot-to-head direction or vice versa).

DTI has been applied to examining brainstem and cortical connectivity related to pain processing (Hadjipavlou et al, 2006). DTI way well find application in the identification of white matter pathways in disease, examination of pathways in congenital disorders and those involved in recovery, advancement of the understanding of localized brain pathology, and directing of interventions.

DTI is limited when exploring areas of fiber crossing, greater complexity, and those involving small pathways. Furthermore, DTI cannot differentiate antegrade from retrograde connections, detect the present of synapses, or determine if a pathway is fucntional (Johansen-Berg and Behrens, 2006). Nonetheless, it offers great potential in brain imaging, and it or some variation of it will be instrumental in the Human Connectome Project of mapping the neural pathways underlying brain function (see Chapter 14).

EEG and MEG

The first studies examining pain-evoked electrical potentials occurred in the 1960s and those involving corresponding magnetic fields in the 1980s. Since then, the use of electroencephalography (EEG) and magnetoencephalography (MEG) has become more common.

As noted by Casey (2000), imaging studies have the capacity to create an image of central neurophysiological processing within a matter of seconds that can be well localized and thus are superior to attempts of analyzing electrophysiological events lasting milliseconds or some transient poorly localized magnetic field. Apkarian et al (2005) have argued, however, that the temporal resolution of EEG and MEG is unsurpassed and that corroborating independent evidence from PET studies confirming EEG and MEG finding has advanced the area of brain imaging. Also, they find MEG to be more the sensitive of the two techniques. However, MEG seems best suited for investigation of superficial cortical areas and may be somewhat limited in its sensitivity to activity in deeper structures.

Optical Intrinsic Signal

Optical intrinsic signal (OIS) is a somewhat less familiar brain neuroimaging technology (Whitsel et al, 2000). When synaptic populations react to specific stimuli or changing physiological conditions, they emit different wavelengths of light within a few hundred milliseconds of the stimulated activity. Specialized near-infrared cameras and optical sensors can detect these changes. The initial signal is referred to as the "intrinsic" signal and is followed immediately by increased CBF.

Advantages of OIS include the following: (a) the intrinsic response is highly correlated with spike discharge activity in cortical neurons; (b) images have high spatial resolution and (c) can be acquired fairly rapidly, that is, three per second; and (d) responses detected by OIS are independent of CBF.

Neurochemistry

The two main approaches to assessing the neurochemistry of pain entail (1) the examination of the metabolic function of the brain in response to specific pharmacological agents, and (2) the direct measures of receptors for neurotransmitters. The second technique involves the introduction of radiotracers that bind to specific receptors. Using kinetic models and binding activity of the radiotracer, receptor sites and enzyme function can be quantified with PET or SPECT. Most studies have examined the activity of the endogenous opioid system, with emphasis on the mu-opioid receptor because of its participation clinically in opioid therapy.

STRUCTURE VS. FUNCTION

Functional neuroimaging studies have begun to unravel the neurobiology of pain. Altered brain chemistry and functional status have revealed a functional reorganization and altered connectivity representative of central plasticity. However, there may be structural or morphological changes as well. It is important to remember that there is no evidence that examining the brain's response to noxious experimental stimuli is predictive of the brain's response in the chronic-pain condition. Extrapolations and generalizations must be made with caution.

Neuroplastic changes (plasticity) relate to alterations in the functional, neurochemical, and structural nature of the peripheral and central nervous systems that may be responsible for acute pain becoming chronic (chronification). Until the advent of neuroimaging technology, studies of morphological changes were limited to the use of autopsy. Modern in vivo imaging using MRI allows for a quantitative analysis of changes in brain structure. Images from an MR scanner generally provide sufficient detail. Images of several individuals can be grouped by mapping them into a coordinated space. Voxel-based morphometry (VBM) using 3D, high-resolution, T1-weighted 1-mm voxels (volumetric picture element) obtained with a 1.5 tesla (T) approach is commonly employed in analyzing structural alterations. Although the exact cause of a lesion or trauma-induced structural change is unknown, examining the changes over time is likely to yield valuable information. A review by Smallwood et al (2013) revealed both decreased and increased gray matter volume (GMV) within and beyond the regions generally considered the pain matrix in patients with chronic pain. Although the precise causes of these structural changes are unclear, May (2008) suggested that decreases in GMV of the brain could result from neuronal destruction, changes in cell size, shrinkage or atrophy of the neurons or glial cells, synaptic loss, or a combination of these factors. The use of this technology makes analyses of cortical thickness, complexity, connectivity, and gyrification index (a measure of the degree of folding or surface of a particular cortical area) possible.

Connectivity involves study of the manner in which various structures in the brain interact (are functionally connected). The advent of fMRI, DTI, and similar technologies has made it possible to not only determine what areas of the brain are activated by nociception and thus considered part of its pain matrix but also how they relate to each other.

For example, Price and colleagues (Craggs et al, 2012) examined connectivity in normal controls (NC) and fibromyalgia (FM) patients. For practical and statistical reasons, they limited their investigation to cortical areas previously demonstrated to be involved in pain processing: the thalamus, S1, S2, posterior insula, and anterior mid-cingulate cortex. Statistical modeling demonstrated that, while not identical, there was considerable similarity in the functional connectivity of these NC and FM patients. Napadow et al (2010) found that spontaneous pain and its intensity in FM patients was related to the strength of the connectivity within the default mode network (DMN) and executive attention network (EAN) and the DMN and the insular cortex.

Ploner et al (2011) demonstrated what they called "flexible functional connectivity." By independently manipulating the emotional and attentional context of the painful stimulus, they were able to observe alterations in the connectivity pattern among the anterior insula and the emotional and attentional networks in the brain resulting in altered pain sensitivity.

Alterations in this functional connectivity have also been found by Benendetti et al (2006) in patients with pain and dementia, and by Mageri et al (2012) and Wolf et al (2011) in patients with borderline personality who had a history of engaging in self-injurious behaviors. The etiology of this change in functional connectivity and whether it represents a cause, consequence, or correlate of these disorders remains unclear.

NEUROIMAGING DATA ON CHRONIC AND PHANTOM PAIN

May (2008) has provided a summary of the research in neuroimaging, organized by location and type of pain. Regarding low back pain (LBP), it was noted that some 70–85% of the U.S. population will experience LBP at some time in their lives. Why and how only a relatively small fraction of these patients develop chronic pain (chronification) remains unclear, although it appears that a combination of predisposing factors, psychological variables, and neuroplasticity is involved. Using VBM, Apkarian et al (2004) were able to detect a significant decrease in cortical GMV in patients with LBP compared to that in similar-aged normal volunteers. Decreases were found in the bilateral dorsolateral prefrontal cortices (DLPFC) and in the right thalamus.

More recently, Mansour et al (2013) studied 46 subjects with first-time low back pain of 4–16 weeks. These subjects were examined with fMRI over a period of a year. Within 2 months of pain onset, differences in the structure and integrity of the white matter distinguished those whose pain persisted from those whose pain began to resolve. At 12 months, structural differences distinguished patients whose pain resolved from those whose pain persisted (became chronic). Patients with chronic pain showed differences in the density of connections (connectivity) between the nucleus accumbens (brain reward, motivation, learning, pleasure, and learning circuit) and the medial prefrontal cortex (involved in decision making, emotional response, and long-term memory).

When compared to (a) non-pain controls and (b) patients with long-standing chronic pain, the brains of patients with newly developed chronic pain had structural abnormalities that mimicked those found in patients with long-standing chronic pain. Such abnormalities were not found in healthy controls and in those whose pain had resolved. White matter normally deteriorates with age. Compared to healthy controls and those whose pain had resolved, the white matter in the subjects whose pain became chronic exhibited 30–50 years of additional aging.

Seifert and Malihofner (2011) summarized studies revealing similar findings, including changes in GVM, in patients with phantom pain, complex regional pain syndrome (CRPS), headache, spinal cord injury, peripheral neuropathic pain, and osteoarthritis. Rodriguez-Raecke et al (2009) and Gwilym et al (2010) examined the effects of hip arthroplasty (replacement) and identified increased volume in DLPFC, ACC, amygdala, brainstem, and thalamus in patients for whom the pain had been eliminated.

Decreases in GMV in the brainstem did appear to correlate with pain intensity and unpleasantness, but not with pain duration. The DLPFC tends to be associated with "top-down" (descending) pain inhibitory activity. Apkarian and Scholz (2006) have speculated on the causes of this neurodegeneration, including the possibility that the constant release of neuroexcitatory neurotransmitters as a result of ongoing nociception (pain) may be toxic to this part of the brain. Whatever the reason, it seems that LBP of sufficient intensity and unpleasantness can cause, or at least is correlated with, a type of neurodegeneration or brain damage. Seminowicz et al (2011) noted enhancement of cortical thickness 6 months post-treatment in a group of LBP patients described as treatment "responders." The clearest change was noted in the DLPFC. Thus, ongoing chronic pain appears to be associated with a neurodegenerative process that potentially can be reversed when the pain is adequately controlled.

Persistent pain following amputation has been described; it has also been observed following the removal of visceral organs, such as the urinary bladder. Even more remarkable is the observation that that stimulation of an unrelated part of the body, such as the lip, in patients with phantom leg pain can occasion the phantom pain. Stimulation of a specific part of the brain is known to produce a sensation in a certain body part, through somatosensory mapping. The more sensitive body parts like the tongue and lips occupy larger cortical areas as depicted by the homunculus. Anatomically connected or adjacent body parts are not necessarily so arranged on the brain. It appears that when a part of the body is removed or its input eliminated, as through spinal cord damage, areas of the brain adjacent to the missing (deafferentated) parts began to grow into (innervate) the deactivated area. It seems that, in a sense, the brain abhors a vacuum and attempts to fill it.

Imaging studies have confirmed this expansion of adjacent cortical representational areas into areas no longer receiving input. The changes tend to occur in the primary somatosensory cortex in painful conditions, but also in the thalamus, posterior parietal, and prefrontal cortices as well as secondary motor cortex in nonpainful conditions. This type of reorganization has been referred to a *maladaptive plasticity*, in contrast to a *functional plasticity*, in which innervation from another area of the brain benefits rehabilitation and recovery of function, such as after a stroke (Cramer et al, 2011). VBM analysis has revealed reductions in gray matter in posterolateral thalamus following traumatic upper and lower amputation. Structural variations were associated with time since amputation, indicating the significant role of the chronic absence of behaviorally relevant input. In general, amputation can cause a structural reorganization of the brainstem, thalamic nuclei, or somatosensory cortex.

In addition to LBP, headache is an all-too-common disorder. Two familiar types of headache are migraine and the chronic daily headache (CDH). Functional imaging studies have revealed changes in activity in areas associated with pain processing, including the cingulate cortex, insular cortex, and thalamus. Hypothalamic and brainstem activity were altered in cluster headache attacks and acute migraine. Such observations tend to support the notion of migraine headache involving complex neurovascular mechanisms instead of the previously hypothesized vascular system only. Structural abnormalities in the emotional processing areas of the brain and the identification of a thicker somatosensory cortex (S1) have lead some to consider the possible involvement of some type of a general "cortical hyperexcitability."

VBM T1-weighted MR images from patients with cluster headache show a co-localization of morphometric alterations and functional activation. That is to say, the areas of the brain that are most active during the migraine headache also show the greatest alteration in structure. Several, but not all, studies have found reduced gray matter density in the ACC, anterior insula, and temporal lobes. Increased density has been reported in the periaqueductal gray matter (PAG) and dorsolateral pons of patients with headache. Areas of the brain specific to migraine, such as the brainstem, appear to be unaffected. However, not all of these studies have agreed on these findings. Differences in the technology employed and patient selection may have contributed to the discrepancies. Nevertheless, there is some agreement regarding the presence of decreased gray matter in traditional pain-processing or pain-transmission structures such as the ACC in patients with migraine headaches. This decrease is similar to that found in LBP and phantom pain patients. One interpretation of these data is that the decrease in cortical gray matter is a consequence of repeated brain insult or damage during these migraine attacks. The changes tend to correlate with pain *duration*, emphasizing the need for early and effective intervention. One intriguing caveat is that many patients with migraine report that their headaches resolve with age. It is unclear if the there is a return to more normal levels of cortical gray matter when the headaches no longer occur.

The second type of headache, chronic daily headache, is defined as having headache 15 or more days out of a month. Morphometric studies of chronic tension-type headaches noted a decrease in gray matter involving the pons, ACC, insular, temporal, orbitofrontal, parahippocampus, and cerebellum. Moreover, the magnitude of the change correlated with the duration of headache. That is, the longer the history of CDH, the greater the decrease in cortical gray matter. Whether this represents a consequence or a cause of the headache pain remains unclear. What appears abundantly clear is that it is difficult to argue that chronic headache is a benign condition.

Standard MRI measures of the anatomical structure and abnormalities in the structure do not always equate to pain. fMRI can be used to assess temporal differences in brain activity in response to stimulation. Magnetic resonance spectroscopy (MRS) is used to identify the level of metabolites present in certain areas of the brain. Siddall et al (2006) used MRS in an effort to determine the accuracy with which they could identify patients with chronic LBP from controls. MR spectra were obtained from 32 patients with LBP and 33 controls without pain. Using a pattern-recognition method developed for biomedical spectroscopy called statistical classification strategy (SCS), they were able to correctly identify 100% of the patients with pain on the basis of ACC spectra, 98.5% from thalamus spectra, and 96.6% from prefrontal cortex spectra.

Fibromyalgia (FM) is characterized by widespread soft-tissue pain, hypersensitivity, and tenderness and stiffness in multiple body areas (Sommer, 2010). Sleep disturbance, fatigue, depression, and anxiety are common comorbidities, though some might argue that these are part of the diagnostic criteria. In order to make the diagnosis of FM, the American College of Rheumatology requires pain in all four body quadrants along with excessive tenderness in 11 of 18 identified muscle-tendon sites and the absence of any clinically demonstrable cause. FM often begins with some type of emotional or physical trauma, with pain occurring initially at a single site and then encompassing other body parts. Historically, because of the absence of a cause, the diagnosis of FM was frequently seen as one of exclusion. Also, the validity of the diagnosis and that of the patient was often overtly questioned. The symptoms of some patients with FM were discounted, while other patients were subjected to overtreatment because of the lack of any therapeutic target.

A series of recent investigations using brain imaging technology has all but revolutionized the way FM is understood (Gracely et al, 2002; Lautenbacher and Rollman, 1997). Brain function has been investigated using fMRI, and morphological and structural changes have been assessed through the use of VBM. When compared to normal controls, patients with FM demonstrate alterations in the medial pain system (affective/motivational component), consisting of the cingulate cortex, frontal cortex and insula cortex, but not in the lateral pain system (sensory/discriminative component).

Kuchinad et al (2007) discovered an average decrease in cortical gray matter volume of 3.7cm^3/year in FM patients compared to 2.4 cm^3/year for normal subjects. The loss in GMV can range from 3.3 to 9.5 times that of controls depending on the duration of the FM. The presence of analgesic medications did not account for these findings, although the duration of medication use was associated with greater changes in the ACC.

Neuroimaging studies have uncovered hypoperfusion in the thalamus of FM patients that is similar to that seen in patients with neuropathic pain secondary to damage in the central or peripheral nervous system (Williams and Gracely, 2006). Dysfunction in the brain's dopaminergic system and decreased binding potential to opioids in the ACC and amygdala have also been discovered (Schweinhardt et al, 2008; Wood, 2004). Consistent with morphometric studies of patients with chronic pain, increases in GMV were not found in any area of the brain. Interestingly, patients suffering from irritable bowel syndrome (IBS), which frequently co-occurs with FM, were also found to have cortical thinning in the ACC, thalamus, and insula cortex (Burgmer et al, 2009).

The question as to whether these pathological findings represent a cause or consequence of FM, and the degree to which genetic and psychological predispositions play a role, has yet to be answered. The issue of whether or not these changes are reversible, as with patients undergoing successful hip arthroplasty, is also unknown. However, what is clear is that what was once considered a questionable diagnosis and thought to be a euphemism for hysteria or hypochondriasis appears to be an abnormality in cortical functioning and processing associated with or possibly causing a type of brain atrophy and neurotransmitter system dysfunction.

The ACC and insula appear to function as integrative structures during the experience and anticipation of pain. The ACC in particular plays a role in pain modulation and analgesia, including placebo analgesia. This effect, however, is mediated via interactions with the orbitofrontal lobe, amygdala, and PAG. The brainstem is also involved in antinociception (suppression of nociceptive input). The decrease in GMV in areas of the brain associated with pain suppression could suggest that chronic pain may be a result of a dysfunction in effective antinociception.

May (2008) noted that (a) pain related physical inactivity and medications do not account for the changes in GVM and (b) the loss of cortical gray matter could represent the neuroanatomical substrate for a "pain memory." The causes of decreased cortical GMV vary and could include a decrease in cell size, cell atrophy (apoptosis), and synaptic loss. Nearly all of the studies mentioned here showed changes in the pain processing matrix. While differences in areas involved were noted, there was significant overlap. The most common finding is a decrease in cortical GMV in cingulate and orbitofrontal cortex, pons, and insula cortex.

The observations discussed here tempt one to consider that the relatively small portion of people who develop chronic pain from an injury or trauma may have structural differences, perhaps genetically related, in the pain-transmission system acting as a diathesis for chronic pain (Mansour et al, 2013). That is, chronification may involve multiple modulatory mechanisms, including nociceptor level, sympathetically mediated pain, wind-up, central sensitization, and descending and ascending central modulation. The influence of the dynamic interaction among neurotransmitters, glial cells, neuronal and endothelial cells, immune systems, and cognitive functions cannot be overlooked when considering the chronification of pain.

ASYMBOLIA FOR PAIN

In 1928, Schilder and Stengel (1928, 1931) described a patient with sensory aphasia and self-mutilating behavior. Over time, they identified some 10 other similar patients. These patients could recognize pain but lacked the proper emotional and motor responses (withdrawal from pain). Furthermore, they appeared oblivious to visual or verbal cues associated with pain. This condition came to known as *asymbolia for pain* (AP). In 1965, Geschwind theorized AP to be a result of "sensory-limbic disconnection." He felt that damage to the insular cortex disrupted the connection and, therefore, the transmission of information from the secondary somatosensory cortex (SII) to the amygdala.

Berthier et al (1988) undertook the detailed examination of six AP patients, which included the use of brain CT scans. Each patient had suffered some type of brain insult, usually a stroke, associated with a rapidly resolving hemiparesis. Lesions were located in the parietal operculum and posterior insular cortex. Pain threshold, tolerance, and endurance were measured by delivering a sequence of electric shocks to the arm. The electric shocks were 2 seconds in duration, 3 seconds apart, beginning at 0.0 mA (milliampers) and increasing by 1.0-mA increments. Superficial pain was assessed by pinprick and thermal stimuli applied to the face, neck trunk, limb, and perineal area. Deep pain was determined by heavy pressure to the tibial, sternal, and supraorbital areas. Withdrawal response, emotional behavior, grimacing, and autonomic reactions were monitored. Responses to visual threats were tested by pretending to slap the face, punch the nose, or prick the eyes with a needle. Finally, reactions to verbal menaces, made by warning of a painful stimulus, for example, "I am going to pinch you hard!", were followed by applying the stimulus. The responses and reactions of these patients were compared to those of a matched group of normal subjects.

The threshold for pain in the AP patients approximated that of the normal subjects, indicating an intact sensory and nociceptive system. However, their pain tolerance and endurance were 2.5 and 6 times that of the normal subjects, respectively. AP patients could discriminate sharp from dull pain but lacked any response to painful stimuli applied to various areas of the body. One patient actually appeared to approach the painful stimulus by extending his arm toward it. Four patients smiled or laughed during the testing. They seemed unaware of their abnormal reactions and unable to learn the appropriate withdrawal and escape behavior. Although their autonomic responses (increased heart rate, sweating, increased blood pressure) suggested physiological distress, none of the AP patients demonstrated or express any anxiety, anger, or unpleasant feelings during testing. Verbal and visual threats failed to elicit any reaction such as a flinch or blinking. CT scans revealed lesions primarily in the insular cortex and parietal opercular cortex rather than solely in SII as suggested by Geschwind (1965). The damage to the insular cortex would also disrupt the insular–amygdala connection. In summary, AP appears to involve a trimodal (somatosensory, visual, and auditory systems) sensory–limbic (insular–amygdala) disconnection driven by damage to the insular and parietal opercular cortex, resulting in a deactivation of the affective-motivational component of pain processing.

These findings appear to illustrate an acquired indifference to pain, as it was brought about by a brain insult later in life. This is in contrast to a dominantly transmitted congenital indifference to pain, described in a 35-year-old mother and her 5-year-old daughter. Although she demonstrated withdrawal reflexes, grimacing, and vocal reactions to pinprick of normal intensity, and both the child and mother showed the typical withdrawal reaction to hot water (43–45°C), neither gave any response to prolonged or repetitive noxious stimulation anywhere on their bodies. Exhaustive clinical and morphological examination of their nerves was unrevealing. All nerves biopsied and examined under light and electron microscopy were normal. In all respects, this mother and child had normal reflexes and sensitivity to other sensory modalities. These two patients and the six described earlier are in sharp contrast to those found to have a congenital insensitivity to pain (CIP) (Bar-On et al, 2002; Landrieu et al, 1990).

Those with CIP lack any awareness of the sensation because of an inherited sensory neuropathy that prevents transmission of nociceptive information from the periphery (see Chapter 12).

DEFAULT MODE NETWORK (DMN)

Although we may rest, the brain does not. Some regions (networks) of the brain show increased activity during task- or goal-directed behavior while others are more active during times of relative quiescence. There are at least four such resting-state networks (RSNs): the default mode network (DMN), salience, sensory/motor engagement, and attention networks. RSNs appear to be involved in attending to environmental (internal and external) stimuli, reviewing past learning and information, preparing for future actions, and memory processing. A reduction or abnormal functioning of this deactivation process has been identified in patients with major depression or cognitive deficits such as in Alzheimer's disease.

Regions of the brain that appear more active during rest include posterior cingulate cortex, precuneus, and medial prefrontal cortex (MPFC). William James suggested that together these brain structures may function like "sentinels." The posterior cingulate cortex and adjacent precuneus continuously monitor and gather sensory information about the external and internal environments. The MPFC tends to be involved in evaluating the salience of this sensory information and the integration of emotional and cognitive processes by incorporating emotional biasing signals (markers) into the decision-making process (Damasio's concept of "somatic markers"; see Chapter 13).

The DMN is one of the most studied of the RSNs (Raichle et al, 2001). It is composed of subsystems of elements of the temporal lobe, MPFC, cingulate cortex, precuneus, and parietal cortex and appears to be influenced by the presence of chronic pain. The right frontal insular cortex (rFIC) may play a role in controlling the switching from a central executive network (CEN) to the DMN. Operationally, these areas involve memory, theory of the mind (see Chapter 11), and integration functions. An adult-like DMN has been noted in children as early as 2 years old (Gao et al, 2009) and is more active during resting than during task performance. It is involved in self-monitoring, pain processing, and salience detection, and when the individual is focused on his or her own internal status, such as remembering the past, prospection, introspection, and self-projection. The brain regions involved show a high level of connectivity characterized by synchronous, coherent neuronal oscillations occurring at a very low rate of 0.1 Hz (one every 10 seconds).

Raichle (2006, 2010a,b) has proposed that the DMN provides a balance of opposing forces to enhance "the maintenance of information for interpreting, responding to, and even predicting environmental demands." He noted that the difference in overall activity between a resting and task-oriented state was a mere 5%. The DMN has been implicated in cognitive processes such as mind-wandering, day-dreaming, and stimulus-independent thoughts. Farmer et al (2012) summarized studies revealing increased functional connectivity between the insular cortex and the DMN in various pain populations and suggested that pain may disrupt the DMN via increased nociceptive input from the insula.

Chronic pain can be considered a highly salient stimulus that continuously taxes the attentional and salience processing networks, thus interfering with cognitive abilities and, more specifically, consuming attentional resources. Foss et al (2006) have suggested that chronic pain can become a "spontaneous percept"—an intrinsic brain activity occurring even in the absence of explicit brain input or output. Prolonged disruption in the normal DMN activity, such as that caused by chronic pain, could result in irreversible changes. Disruptions in the DMN include spontaneous bursts of activity and altered functional connectivity. Altered activity in the DMN may result in increased inhibitory drive and asynchronous neuronal firing. Seifert and Malihofner (2011) have provided a review that identifies a number of DMN aberrations in pain patients, including reduced deactivation, altered thalamocortical connectivity, aberrant temporal and spatial activity, and altered network connectivity. These abnormalities were particularly evident in complex regional pain syndrome.

Cauda et al (2010) compared patients with diabetic neuropathic pain (NP) to individuals without pain and concluded "that the parieto-fronto-cingulate network controlling attention to external stimuli was impaired in the NP group and that chronic pain can disrupt the synchrony of a common pool of brain areas, involved in self-monitoring, pain processing and salience detection" (p. 806). Increased connectivity among the brain regions of the DNM was noted in patients with fibromyalgia. Bluhm et al (2007) noted that schizophenics also tend to demonstrate unusual patterns of activity in the DMN. Abnormal connectivity was reported to correlate with higher levels of dissociation, impulsiveness, self-injurious behavior, and overall psychopathology in patients diagnosed with borderline personality disorder. DMN abnormalities have also been identified in patients diagnosed with autism, Alzheimer's disease, depression, schizophrenia, and attention deficit hyperactivity. All of this suggests that chronic pain may indeed share a common mechanism with a variety of well-known neurological conditions that manifest emotional, cognitive, and behavioral dysfunction.

Farmer et al (2012) summarized studies revealing increased functional connectivity between the insular cortex and the DMN in various pain populations and suggested that pain may disrupt the DMN via increased nociceptive input from the insula. Seminowicz et al (2011) examined changes in the RSN when acute pain was presented to healthy subjects. The pattern of response was opposite that observed by Baliki et al (2008) in patients with chronic LBP. This differential effect of acute pain on brain activity in healthy vs. chronic pain subjects emphasizes the change in brain dynamics. It also puts into question the usefulness of studying the effects of acute pain on normal populations as a means of understanding clinical populations.

DMN activity has also been linked to consciousness. Vanhaudenhuyse et al (2010) found that connectivity strength within the DMN was proportional to the level of consciousness in brain-damaged patients and could be used to differentiate patients in a coma or vegetative state from those in a minimally conscious state and those with locked-in syndrome. Furthermore, levels of connectivity followed a nonlinear pattern. The relationship of the posterior cinglate cortex and precuneus was found to have the greatest degree of significance in correlating DMN connectivity and consciousness. Furthermore, Fingelkurts et al (2012) hypothesized that EEG operational synchrony within the DMN (strength of the DMN EEG connectivity) is a key component of self-awareness and, thus, consciousness. They were able to demonstrate a significant reduction in, and in some cases the absence of, DMN EEG operational synchrony in patients in a vegetative state compared to that in normal individuals. In addition, the decoupling of operations performed by the neuronal assemblies in the DMN was greatest for those in the vegetative state, medium for those in a minimally conscious state, and nominal for normal subjects.

Given the complex and emergent nature of consciousness (Kupers et al, 2011), the DMN is likely to be a necessary but surely not a sufficient component. It probably serves an intermediate role in processing and integrating information from external (sensory) and internal (cognitive) sources. A dyssynchronis and decoupled DMN would likely be associated with an absence of pain experience as ordinarily conceptualized. However, maintenance of functional connectivity in patients in a minimally conscious state along with activation of the pain matrix compelled Schnakers et al (2010) to reconsider presence of the experience of pain in patients unable to communicate their sensations, along with possible use of analgesics in such patients.

DIFFUSE NOXIOUS INHIBITORY CONTROLS (DNIC)

DNIC involves the assessment of the degree to which a painful tonic (test) stimulus is affected by a second painful phasic (conditioning) stimulus presented to a remote part (heterotopic) of the body (Van Wijk and Veldhuijzen, 2010). Ordinarily, the pain threshold, intensity, and/or tolerance produced by the test stimulus are improved in the presence of the conditioning stimulus. Presumably, this effect is created by activating the endogenous central nervous system pain-inhibitory system. This process has also been referred as "counterstimulation," "counterirritant," "pain inhibits pain," or "heterotopic noxious conditioning stimulation" (HNCS). A group headed by Yarnitsky (2010) recommended using the term *conditioned pain modulation* (CPM).

In 1992, Le Bars and colleagues noted that some of the neurons in the dorsal horn were strongly inhibited by a painful stimulus applied to any part of the body outside of their respective receptive fields. This was referred to DNIC and was thought to involve a spinal–brainstem–spinal mechanism. The function of the DNIC system appeared to be to inhibit ongoing pain in remote areas when a new pain is introduced, and was thought to involve aspects of the descending inhibitory system. DNIC only influenced convergent neurons. The inhibitory effect is only created by so-called conditioning stimuli that are nociceptive in nature—activating A-delta or A-delta and C-peripheral fibers. The inhibitory effects can outlast the duration of the conditioning stimulus by several minutes. Lesions in the subnucleus reticularis dorsalis (SRD) in the caudal medulla suppress the DNIC effect. Input to the SRD arrives from heterotopic noxious stimuli, resulting in the activation of projections that extend back down to the dorsal horn of the spinal cord.

Yarnitsky (2010; Yarnitsky et al., 2010) has summarized some of the clinical research on DNIC (CPM). When compared to DNIC (CPM) of normal individuals, decreased DNIC (CPM) efficiency was found in patients with IBS, temporomandibular disorders, sleep disorders, tension headache, fibromyalgia, polymorphism of the dopamine-3-receptor, depression, chronic pancreatitis, and painful osteoarthritic knees, and in those treated with opioids. The opioid effect, however, was only significant in men. It was suggested that this was in accordance with previous laboratory-based literature showing that opioids decrease the activity of the descending inhibition pathways. This might expose patients to increased nociceptive activity and provide a mechanism for opioid-induced hyperalgesia.

Minimal decrease was found with atypical facial pain. There appeared to be no changes among patients with Parkinson's disease, schizophrenia, trapezius myalgia, or rheumatoid arthritis. There was a significant negative correlation between DNIC (CPM) efficiency and chronic post-thoracotomy pain scores.

The role of the DNIC (CPM) effect as a predictor of analgesic efficacy has not been studied. There was no correlation between symptom severity and changes in the DNIC. The potential relationship between DNIC and the dopamine system is unclear. Theoretically, analgesics that augment the descending inhibition, such as selective nor-epinephrine reuptake inhibitors (SNRIs), should be more effective in patients with less efficient DNIC (CPM) than in those with an already efficient DNIC (CPM) prior to the analgesic. The effect of pain attenuation through expectation was found by Goffaux et al (2009) to supersede that of DNIC (CPM), suggesting different mechanisms of action for expectation of pain relief and for DNIC (CPM).

The nonadditive (nonlinear) properties of DNIC (CPM) have been highlighted by Lautenbacher et al (2007). Bodily pains at remote locations summate to produce a sensation greater than either one presented separately. Two pains are clearly greater than one, but the relationship is nonlinear. For example, an electrical stimulus rated as 67 and a thermal one as 64 combine to produce 79; electrical and thermal stimuli each at 70 combine for an 87; a highly painful thermal stimulus of 82 is unchanged by adding an electrical or a non-noxious stimulus; adding a barely noxious stimulus (67) produced an 88; adding the most intense stimulus (79) produced a 93. The authors concluded, "In essence, slightly to moderately noxious stimuli combine far from additively to produce a quite painful experience. Strong pain experiences, particularly when induced by tonic heat, are only moderately influenced by the addition of a second stimulus" (p. 197).

These findings are thought to demonstrate a pathophysiological role for DNIC (CPM) in the development of clinical pain, suggesting that a pronociceptive state may be a causative factor in the generation of chronic pain disorders, particularly those considered to have medically unexplained symptoms (MUS; see Chapter 7). The situation for neuropathic and inflammatory states is less clear, but it seems that, at least in some conditions, clinical pain intensity might be affected by DNIC (CPM). A study by Kosek and Ordenburg (2000) reported reduced inhibitory efficiency in osteoarthritis patients with pain. However, improvement in DNIC (CPM) efficiency was associated with pain relief after surgery. To that end, a variety of other conditioning stimuli could have been used, including stress and hypnotic suggestion. The common use of a painful stimulus as the means of conditioning is due to it being an easy and quick way to induce activity in the descending pain modulatory pathways.

Edwards (2005; Edwards et al, 2003) speculated that a deficient endogenous pain inhibitory pathway (DNIC system), especially in a pain-sensitive individual, may be a risk factor for the development of chronic pain. A pronociceptive state can be expressed by either decreased inhibition or enhanced summation, or both. Pronociceptive systems seem to be more prone to acquiring one or more of the idiopathic pain syndromes. Pain-sensitive patients demonstrated a relatively low pain threshold and tolerance as well as enhanced temporal summation. According to Yarnitsky (2010, Yarnitsky et al., 2010), most of the work in this area has been done on the idiopathic pain syndromes, such as IBS, temporomandibular disorders, fibromyalgia, and tension-type headache. A review article by Lewis et al (2012) noted that age, gender, menstrual cycle phase, psychosocial factors, caffeine, various pharmacological agents, and time of testing can influence the effect. Females with chronic pain tended to show greater impairment than males. Nevertheless, 70% of the 40 controlled studies reviewed found clinically meaningful impairment in the chronic pain population and concluded "conditioned pain modulation is impaired in populations with long-term pain conditions" (p. 941). The degree to which this represents a cause–effect relationship is yet to be determined.

THE BRAIN, SYSTEMS THEORY, AND PAIN

Coherence is the strength of the linear relationship between two signals. It reflects the degree to which phases and amplitudes are distributed at a given frequency. This relationship is assessed at every frequency or specific time period (epoch). The coherence value can range from 0% (phase and amplitudes are randomly distributed at all epochs) to 100% (perfect coherence). Perfect coherence indicates that there is a constant phase difference and amplitude ratio (the two signals are completely phase locked) at a given frequency. The usual frequency bands included delta 1–3 Hz (hertz; cycles per second), theta (θ) 4–8 Hz, alpha (α) 9–13 Hz, beta (β) 14–30 Hz, and gamma (γ) 31–100 Hz.

Oscillation is repetitive variation, usually in time or between two or more states, as in a swinging pendulum. In general, oscillations can be characterized by their frequency, amplitude, and phase. Neural oscillations occur throughout the central nervous system, the most evident of which may be the large-scale oscillations measured by EEG. In large-scale oscillations, amplitude changes are considered to result from changes in synchronization within a neural ensemble, also referred to as *local synchronization*. In addition to local synchronization, oscillatory activity of distant neural structures (single neurons or neural ensembles) can synchronize. Neural oscillations and synchronization have been linked to a number of cognitive functions, such as information transfer, perception, motor control, and memory.

Neural oscillations have been most widely studied in neural activity generated by large groups of neurons. In general, EEG signals have a broad spectral content but also reveal oscillatory activity in specific frequency bands. The best-known frequency band is alpha-activity (8–12 Hz) that can be detected from the occipital lobe during relaxed wakefulness and increases when the eyes are closed. Faster rhythms such as gamma (30–70 Hz) activity have been linked to cognitive processing. EEG signals change dramatically (phase shift) during sleep and show a transition from faster frequencies such as alpha waves to increasingly slower frequencies. Different sleep stages are commonly characterized by their spectral content. Thus, neural oscillations have been linked to cognitive states, including awareness and consciousness.

Baria et al (2011) noted a correlation between pain perception and a shift toward higher frequency oscillation in DMN in patients with chronic LBP. Gross et al (2007) found that 60–95 Hz gamma oscillations in the primary somatosensory cortex was associated with nociceptive stimulation. Moreover, the amplitude of these oscillations was positively correlated with pain intensity and was stronger when compared to those generated by unperceived stimuli of the same intensity.

Synchronicity involves the simultaneous occurrence of two or more events. These events are generally considered to be causally unrelated, therefore very unlikely to occur together, even by chance. Yet, within the concept of synchronicity, events are experienced as occurring together in a meaningful way. C.G. Jung (1960) introduced the term *synchronicity* in the 1920s. Jung coined the term as a means of describing what he called "temporally coincident occurrences of acausal events." He issued a variety of other descriptive phrases, including "acausal connecting principle," "meaningful coincidence," and "acausal parallelism." In general, synchronicity does not question the issue of causality but asserts that, in the same manner that events may be grouped by cause, they may also be grouped by meaning. A grouping of events by meaning need not have an explanation in terms of cause and effect. Synchronistic events reveal an underlying pattern, a conceptual framework that encompasses but is larger than any of the systems that display the synchronicity. Synchronization requires the coordination of events to operate a system in unison. Systems operating with all their parts in synchrony are said to be *synchronous* or *in sync*. For example, an orchestra playing in sync will reveal the underlying musical score and the actions of the conductor.

Although not frequently encountered in the literature, these concepts may be very relevant to pain. Some chronic pain syndromes, particularly neuropathic pain, have been associated with dysrythmic or uncoordinated cortical activity. For example, patients with chronic neurogenic pain demonstrate excessive EEG oscillations in the 4- to 9-Hz (theta) frequency band compared to those in healthy controls. According to Sarnthein and Jeanmonod (2008), the origin of this excess theta-frequency activity appears to be the cortical pain matrix, in particular, the interaction between the thalamus and cortex. At the network level, temporal and spatial patterns of activity in cortical and thalamic areas demonstrate wide variability, suggesting that the reverberating thalamocortical circuit supports a wide range of dynamic interactions necessary for input analysis. Indeed, the concept of thalamocortical dysrhythmia (TCD) has been put forth as a mechanism to explain neurogenic pain. They cite the following as supportive evidence: (a) a therapeutic lesion in the central lateral nucleus (CL) relieves neurogenic pain in the clinical setting; (b) low-threshold calcium spike (LTS) bursts are present in the somatosensory thalamus and in the CL; and (c) enhanced 4–9 Hz (theta) frequency activation occurs in patients with neurogenic pain. Abnormal thalamocortical interactions (TCD) set the stage for the persistence of slow-wave cortical activity.

It is thought that thalamic neurons become hyperpolarized secondary to deafferentation or excessive inhibition. This hyperpolarization causes the activation of low-threshold Ca^{2+} current, along with spontaneous low-threshold spiking activity and bursts of fast Na^+-dependent action potentials. The presence of this low-frequency activity alongside the higher frequency (gamma) activity creates an "edge effect" secondary to lateral inhibition. The consequence of this lateral inhibition is aberrant gamma activity and the associated experience of pain in the absence of any noxious peripheral stimulus.

Hippocampus

Another example of the importance of synchronicity comes from the activity of the hippocampus. The hippocampus is part of the limbic system and instrumentally involved in learning, memory, and emotions. In particular it performs the function of consolidating information and short-term memories into long-term ones. The hippocampal formation aids in the understanding of the context of pain as well as learning and memory in pain pathways. According to Buzsaki (1996), when isolated from its sources of input and output, the hippocampus operates in a type of transition phase between a quiescent state and an abnormally active (epileptic) state—the edge of chaos. Two cooperative states exist between hippocampal neurons and their associated networks: theta/gamma oscillation found during exploratory behavior, and SPW (sharp wave)/200 Hz ripple bursts seen during consummatory behavior. These SPW-burst events "compress time and allow temporarily distinct neuronal representations, acquired during explorative behavior, to be combined into a coherent whole."

Buzsaki (1996) views the hippocampus as an "appendage" of the neocortex and engaging in regular dialogue with it. Information regarding the internal and external world tends to be gathered and passed on to the hippocampus in a rather haphazard fashion. He states that

the main function of the hippocampal formation is to modify its inputs by feeding back a processed 'reafferent copy' to the neocortex....[T]he neocortico-hippocampal transfer of information and the modification process in neocortical circuitries by the hippocampal output take place in a temporally discontinuous manner and might be delayed by minutes, hours, or days. Acquisition of information may happen very fast during the activated state of the hippocampus associated with theta/gamma oscillations. Intrahippocampal consolidation and the hippocampal-neocortical transfer of the stored representations, on the other hand, is protracted and carried by discrete quanta of cooperative neuronal bursts during slow-wave sleep. (Buzsaki, 1966, p. 81)

Reduced hippocampus volumes have been noted in patients with chronic LBP and complex regional pain syndrome but not those diagnosed with osteoarthritis. Furthermore, reduced neurogenesis (the process of generating new neurons that integrate into existing circuits) in the hippocampus has been associated with neuropathic pain conditions. Baliki et al (2011) note that these data suggest that different pain conditions may have different "brain signatures."

The hippocampus became very important to Apkarian's research (Mutso et al, 2012) because of his emphasis on the role of conditioning and extinction in the creation and maintenance of chronic pain conditions. Ordinarily, if one strains one's back performing an activity, the problem improves with proper treatment. The person repeats that activity but in a fashion that minimizes the chance of pain. Over time, the accompanying emotional (fear) and physiological reactions associated with the activity dissipate and undergo extinction. However, in the setting of chronic pain, any and all activity produces aversive consequences, and the associated emotional and physiological responses are strengthened. In the setting of neuropathic pain conditions, apparently random, unpredictable paroxysms of pain occur, further strengthening the association with various environments (contexts). Therefore, there is no opportunity for extinction to take place, and the pain persists. Mutso et al "hypothesize that chronic pain can be redefined in terms of context conditioning and extinction, and viewed as a state of continual learning through which aversive emotional associations are constantly made with otherwise incidental events due to the persistent presence of a patient's pain. Moreover, due to the constant presence of the pain, such chronic pain patients may become unable to extinguish the conditioned event since at each re-exposure pain may still be present" (Mutso et al, 2012, p. 5747). Given the unique role of the hippocampus in contextual-dependent learning, it is thought that this process becomes "dysregulated."

Protein kinase, in particular extracellular signal-related kinase (ERK), in the hippocampus appears to be crucial to contextual-fear extinction. Decreases in ERK1 and ERK2 phosphorylation (the process that turns protein enzymes on and off, thus affecting their activity and function) and in *ERK2* gene expression were discovered in animal models of neuropathic pain. Diminished ERK activity also results in a reduction of short-term synaptic plasticity in the hippocampus. Furthermore, a reduction in the number of newly born cells in the hippocampus might explain the reduction in hippocampal volume. This would also impact neurogenesis and, by extension, the mechanism underlying learning, memory, and contextual extinction. Taken together, the decrease in neurogenesis and short-term synaptic plasticity may account, in part, for the emotional and cognitive deficits seen in chronic pain conditions. These findings have been shown to be a consequence of ongoing pain vs. generalized stress or anxiety.

In summing up the brain's involvement in the experience of pain, Apkarian and his colleagues note: "If one assumes the simple notion that the brain is a dynamical network, wherein detailed connectivity is constantly modified by the instantaneous experience of the organism, then it should be evident that quantifying chronic pain as an outflow of spinal cord processing (and primarily focusing on spinothalamic pathway transmission), is simplistic and inadequate" (Apkarian et al, 2009, p. 95).

Avalanches

In systems theory, the term *avalanche* is used to refer to a sudden and sometimes cataclysmic change, such as an earthquake. It is the antithesis of a smooth, gradual, and linear change in the system. The sandpile model is often used as an illustration.

Ultimately, the sandpile, created by dropping handfuls of sand on a relatively flat surface, reaches a point of "self-organized criticality," such that adding even a small amount of sand could (a) have no effect, (b) role down the side of the pile and stop, (c) displace or knock a few grains down, or (d) cause a huge avalanche and cave in the entire side of the pile.

This concept is played out in the central nervous system during neuronal processing when a single or small number of neurons are integrating the input from thousands of other neurons. This basic process of integration and redistribution of information back to the network is a common characteristic of complex systems. The activity is modulated by the ever-present facilitator and inhibitory mechanisms. A disruption in this balance could produce an avalanche of activity, such as that seen in epileptic behavior. Clinically, this could reveal a patient that has "decompensated" into their pain, manifesting all of the well-recognized behavioral, cognitive, emotional, and physiological components. Unlike a fork in the road, where one can return to the point of bifurcation and take the other direction, an avalanche is more like going over the precipice—the point of no return. This might explain why many patients with chronic pain and chronic pain conditions are so recalcitrant to otherwise effective treatments; the system has changed.

CONCLUSION

As a sensory phenomenon, pain has been interpreted as being directly explainable by the functional properties of receptors, afferent nerve fibers, and the central sensory system. This linear approach to pain held sway for many centuries. Some remnants remain, as evidenced by the continued use of numerical rating scales to measure pain. Pain as a perception, by contrast, embodies the total psychological experience of the complex, dynamic, and holistic aspects of the sensory stimuli. Fortunately, this sensation–perception dichotomy has been abandoned by most researchers. Contemporary theories recognize and elaborate on the complex and dynamic aspects of the sensory and perceptual processes involved. Furthermore, the presence of neural oscillations, coherence, and synchronization, especially in spatially separated cortical structures, may reflect a type of quantum entanglement and should encourage expanding future investigations of brain function to include elements of quantum theory and mechanics.

Systems theory specifies that many systems of interconnected and nonlinear elements evolve over time into a critical state. This process of evolution is an emergent property of the system in that it can take place without any external signal or direction. Efforts to advance and expand the understanding of pain, especially chronic pain, will benefit from considering this aspect of systems theory. The ongoing and spontaneous activity of networks in the brain, such as the DMN, has been well documented. The mere activation of a peripheral nociceptor may be of little consequence. However, as the information is transmitted to various subcortical and cortical structures the impact becomes more defined. In the physically and emotionally vulnerable individual in whom "the system" is at the edge of chaos and demonstrates criticality, a usually small perturbation can result in the system collapsing into chronic pain.

The ontological development of the brain must be considered within the context of the organism's experience; there is substantial interplay between the external and internal worlds. The brain should be seen as an organ that establishes boundaries and limitations (an organ of capacity), not from a deterministic perspective. In much the same way that certain body types and composition make it more or less difficult to accomplish specific feats, they do not guarantee that these feats will be accomplished. The brain has its own complex set of dynamic circuits whose architecture, structure, and function are susceptible to modification. Despite the apparent intricacies of brain function and structure, the discussion is incomplete until considered in the context of the "mind" and consciousness (see Chapter 13). Because of the enormity of the subject, this topic can only be addressed in the most superficial manner. But, to ignore it can leave one with an illusion regarding the depth of our understanding of the genesis of our thoughts, perceptions, emotions, and behavior.

REFERENCES

Apkarian AV, Baliki MN, Geha PH. Towards a theory of chronic pain. *Prog Neruobiol.* 2009;87:81–97.

Apkarian AV, Bushnell MC, Treede RD, Zubueta JK. Human brain mechanisms of pain perception and regulation in health disease. *Eur J Pain.* 2005;9:463–484.

Apkarian AV, Scholz J. Shared mechanisms between chronic pain and neurodegenerative disease. *Drug Discovery Today: Disease Mechanisms.* 2006;3(3),319–326.

Apkarian AV, Sosa Y, Krauss BR, et al. Chronic pain patients are impaired on an emotional decision-making task. *Pain.* 2004;108(1-2):129–136.

Baliki MN, Geha PY, Apkarian AV, Chialvo DR. Beyond feeling: chronic pain hurts the brain, disrupting the default-mode network dynamics. *J Neurosci.* 2008;28(6):1398–1403.

Baliki MN, Schnitzer TJ, Bauer WR, Apkarian AV. Brain morphological signatures for chronic pain. *PLoS ONE.* 2011;6(10):e26010.

Baria AT, Baliki MN, Parrish T, Apkarian AV. Anatomical and functional assemblies of brain BOLD oscillations. *J Neurosci.* 2011;31:7910–7919.

Bar-On E, Weigl D, Parvari R, Katz K, Weitz R, Steinberg T. Congenital insensitivity to pain: orthopedic manifestations. *J Bone Joint Surg.* 2002;84-B:252–257.

Benedetti F, Arduino C, Costa S, et al. Loss of expectation-related mechanisms in Alzheimer's disease makes analgesic therapies less effective. *Pain.* 2006;121:131–144.

Berthier M, Starkstein S, Leigyards R. Asymbolia for pain: a sensory-limbic disconnection syndrome. *Ann Neurol,* 1988;24:42–49.

Blankenberg F, Ruff CC, Deichmann R, Rees G, Driver J. The cutaneous rabbit illusion affects human primary sensory cortex somatotopically. *PLoS Biol.* 2006;4(3):0459–0466.

Bluhm RL, Miller J, Lanius RA, et al. Spontaneous low-frequency fluctuations in the BOLD signal in schizophrenic patients: anomalies in the default network. *Schizophren Bull.* 2007;33(4):1004–1012.

Burgmer M, Gaubitz M, Konrad C, et al. Decreased grey matter volume in the cingulo-frontal cortex and the amygdala in patients with fibromyalgia. *Psychosom Med.* 2009;71:566–573.

Buzsaki G. The hippocampus-neocortex dialogue. *Cereb Cortex.* 1996;6:81–92.

Casey KL. The imaging of pain: background and rationale. In KL Casey, MC Bushnell, eds. *Pain Imaging: Progress in Pain Research and Management,* Vol 18. Seattle: IASP Press; 2000:1–29.

Casey KL, Bushnell MC. *Pain Imaging: Progress in Pain Research and Management,* Vol. 18. Seattle: IASP Press; 2000.

Cauda F, D'Agata F, Sacco K, et al. Altered resting state attentional networks in diabetic neuropathic pain. *J Neurol Neurosurg Psychiatry.* 2010;81:806–811.

Craggs JG, Staud R, Robinson ME, Perlstein WM, Price DD. Effective connectivity among brain regions associated with slow temporal summation of C-fiber-evoked pain in fibromyalgia patients and healthy controls. *J Pain.* 2012;13(4):390–400.

Craig AD, Bushnell MC. The thermal grill illusion: unmasking the burn of cold pain. *Science.* 1994;265:252–255.

Cramer SC, Sur M, Dobkin BH, et al. Harnessing neuroplasticity for clinical applications. *Brain.* 2011;134:1591–1609.

deCharms RC, Christoff K, Glover GH, Pauly JM. Learned regulation of spatially localized brain activation using real-time fMRI. *Neuroimage.* 2004;21:436–443.

deCharms RC, Maeda F, Glover GH, et al. Control over brain activation and pain learned by using real-time functional MRI. *Proc Natl Acad Sci U S A.* 2005;102:18626–18631.

Edwards RR. Individual differences in endogenous pain modulation as a risk factor for chronic pain. *Neurology.* 2005;65:437–443.

Edwards RR, Ness TJ, Weignent DA, Fillingim RB. Individual differences in diffuse noxious inhibitory controls (DNIC): association with clinical variables. *Pain.* 2003;106:427–437.

Farmer MA, Baliki MN, Apkarian AV. A dynamic network perspective of chronic pain. *Neurosci Lett.* 2012;520:197–203.

Fingelkurts AA, Fingelkurts AA, Bagnato S, Boccagni C, Galardi G. DMN operational synchrony relates to self-consciousness: evidence from patients in vegetative and minimally conscious states. *Open Neuroimaging J.* 2012;6:55–68.

Foss JM, Apkarian AV, Chialvo DR. Dynamics of pain: fractal dimension of temporal variability of spontaneous pain differentiates between pain states. *J Neurophysiol.* 2006;95:730–736.

Gallagher HL, Firth CD. Functional imaging of "theory of mind." *Trends Cogn Sci.* 2003;7:77–83.

Gao W, Zhu H, Giovanello KS, et al. Evidence on the emergence of the brain's default network from 2-week-old to 2-year-old healthy pediatric subjects. *Proc Natl Acad Sci U S A*. 2009;106:6790–6795.

Geldard FA, Sherrick CE. The cutaneous "rabbit": a perceptual illusion. *Science*. 1972;178:178–179.

Geschwind N. Disconnection syndromes in animals and man. *Brain*. 1965;88:237–294.

Goffaux P, de Souza JB, Potvin S, Marchand S. Pain relief through expectation supersedes descending inhibitory deficits in fibromyalgia patients. *Pain*. 2009;145:18–23.

Gracely RH, Petzke F, Wolf JM, Clauw DJ. Functional magnetic resonance imaging evidence of augmented pain processing in fibromyalgia. *Arthritis Rheum*. 2002;46:1333–1343.

Gross J, Schnitzler A, Timmermann L, Ploner M. Gamma oscillations in human primary somatosensory cortex reflect pain perception. *PLoS Biol*, 2007;5:e123.

Gwilym SE, Filippini N, Douaud G, Carr AJ, Tracey I. Thalamic atrophy associated with painful osteoarthritis of the hip is reversible after arthroplasty: a longitudinal voxel-based morphometric study. *Arthritis Rheum*. 2010;62:2930–2940.

Hadjipavlou G, Dunckley P, Behrens TEJ, Tracey I. Determining anatomical connectivities between cortical and brainstem pain processing in humans: a diffusion tensor imaging study of healthy controls. *Pain*. 2006;123(1-2):169–178.

Johansen-Berg H, Behrens TEJ. Just pretty pictures? What diffusion tractography can add in clinical neuroscience. *Curr Opin Neuroimaging*. 2006;19(4):379–385.

Jung C. *The Structure and Dynamics of the Psyche* (Collected Works of C.G. Jung, Vol 8). Adler G, Hull RFC, trans. Read H, Fordham M, Adler G, McGuire W, eds. Princeton, NJ: Princeton University Press; 1960.

Koch C, Laurent G. Complexity and the nervous system. *Science*. 1999;284(5411):96–98.

Kosek E, Ordenburg G. Lack of pressure pain modulation by heterotopic noxious conditioning stimulation in patients with painful osteoarthritis before, but not following surgical pain relief. *Pain*. 2000;88:69–78.

Kuchinad A, Schweinhardt P, Seminowicz DA, Wood PB, Chizh BA, Bushnell MC. Accelerated brain grey matter loss in fibromyalgia patients: premature aging of the brain? *J Neurosci*. 2007;27(15):4004–4007.

Kupers R, Pietrini P, Ricciardi E, Ptito M. The nature of consciousness in the visually deprived brain. *Front Psychol*. 2011;2:1–14.

Landrieu P, Said G, Allaire C. Dominantly transmitted congenital indifference to pain. *Ann Neurol*. 1990;27:574–578.

Lautenbacher S, Prager M, Rollman GB. Pain addictivity, diffuse noxious inhibitory controls, and attention: a functional measurement analysis. *Somatosens Mot Res*. 2007;24(4):189–201.

Lautenbacher S, Rollman GB. Possible deficiencies of pain modulation in fibromyalgia. *Clin J Pain*. 1997;13:189–196.

Le Bars D, Villanueva L, Willer JC, Bouhassira D. Diffuse noxious inhibitory controls (DNIC) in animals and in man. *Patol Fiziol Eksp Ter*. 1992; Jul-Aug (4):55–65.

Lewis GN, Rice DA, McNair PJ. Conditioned pain modulation in populations with chronic pain: a systematic review and meta-analysis. *J Pain*. 2012;13(10):936–944.

Mageri W, Burkart D, Fernandez A, Schmidt LG, Treede R. Persistent antinociception through repeated self-injury in patients with borderline personality disorder. *Pain*. 2012;153:575–584.

Mansour AR, Baliki MN, Huang L, Torbey S, Hermann KM, Schnitzer TJ, Apkarian AV. Brain white matter structural properties predict transition to chronic pain. *Pain*. 2013;154(10):2150–2159.

May A. Chronic pain may change the structure of the brain. *Pain*. 2008;137:7–15.

Minoshima S, Cross DJ, Koeppe RA, Casey KL. Brain activation studies using PET and SPECT: execution and analysis. In Casey KL, Bushnell MC, eds. *Pain Imaging. Progress in Pain Research and Management*, Vol 18. Seattle: IASP Press; 2000:48–95.

Mutso AA, Radzicki D, Baliki MN, et al. Abnormalities in hippocampal functioning with persistent pain. *J Neurosci.* 2012;32(17):5747–5756.

Napadow V, LaCount L, Park K, As-Sanie S, Clauw DJ, Harris RE. Intrinsic brain connectivity in fibromyalgia is associated with chronic pain intensity. *Arthritis Rheum.* 2010;62(8):2545–2555.

Ploner M, Lee MC, Wiech K, Bingel U, Tracey I. Flexible cerebral connectivity patterns subserves contextual modulations of pain. *Cereb Cortex.* 2011;21:719–726.

Raichle ME. The brain's dark energy. *Science.* 2006;314:1249–1250.

Raichle ME. Neuroscience: the brain's dark energy. *Sci Am.* 2010a;302(3):44–49.

Raichle ME. Two views of brain function. *Trends Cogn Sci.* 2010b;14(4):180–190.

Raichle ME, MacLeod AM, Snyder AZ, PowersWJ, Gusnard DA, Shulman GL. A default mode of brain function. *Proc Natl Acad Sci U S A.* 2001;98(2):676–682.

Raij TT, Numminen J, Närvänen S, Hiltunen J, Hari R. Brain correlates of subjective reality of physically and psychologically induced pain. *Proc Natl Acad Sci U S A.* 2005;102(6):2147–2151.

Rodriguez-Raecke R, Niemeier A, Ihle K, Ruether W, May A. Brain grey matter decrease in chronic pain is the consequence and not the cause of pain. *J Neurosci.* 2009;29:13746–13750.

Roy CS, Sherrington CS. On the regulation of the blood-supply of the brain. *J Physiol.* 1890;11:85–108.

Sarnthein J, Jeanmonod D. High thalamocortical theta coherence in patients with neurogenic pain. *Neuroimage.* 2008;39:1910–1917.

Schilder P, Stengel E. Schmerzasymbolie. *Zeitschrift für die gesamte Neurologie und Psychiatrie.* 1928;113(1):143–158.

Schilder P, Stengel E. Asymbolia for pain. *Arch Neurol Psychiatry.* 1931:25(3):598–600.

Schnakers C, Chatelle C, Majerus S, Gosseries O, De Val M, Laureys S. Assessment and detection of pain in noncommunicative severely brain-injured patients. *Expert Rev Neurother.* 2010;10(11):1725–1731.

Schweinhardt P, Sauro KM, Bushnell MC. Fibromyalgia: a disorder of the brain? *Neuroscientist.* 2008;14(5):415–421.

Seifert F, Malihofner C. Functional and structural imaging of pain-induced neuroplasticity. *Curr Opin Anesthesiol.* 2011;24:515–523.

Seminowicz DA, Jiang LI, Ji Y, Xu S, Gullapalli RP, Masri R. Thalamocortical asynchrony in conditions of spinal cord injury in rats. *J Neurosci.* 2012;32(45):15843–15848.

Seminowicz DA, Wideman TH, Naso L, et al. Effective treatment of chronic low back pain in humans reverses abnormal brain anatomy and function. *J Neurosci.* 2011;31(20):7540–7550.

Siddall PJ, Stanwell P, Woodhouse A, et al. Magnetic resonance spectroscopy detects biochemical changes in the brain associate with chronic low back pain: a preliminary report. *Anesth Analg.* 2006;102:1164–1168.

Simner J. Defining synaesthesia. *Br J Psychol.* 2012;103(6):1–15.

Smallwood RF, Laird AR, Ramage AE, et al. Structural brain anomalies and chronic pain: a quantitative meta-analysis of gray matter volume. *J Pain.* 2013;14(7):663–675.

Sommer C. Fibromyalgia: a clinical update. *IASP Pain Clinical Updates.* 2010;18(4):1–4.

Stephenson DT, Arneric SP. Neuroimaging of pain: advances and future prospect. *J Pain.* 2008;9:567–579.

Thompson SJ, Bushnell MK. Rodent functional and anatomical imaging of pain. *Neurosci Newslett.* 2012;520(2):131–139.

Thunberg T. Förnimmelserne vid till samma ställe lokaliserad, samtidigt pågående köld-och värmeretning. *Uppsala Läkfören Förh.* 1896;1:489–495.

Tracey I, Mantyh PW. The cerebral signature for pain perception and its modulation. *Neuron.* 2007;55:377–391.

Vanhaudenhuyse A, Noirhomme Q, Tshibanda L, et al. Default network connectivity reflects the level of consciousness in non-communicative brain-damaged patients. *Brain.* 2010;133:161–171.

Van Wijk G, Veldhuijzen DS. Perspective on diffuse noxious inhibitory controls as a model of endogenous pain modulation in clinical pain syndromes. *J Pain.* 2010;11(5):408–419.

Whitsel BL, Tommerdahl M, Kohn A, Vierck CJ, Favorov O. The S1 response to noxious skin heating by optical intrinsic signal imaging. In Casey KL, Bushnell MC, eds. *Pain Imaging. Progress in Pain Research and Management*, Vol 18. Seattle: IASP Press; 2000:32–47.

Williams DA, Gracely RH. Biology and therapy of fibromyalgia. Functional magnetic resonance imaging findings in fibromyalgia. *Arthritis Res Ther.* 2006;8(6):224.

Wolf BC, Sambatari F, Vasuc N, et al. Aberrant connectivity of resting-state networks in borderline personality disorder. *J Psychiatry Neurosci.* 2011;36(6):402–411.

Wood PB. Stress and dopamine: implications for the pathophysiology of chronic widespread pain. *Med Hypotheses.* 2004;62(3):420–424.

Yarnitsky D. Conditioned pain modulation (the diffuse noxious inhibitory control-like effect): its relevance for acute and chronic pain states. *Curr Opin Anesthesiol.* 2010;23:611–615.

Yarnitsky D, Arendt-Nielsen L, Bouhassira D, et al. Recommendations on terminology and practice of psychophysical DNIC testing. *Eur J Pain.* 2010;14:339.

5 Pain Processing: Some Theories

The brain is not color-coded, its internal connections are not readily visible, its physiological operations are ephemeral, and it is organized in a series of processing areas and nested hierarchies that form networks, so it is difficult to analyze.
–A.D. Craig (2008, p. 272)

INTRODUCTION

The fundamentals of specificity, pattern, intensity, and summation theories (see Chapter 2) will not be reiterated here. Rather, the emphasis will be on more contemporary approaches. The work associated with Melzack will be highlighted because of its historical meaningfulness, impact on the current view of pain, and heuristic value. Melzack's neuromatrix theory (Melzack, 2001) attempted to account for phantom pain in congenitally absent limbs (Melzack et al, 1997), but also laid the foundation for understanding how pain could emerge from within a system of cortical networks. Price's model expanded on the role of cortical structures and emphasizes the notion of threat perception and unpleasantness. The importance of patients' interpretation of sensory input became a critical component of the process. Craig's model represents a shift toward viewing pain within the context of a homeostatic processing system. The pain processing system is my interpretation of the interaction among the affective/cognitive and nociceptive aspects of pain and overall stress of the system (individual). It also illustrates how the concept of phase transition may be incorporated.

The different theories of pain processing share a common feature of incorporating both the affective and sensory components of pain. They differ with respect to the amount of emphasis given to the periphery and the central/cortical mechanisms.

Psychosocial theories, for example, spend relatively little time in the periphery, compared to mechanistic theories, such as that outlined by Woolf (Woolf, 2004; Woolf and Max, 2001). Furthermore, it is important to remember that pain does not appear to be a unitary concept. There are several types of pain (see Chapter 3), each with its own neurochemical and physiological identity (Honore et al, 2000; Mannion and Woolf, 2000). It remains to be seen if an all-encompassing theory of pain will emerge.

GATE CONTROL THEORY (GCT)

Prior to the GCT (Melzack and Wall, 1965), the specificity theory and pattern theory held sway as the predominating explanations for pain. Several clinical observations led Melzack and Wall to question specificity and patterns theories. For example, these theories did not seem to be able to adequately account for (a) pain after amputation (phantom pain), (b) pain following peripheral nerve infections or diseases (peripheral neuralgias), and (c) the burning pain after partial lesioning of the peripheral nerve (causalgia). Four common features of these syndromes were especially bothersome. First, surgical lesions in the central and/or peripheral nervous systems failed to relieve the pain. Even after such operations, stimulation below the level of the lesion could elicit still more severe pain. Second, non-noxious stimulation, including gentle touch, could trigger excruciating pain. At times there could be paroxysms of spontaneous pain. Third, new "trigger zones" emerged unpredictably and in areas where no damage existed. Finally, pain in hyperalgesic skin (pain disproportionate to the stimulus) occurred after long delays and continued well after the stimulus was removed.

Furthermore, specificity and pattern theories did not explain the variety of observations that suggested the influence of psychological factors. For example, Beecher (1959) reported on the relative absence of pain or the need for morphine by extensively wounded American soldiers at the Anzio beachhead, presumably because they were overjoyed at having survived and at the prospect of returning home. That they, indeed, could still feel pain was evident by their demonstrating a painful response to procedures such as drawing blood. Similarly, S. Weinstein (reported in Melzack and Casey, 1968) described how, during a previous war, he was doused with gasoline and set on fire. Fortunately, he was able to extinguish the flames within 30 seconds. During this time he was completely aware of the flames engulfing his body. However, he denied having the slightest tactile sensation and did not experience any pain. In addition, others (Murphy, 1951) had observed that patients undergoing frontal lobotomies continued to report pain, but declared that it was not bothersome. Finally, there were the data from the experiments of Ivan Pavlov, who is most recognized for demonstrating the principles of classical conditioning (1927). Using these principles, Pavlov demonstrated that when an electric shock, a cut, or burn was immediately and consistently followed by the presentation of food to a partially food-deprived dog, over time the animals responded to these insults as signals for food and failed to show even the smallest pain responses. Taken literally, this might seem to some to reflect a type of "nonpainful pain."

Melzack and Wall (1965) proposed that the experience of pain resulted from an interaction involving three systems: (a) substantia gelatinosa, (b) dorsal column, and (c) the first central transmission cell (T cell). The *substantia gelatinosa* is the area of the dorsal horn of the spinal cord that receives afferent input from the skin via A-delta (large-fiber) and C-afferent (small-fiber) nerves. The GCT theory states that the substantia gelatinosa functions as a kind of gate-control system. The large-fiber activity tends to open the gate and small fibers to close it. Thus, these incoming afferent patterns are modulated before they influence the T cell. Furthermore, the afferent patterns in the dorsal column system activate certain brain processes which in turn can influence the modulatory activity of the gate-control system via efferent inputs. Therefore, the number of impulses transmitted by the T cell over a given period of time is determined by the interaction of inputs from A-delta (large fibers), C-fibers (small fibers), and descending input from the brain. When the output activity of the T cell reaches or exceeds a critical level, an action system(s) is triggered.

The incorporation of a descending system from the brain was critical. It provided a mechanism by which psychological and cognitive factors such as attention and anxiety, previously ignored or at least left unaccounted for, could impact the experience of pain. Suddenly, the ability of wounded soldier's intense emotions of relief and joy at surviving the injury and the prospect of returning home to loved ones to overwhelm the expected pain from his physical injuries made sense. Although not recognized as such at the time, the GCT also ushered in an appreciation for the involvement of a systems approach to the experience of pain. Pain began to be understood as a process and not an event or state.

In 1968, Melzack and Casey expanded on the central control systems involved in modulating pain. They highlighted two major components of pain, the *sensory-discriminative* and the *motivational-affective*. The sensory-discriminative system processed the spatial and temporal aspect of the stimulus and involved the neospinothalamic system, including the ventrobasal thalamus. The ventrobasal thalamus is somatotopically organized. Input to the ventrobasal thalamus is received via the dorsal column lemniscal pathways, which are predominately contralateral to the site of stimulation. Thus, the sensory-discriminative system enables one to provide a precise description of the location of the stimulation—the little finger, big toe—and its qualitative characteristics, such as burning, sharp, or dull.

The motivational-affective component consisted of the paramedial, reticular, and limbic systems. The *paramedial ascending system* included the spinoreticular, spinomesencephalic, and paleospinothalamic pathways. The medial thalamus rather than the ventrobasal thalamus is involved. The medial thalamus receives mixed sensory input and is not somatotopically organized like the ventrobasal thalamus. The *limbic system* included the frontal cortex, hippocampus, reticular activating system, and amygdala. Stimulation at the mesencephalic level was known to produce a strong drive to avoid aversive stimulation. A fear-like response associated with escape behavior occurred when of the medial thalamus was stimulated. Aversive drive and escape behavior was also noted when limbic structures, such as the hippocampus and amygdala, were stimulated. When the amygdala or cingulum bundle, which connects the posterior frontal cortex to the hippocampus, was deactivated, the previously observed negative affect or emotional response to intense stimulation disappeared.

In some cases there seemed to be an overlapping of brain areas associated with aversive drive and approach responses. Leknes and Tracey (2008) have described a common neurobiology for pain and pleasure involving the opioid and dopamine systems. This overlap between approach and avoidance or aversive structures may explain why an aversive response to a noxious stimulus can be blocked or overcome by stimulation of the reward system. For example, Pavlov's dogs appeared to be unaffected by previous painful stimulation after it had been paired with food. Also, Doleys and

Davidson (1976) demonstrated that pigeons acted as though more intense stimulation (brief electric shock) was desirable when it was associated with the appearance of food, but only up to a certain intensity, after which the brief electric shock again seemed aversive (painful). The relationship of shock intensity and shock aversiveness formed a U-shaped (quadratic) rather than a linear function. Melzack and Casey (1968) were convinced that the neural structure comprising the paramedial, reticular, and limbic system, in fact, controlled the motivational (approach or avoid) and affective aspects of pain.

In general, Melzack and Casey proposed that brain structures forming the motivational-affective system served as a central intensity monitor. The intensity of the T-cell output, determined in part by the number of large and small fibers activated and their rate of firing, activated these motivational-affective structures, the medial brainstem in particular. Output from the medial brainstem could be enhanced by spatial and temporal summation and provided a measure of stimulation intensity. Up to some critical level, which could be modified by various circumstances, the output activated positive and approach mechanisms. Beyond this critical level, avoidance, aversive, and negative affective mechanisms would be activated. Melzack and Casey (1968) also recognized the contribution of anticipation, prior experience, attention, anxiety, cultural background, and conditioning to the experience of pain and associated responses. Cognitive and higher level activities were noted to affect both the sensory and motivational systems. Taken together, they felt there was evidence to demonstrate that "input was localized, identified in terms of its physical properties, evaluated in terms of present and past experience, and modified before it activates the sensory or motivational systems" (p. 433).

Melzack and Wall (1965) had previously suggested that the dorsal column and dorsolateral projection pathways severed as a central-control-trigger. These pathways allowed information regarding the location and nature of a stimulus to be transmitted rapidly to the cortex, thus activating the central control processes. This in turn provided a mechanism for the modulation of the input via activation of (a) the sensory-discriminative system and (b) a descending inhibitory system that exerts its influence at the level of the spinal cord. Therefore, the input was actually modulated before it was transmitted to the sensory-discriminative and motivational-affective systems. The frontal cortex received its input from intracortical fibers rather than peripherally and then projected it to reticular and limbic structures and was found to mediate between the cognitive and the motivational-affective aspects of pain. The lack of an aversive drive (desire to withdraw from a stimulus), and the typical negative emotional response to an intense stimulus following a lobotomy, may be explained by the deactivation of these central control processes.

The word *pain* was thus considered to be a label encompassing a variety of different and unique experiences. As Melzack and Casey (1968) state,

Pain varies along both sensory-discriminative and motivation-affective dimensions. The magnitude or intensity along these dimensions, moreover, is influenced by cognitive activities, such as evaluation of the seriousness of the injury. If injury or any other noxious input fails to evoke aversive drive, the experiences cannot be labeled as pain. Conversely, anxiety and anguish without somatic input is not pain. Pain must be defined in terms of its sensory, motivational and central control determinants. Pain, we believe, is a function of the interactions of all three determinants and cannot be ascribed to any one of them. (p. 434)

The therapeutic implications were immediately obvious. Emphasis was shifted away from merely attempting to reduce the sensory input by surgical or pharmacological means to altering motivational, affective, and cognitive factors. Although not recognized and discussed as such until sometime later, the nonlinear aspects of the system were beginning to emerge. That is, the pain experienced was not proportional to the nociceptive input. The difference between a nerve impulse and pain was beginning to be understood (Wall and McMahon, 1986). Furthermore, this central-control processing system was very dynamic, in that it was constantly influenced by and responsive to a host of physical and psychological variables.

PATTERN-GENERATING MECHANISM AND PHANTOM PAIN AND SENSATION

In 1978, Melzack and Loeser proposed the existence of a central pattern-generating mechanism to explain phantom pain. *Phantom body pain* is defined as pain felt in an area of the body where there is complete loss of sensory input. The term *phantom limb* was coined by Silas Weir Mitchell in his 1872 book, *Injuries of Nerves and Their Consequences*. In this book he chronicled his observation as a physician during the Civil War. He recorded numerous reports of soldiers describing a tingling sensation and the continued presence of a part of the body that had been lost in battle or amputated. Often the sensations mimicked those experienced prior to amputation. At first the phantom felt normal in size. Later the shape could begin to change and might even shrink and telescope into the stump or perhaps disappear. Some of the more unfortunate individuals also suffered from a feeling of horrific burning pain in the phantom.

Surveys in the early 1980s estimated that 72% of amputees have phantom pain 8 days after amputation, 65% at 6 months, and as many as 60% at 2 years (Jensen et al, 1983, 1985; Katz and Melzack, 1990). There have been some reports of patients not developing phantom pain until years later, when the stump was exposed to a noxious event such as an injection or surgical revision.

Phantom body pain is reported by about 5–10% of paraplegics suffering from damage to the spinal cord. In some cases the pain is noted immediately after the injury; in other instances, phantom pain was not reported until 11 years later. Efforts to treat this type of pain have included cordectomies (removal of a section of the spinal cord). Although this approach virtually eliminates any possibility of input from the periphery, it has proved unsuccessful. Often the spinal cord is completely severed, making it impossible for any peripheral stimulation to be transmitted to the brain (deafferentation). The question then becomes how could one experience pain in the absence of any input from A-delta and C-fibers in the periphery, which plays such a crucial role in pain processing?

Melzack (1989; Katz and Melzack, 1990) considered phantom pain that reproduced the experience of preamputation pain to represent a somatosensory memory. In some instances, such as a brachial plexus avulsion injury, the limb remains but the patient experiences it in a different and often painful position. Imagine looking down at an arm that you cannot feel, but the one you do feel, you cannot see. Not all phantom sensations are painful. Painful and nonpainful phantom sensations have been reported upon removal or deafferentation of breasts, teeth, bladder, eye, ulcers, and rectum. For instance, two young female patients I interviewed underwent removal of their urinary bladders secondary to severe interstitial cystitis only to continue to feel the painful sensation of the bladder filling and the urgent need to void.

Volleys of nerve impulses following termination of an aversive or noxious stimulus are referred to as *afterdischarges* and are associated with normal pain. High-frequency firing during exposure to a noxious stimulus followed by afterdischarge bursts, sometimes lasting several minutes after cessation of the noxious stimulus, have been recorded in spinal cord cells and the brainstem reticular formation. Likewise, deafferentation has been associated with a variety of activities involving central neurons. In one study, cutting of the dorsal roots in the cat was followed by abnormal bursts of cell firing in the dorsal horn lasting as long as 180 days after the fact. Single shock impulses to adjacent intact roots also produced prolonged firing. High-frequency burst firing patterns could be produced by non-noxious stimulation. Furthermore, this abnormal activity was found to occur in lamina-V cells thought to be involved in the transmission process related to pain. Melzack and Loeser (1978) reasoned that if these high-frequency bursts were part of the pain signaling pattern, then any pathology that led to prolonged bursting patterns might also produce the experience of pain in the associated body part in the absence of any peripheral input from that body part.

The fact that bladder and bowel distention, as well as prolonged pressure due to sitting, could intensify the pain, suggested that visceral afferents ascending in the sympathetic chain running parallel to but outside the spinal cord could be transmitting signals to the spinal cord at levels above the transaction. However, temporarily blocking bilateral sympathetic activity via the use of an anesthetic or performing a sympathectomy proved futile. Furthermore, spinal cord transections in the thoracic spine at levels well above those receiving input from visceral afferents serving the lower body produced disappointing results. Although evidence existed showing the modulating effects of emotional states such as anxiety, hostility, frustration, and depression, there was no evidence that phantom body pain was caused by psychological factors.

From these findings Melzack and Loeser (1978) concluded the following:

(1) Paraplegic patients experience phantom body pain in body parts below the level of spinal cord damage.
(2) The pain is not relieved by spinal cord cordectomy or blocking of other possible routes, such as the sympathetic nervous system.
(3) Peripheral input is not the cause of the pain.
(4) The mechanism causing the pain must be central to the level of the cord transaction.
(5) Loss of input to the central structures as a result of deafferentation may play a role in producing the pain.

Their theory rested on the assumption, based on the gate control theory, that "pain occurs when the number of nerve impulses per unit time from the somatic projection systems to the brain area that subserve pain exceeds a critical level. Injury or noxious stimulation may produce such a level." They proposed "that a similar suprathreshold level may occur either directly or secondarily as a result of loss of input" (Melzack and Loeser, 1978, p. 223).

Melzack and Loeser proposed the existence of neuron pools (the entire "gate"). Such neuron pools and other nuclei are located at many levels of the spinal cord and brain along the path of the major somatosensory projection system and function as pattern- generating mechanisms. Ordinarily, the activity of these neurons is under the control of sensory input and descending brain mechanisms. Of necessity, the pattern-generating mechanism in paraplegics who experience phantom body pain must be above the level of the transaction and project to areas of the brain responsible for localization of sensory input. Moreover, the prolonged bursting activity of these pattern-generating mechanisms can be modulated by a variety of autonomic, visceral, psychological, and environmental variables.

The authors further speculated that loss of segmental input to the brain affected the brain's inhibitory system, resulting in a decrease in descending inhibition. The absence of descending inhibition would make it easier for non-noxious stimuli to trigger the abnormal bursting patterns. The neural substrates underlying memories for previous pain could thus be activated, resulting in the phantom body pain. Diminished inhibition would also enable the abnormal bursting to persist for an extended period and to recruit other nearby neurons into the pool. This enlargement of the abnormally firing neuron pool would manifest itself by intensification of pain and a sensation of the pain spreading. However, the explanation for the fact that only 5–10% of paraplegics manifest phantom body-pain remains unclear.

RONALD MELZACK: NEUROMATRIX THEORY

Some years after the GCT was proposed and elaborated, Melzack (1989, 1999) enumerated a number of general observations regarding pain:

(1) There is a general lack of correlation between the degree of pain and the severity of injury as reported by soldiers and patients in emergency rooms.
(2) Phantom pain has been reported by persons with a congenitally absent limb.
(3) Pain is associated with depression.
(4) Pain persists after blocking the "involved" nerve with an anesthetic.
(5) Somatic delusions are present in psychologically normal persons.
(6) There is increased pain without increased peripheral stimulation (i.e., emotional, psychological, visual).
(7) Persons with early childhood trauma report relatively greater pain than that among those without such trauma.
(8) Patients have reported identical or near-identical pain after the pain generator has been removed or disabled.

These observations became puzzling and appeared to defy explanation, even in the context of the GCT. His considerable research into phantom pain led to several conclusions. First, as the phantom feels so real, it is reasonable to speculate that the body we usually feel involves the same or very similar "neural processes in the brain." These brain processes are normally activated and modulated by moment-to-moment inputs from the body, but these processes can also produce the sensation of a body part without any peripheral input. Second, all of the qualities we normally feel from the body, such as pain, can be felt without any input from the body. Therefore, the true origin of these experiences must lie in the various *neural networks* in the brain. It follows that stimuli may trigger these built-in sensations, or neural networks, but do not produce them. Third, the body is perceived as a unity, identified as the "self," distinct from others and the surrounding environment. The sense of "unity" and of "self," as a point of reference, is produced by central neural processes and is not a result of input from the peripheral nervous system or the spinal cord. And fourth, the brain processes that underlie the "body-self" are built in genetically but are modifiable by experience.

Melzack felt that there was a neural system which existed in the brain that is capable of creating many of our painful experiences, even when input form the body is cut off, as in the case with amputation, nerve avulsion, or deafferentation. Indeed, he stated, "we don't need a body to feel a body" (1989, p. 4). What we experience as our body, in fact, is produced by various neural networks within the brain. These various networks are normally triggered or modulated by inputs from the body. This notion contrasted sharply with specificity theory, in which the sensations experienced are said to be inherent in the peripheral nerve fiber or some specific center of the brain. Indeed, Mezack stated that "pain is not injury" (1989, p. 9). Temperature changes occur "out there," but the experience of warmth and cold are not "out there." Similarly, the experiences of itching, stinging, smarting, or tickling have no external equivalents. Rather, these qualities, like that of pain experiences, are produced by built-in neuromodules whose neurosignatures innately produce these qualities. This idea led to the development of the neuromatrix theory (Melzack, 1999, 2001).

The key components of Melzack's neuromatrix theory are the neuromatrix, cyclical processing and synthesis, neurosignature, and sentient neural hub. The *neuromatrix* is described by Melzack as a large, widespread network of neurons consisting of loops between the thalamus and cortex, cortex and limbic system, and somatosensory system. This network of neurons is (a) spatially distributed throughout the brain, (b) initially determined genetically, and (c) specifically programmed to produce signature patterns. These patterns are referred to as *neurosignatures* and they originate or take form within the neuromatrix. This is in keeping with Webster's definition of a matrix as "that within which, or within and from which, something originates." The term *phylomatrix* describes the network of neurons whose synaptic connections and output pattern (neurosignature) were genetically determined, and *ontomatrix*, those patterns that are modified during the course of development or by sensory experience.

The neuromatrix thus becomes a psychologically meaningful unit, developed by both heredity and learning, that represents an entire unified entity or "body-self." The point at which the neuromatrix or any part of it (neuromodule) becomes active and susceptible to modification is genetically determined. Multiple inputs act upon the neuromatrix programs and contribute to the output neurosignature, including (1) sensory input (visceral, cutaneous), (2) visual and other sensory inputs that influence the cognitive interpretation, (3) phasic and tonic cognitive and emotional inputs from other areas of the brain, (4) intrinsic neural inhibitory modulation inherent in all brain function, and (5) activity of the body's stress-regulatory system (cytokines, endocrine, autonomic, immune and opioid systems). These inputs influence which set of synaptic connections survive, grow, or die off. Certain of these modified synaptic configurations become permanent and impart distinct patterns to the neurosignature. Thus, the phylomatrix pattern produces the experience of "a" body. The various influences mentioned sculpt the phylomatrix to produce the ontomatrix, that is, the unique body-self of the individual. In this way, the individual can experience the presence of a limb, even when it never did or no longer does exist.

The neuromatrix was conceptualized to have a variety of different components or loops. The various thalamocortical and limbic-cortical loops within the neuromatrix diverge, allowing for parallel processing. The sensory dimension is assumed to be subserved by the portion of the neuromatrix that lies in the sensory projection areas of the brain. Similarly, the affective dimensions are subserved by areas in the brainstem and limbic system. Melzack proposed the existence of *neuromodules*—specific parts of the neuromatrix determined by genetic factors but modified by experience—to subserve the major psychological dimensions or qualities of experience. These neuromodules constitute a distinct portion of the neurosignature in the same way that different instruments (modules), though each unique, together make up the orchestra (neruosignature). Indeed, Melzack proposed that this parallel processing occurs simultaneously in the known and identifiable somatosensory projection systems. However, these loops also converge repeatedly to permit interactions among the outputs of this processing. Melzack referred to this as repeated *cyclical processing and synthesis* (CPS) of nerve impulses through the neuromatrix. The product or output of this cyclical processing and synthesis was a neurosignature. It is this cyclical processing and synthesis that imposes constancy on the inputs.

Neurosignatures are nerve-impulse patterns that are experienced as the body and all of the various somatosensory qualities we feel. They are a product of genetic and sensory influences and are determined by the synaptic architecture of the neuromatrix. Its components subserve the sensory-discriminative, affective-motivational, and evaluative-cognitive dimensions of pain experience. The neurosignature is produced by patterns of synaptic connections within the neuromatrix and is imparted on all the nerve impulse patterns that flow through the neuromatrix. The pattern of nerve impulses of varying temporal and spatial dimensions is produced by neural programs genetically built into the neuromatrix and determines the particular qualities and other properties of the pain experience and behavior. Although the neurosignature can be triggered or modulated by various types of inputs, including sensory, cognitive, and physical or psychological stress, it emanates from within the neuromatrix.

The neurosignature is a continuous outflow from the neuromatrix and is projected to areas in the central core of the brainstem, the sentient neural hub. It is here that this stream of neural impulses is converted or transduced into a continually changing stream of consciousness, awareness, and movement. Two primary neurosignatures include one for the body-self and another for three-dimensional space. These are always present in the intact person and represent constant qualities in the continuous flow of experience. A particular neurosignature pattern can flow through the body-self neuromatrix that produces movement. These signature patterns bifurcate such that one pattern proceeds to the sentient hub and the other to the neuromatrix. The pattern proceeding to the sentient hub is converted into the experience of movement, while that through the neuromatrix activates spinal cord neurons, creating the actual physical movement. Therefore, even if input from a body part is absent, as in the case of an amputation or nerve lesion, the neurosignature provides information as though the body were intact. This may also explain how a phantom body part that has disappeared shortly after amputation can be evoked years later.

Reponses (action patterns) to sensory inputs occur only after these inputs are analyzed and synthesized thoroughly enough to produce a meaningful experience. For example, when one responds to pain by withdrawing or by seeking help, the response is to an experience that has sensory qualities, affect, and meaning (dangerous or potentially dangerous) to the body-self. After inputs undergo transformation in the neuromatrix for the body-self, appropriate action patterns are activated concurrently with the neuromatrix from experience. Large-diameter, fast-conducting fibers (A-delta and C-fibers) activate the CPS mechanism, which rapidly identifies the type of input (i.e., the self, others, objects). Several response options (action-neuromodules) are also activated by this input and remain available until the CPS completes its synthesis of the neurosignature for experience. Response options are eventually narrowed to the best one as the input becomes better defined and evaluated. According to Melzack, "in the neuromatrix for action patterns, the CPS produces activation of several possible patterns and their successive elimination until one particular pattern emerges as the most appropriate for the circumstances at the moment. In this way, input and output are synthesized simultaneously, in parallel, and not in series" (Melzack, 1989, p. 13).

The human stress-regulatory system is made up of a variety of homeostasis-regulation patterns designed to maintain the organism in a balanced (homeostatic) state. Stresses, such as injury to bone, muscle, or nerve, contribute to the neurosignature pattern creating chronic pain. Thus, the neuromatrix theory of pain not only incorporates genetic contribution, neural-hormonal stress mechanisms, and neural mechanisms of sensory transmission into the system but also treats them as having equal importance.

Melzack admits to building his theory on a highly conceptual nervous system. However, considering an estimated 100 billion nerve cells in the brain and that each neuron may have synaptic connections with hundreds or thousands of other neurons as they project from superficial to deep and back to the more superficial layers again, it would be difficult to build a theory any other way. The limits of the scientific knowledge then, more than 25 years ago, and now, despite its phenomenal growth, imposes significant constraints on building a comprehensive theory based solely on what is known.

In the tradition of Hebb (1955), Melzack reached beyond the data in an effort to provide "global answers to major problems" (1989, p. 6). As any good theory should, it provides a plausible explanation for the clinical observations. Equally important to Melzack,

the neuromatrix theory guides us away from the Cartesian concept of pain as a sensation produced by injury, inflammation, or other tissue pathology and toward the concept of pain as multidimensional experience produced by multiple influences. These influences range from the existing synaptic architecture of the neuromatrix—which is determined by genetic and sensory factors—to influences from within the body and from other areas of the brain. Genetic influences on synaptic architecture may determine, or predispose toward, the development of chronic pain syndromes.... [T]he neuromatrix, as a result of homeostasis-regulation patterns that have failed, produces the destructive conditions that may give rise to many of the chronic pain that so far have been resistant to treatments developed primarily to manage pains that are triggered by sensory inputs. (Melzack, 1999, p. S125)

DONALD D. PRICE'S MODEL

Price (1999; 2000) emphasized the importance of considering pain unpleasantness as well as pain intensity. His view encouraged recognition of the affective-emotional component of pain. Indeed, as will be discussed later, the two components, affective and sensory (intensity), can be independently manipulated. An obvious everyday example is provided by those who exercise vigorously. The aching or burning sensation brought on by an intense workout is accompanied by a sense of satisfaction or even joy. The same sensations brought on by disease would be regarded very differently. It is important to differentiate between what happens to the body (nociception) and one's reaction to it (affective response). Indeed, Price (1999) proposed a new definition of pain as "a somatic perception containing (1) a bodily sensation with qualities like those reported during tissue-damaging stimulation, (2) an experienced threat associated with this sensation, and (3) a feeling of unpleasantness or other negative emotions based on this experienced threat" (pp. 2–3).

Price describes nociceptive input as initiating (a) nociceptive sensations (encoded in the primary and secondary somatosensory cortex, with possible involvement of the posterior parietal complex and insular cortex), and (b) arousal, autonomic and somatomotor activation (reticular formation, amygdala, hypothalamus, and supplemental motor areas). The combined effect of this sensory awareness and arousal/activation is a perceived intrusion or threat, which is followed by immediate pain-unpleasantness (anterior cingulate cortex). Immediate pain-unpleasantness stimulates a process of "reflection" on the meaning of the pain in terms of its impact on life function, ability to endure, and the future (prefrontal cortex). This reflection results in the secondary pain affect (depression, anxiety, suffering) and a behavioral response or responses.

In Price's model, pain is made of both sensory and affective components. Pain unpleasantness (unpleasant emotional feelings) is part of the affective dimension of pain, made up of feelings and emotions relating the present or short-term experiences, such as distress and fear. In the presence of persistent nociception or stimulation, another component of the affective dimension, secondary pain affect emerges and is defined by one's emotional feelings toward the long-term implications of pain, such as depression, anxiety, and suffering. Sensory attributes known to influence pain unpleasantness include intensity, persistence, and spread. Sensory characteristics such as persistent burning, stinging, and aching dispose the individual to perceive pain as invasive and intrusive to the body and consciousness. Not unlike Damasio's neurological view of emotional mechanisms (see Chapter 13), pain unpleasantness is seen as a product of pain sensation, arousal, and autonomic and somatomotor responses in relation to the meaning and context of the pain itself. The interaction of pain unpleasantness and pain sensation is shown by the presence of increased pain-unpleasantness in subjects undergoing painful stimulation in an ischemia-pain or cold-presser test in which the duration is not specified, compared to a 5-second heat or electrical shock, where the brevity of stimulus is guaranteed. Hypnotic suggestion has also been used to explore the relationship between pain unpleasantness and pain sensation.

This model, as much or more than any other, has spawned interest in treatments that affect the unpleasant (affective) component of pain without necessarily influencing the sensory component. The affective component is a product of a dynamic and complex interaction involving a network of cortical structures. Price's model addresses the question of why pain hurts. There is the implication that the sensory component may well be hard-wired. Effective pain control emanates from altering the manner in which the sensory information is interpreted and responded to—a type of self-directed neuroplasticity (see Chapter 14).

The pain processing system model emerged as a result of considering observations in the clinical setting. It represents more of a functional approach to the dynamic interaction between nociceptive intensity and the patient's combined affective/cognitive ability to cope, rather than a neurophysiological model of pain processing. Several factors had to be accounted for. First, although pain can exist without peripheral stimulation, in most instances there is some degree of nociceptive drive. Even though the initial injury leading to nociceptive activity often resolves, the nociceptive drive frequently continues because of peripheral and/or central sensitization.

Second, affective variables such as depression, anxiety, and fear, along with cognitive variables including appraisals and expectations, can significantly influence the degree of pain and suffering experienced in response to nociception. This was illustrated by a case involving a female patient with terminal cancer. Her pain was severe enough that it could not be controlled unless she was heavily sedated. This prevented any meaningful interaction with her family during her final days of life. A procedure deactivating her anterior cingulate was performed. This effectively eliminated her affective (emotional) response to nociception. Thereafter, she continued to report the same physical or nociceptive sensations, and although her emotional response, in general, was blunted, she was able to interact with her family.

Third, the interaction between the affective/cognitive and nociceptive (sensory/discriminative) systems is very dynamic. Finally, the model should take into account the negative consequences that can occur as a result of this ongoing processing, particularly if associated with high levels of persistent nociceptive input.

Figure 5.1 illustrates such a model. The x, or vertical, axis represents the degree of affective/cognitive competence (acc) in coping with pain. The y, or horizontal, axis represents the degree of nociceptive stimulation (ns). The "output" of the system is determined by the interaction of acc and ns. This interaction can be very dynamic and change moment to moment. For example, ns input can be suddenly increased by injury, disease, or infection, or decreased by the application of modality therapy (heat or ice) or medication. In this model, whenever A is greater than B (A > B), the output is interpreted as tolerable or nonpainful. If B is greater than A (B > A), the output is considered as pain.

The model also recognizes that there can be quantitative differences in the degree to which A is less than or greater than B. The greater the difference between A and B, wherein A is less than (<) B, the greater the degree of "pain and suffering" experienced by the patient. When A is greater than (>) B, the patient is aware of the ns, but does not experience it as painful, in the ordinary sense of the word. Therefore, A >> B might produce an output that is considered detectable; A > B = tolerable; A < B = pain; A << B severe pain and suffering.

By way of an example, assume a treatment is introduced that reduces the level of ns input to the brain (B1 is reduced to level B2) but, the level of acc (A1) remains unchanged. The level of A1 is now greater than (>) B2, rendering the B2 ns tolerable. By contrast, if the level of acc (A2) improved without affecting the ns (B1), a previously painful stimulus (A1 < B1) is now tolerable (A2 > B1). The ideal situation would be a treatment that reduces ns (B1 to B2) and increases acc (A1 to A2). The magnitude of the difference between A2 and B2 is much greater than that between A1 and B2. Therefore, although the ns (B2) is the same in both scenarios, it would be minimally detectable in the A2 situation, and more intense but tolerable and potentially nonpainful in the A1

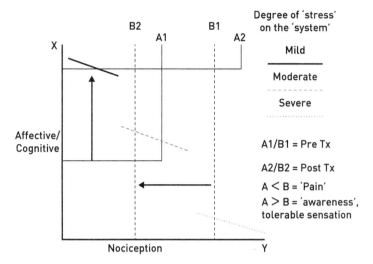

FIGURE 5.1

Pain processing system. See text for details.

situation. According to the model, the output of the interaction acc and ns would not be experienced as pain by the patient. The functional threshold or level at which one would expect increased activity would be A > B. However, improved functioning might be compromised by factors unrelated to pain, such as deconditioning.

It seems evident that the model would also have to take into account the differential demand on the system when both acc and ns are low compared to when they are high, especially if ns (B) is higher than acc (A). This demand is illustrated by the diagonal sloping lines. If both acc and ns fall in the solid-line area, the demand would be mild, moderate if in the range of the middle dashed-line, and severe if in the zone represented by the dotted-line closest to the Y axis. The greater the demand on the system, as reflected by altered physiological processing, anatomical deformities, release of substances at "toxic" levels, and major psychological disorders, the more likely the system is to default and lose its ability to adjust and adapt (decomplexification). The ultimate consequence is that the patient decompensates into chronic pain. In the most extreme of cases the ns could be so severe as to cause loss of consciousness, as indicated by the terminal point of the dotted line approaching the maximum level of ns.

The levels of stress on the system are purposely not connected in a linear fashion, in order to reflect qualitative and quantitative differences between mild, moderate, and severe. In a sense, going from one level to another represents a phase transition. This is supported by data suggesting the presence of significant clinical differences in symptom constellations, quality of life, and function among patients described as having pain in the mild, moderate, and severe ranges. The slight decreasing angle of each level suggests that while changes can occur within a level and may reach statistical significance, clinically relevant changes tend to occur only when the patient progresses from one level (phase) to another (see Chapter 6).

PAIN AS A HOMEOSTATIC EMOTION

The recent history of trying to understand pain has included an ongoing debate between those believing it to be a specific sensation involving specialized structures in the peripheral and central nervous system (specificity theory) and those viewing it as an integrated state resulting from the processing of somatosensory activity within a distributed neural network or matrix (convergence theory). Craig (2002, 2003a,b, 2009), however, views pain as

represented by the forebrain integration of both specific labeled lines and convergent somatic activity in a well-organized, hierarchical system that subserves homeostasis. In this view, pain is one aspect of the representation of the physiological condition of the body (interoception)—as distinguished from fine touch (exteroception)—and it is a homeostatic emotion, that is, both a feeling and a motivation like temperature, itch, thirst, and hunger. (Craig, 2003b, p. 4)

In this context, *homeostasis* is defined as a dynamic and ongoing process involving many integrated mechanisms that maintain an optimal balance in the physiological condition of the body for the purpose of survival. In mammals, these mechanisms include autonomic, neuroendocrine, and behavioral. A *homeostatic emotion* is defined as the human perception of the combination of a feeling and a motivation. In addition, Craig proposes the existence of a homeostatic sensory condition in the body that guides energy utilization or energy acquisition. According to Craig, homeostasis, rather than mere nociception, is the fundamental role of the small-diameter afferent fibers and the lamina I system, and is the essential nature of pain.

Small-diameter primary afferent A-delta and C-fibers are traditionally seen as nociceptive fibers transmitting information to the lamina I of the spinal cord. It is the summated activity of C-nociceptors that is associated with the conscious perception of pain in humans. However, only a portion of these fibers are characterized as nociceptors. Others carry an unprovoked and ongoing slow discharge that is not perceived. These fibers innervate nearly all of the tissues of the body and thus carry all types of information regarding the physiological condition of the body, including that which is related to mechanical, thermal, chemical, metabolic, hormonal, muscle, joint, and visceral activity.

Lamina I neurons make up a number of modality-selective classes that transmit distinct feelings from the body, such as first (sharp) pain, second (burning) pain, cool, warm, itch, sensual touch, muscle ache and cramp. Each class consists of a morphologically, physiologically, and biochemically distinct type of neuron that receives input from a specific subset of small-diameter afferents. As such, these classes are considered to be labeled lines. These labeled lines relay ongoing information relating to the external (exteroceptive) and internal (interoceptive) physiological status of the body to lamina I. By virtue of being sensitive to cytokines, opioids, steroids, hormones, and other local and circulating immune modulators, many of these small-diameter afferents have a homeostatic role similar to that of the sympathetic and parasympathetic autonomic efferents in the regulation of immune and neuroendocrine functions.

Craig distinguishes these neurons from those found in the deeper layers, especially lamina V, of the dorsal horn (wide-dynamic range [WDR] neurons), which tend to be more modality ambiguous. The integration of afferent input into the dorsal horn is marked by WDR neuron activity. The lamina I neurons then provide ongoing information to subcortical and cortical structures and not just signals relating to acute or emergency situations. Sherrington (1900) had limited the interoceptive system to that involving only the viscera. Craig, however, has extended the interoceptive system to include information regarding any and all activity concerning the internal status of the organism, including immunological, hormonal, and autonomic activity. Furthermore, these lamina I neurons have been shown to project to "major homeostatic integration sites" in the brainstem (see Figure 5.2). By virtue of the fact that these interoceptive pathways (a) reflect all aspects of the physiological condition of the body, (b) are associated with autonomic motor control, (c) are distinct from the exteroceptive system,

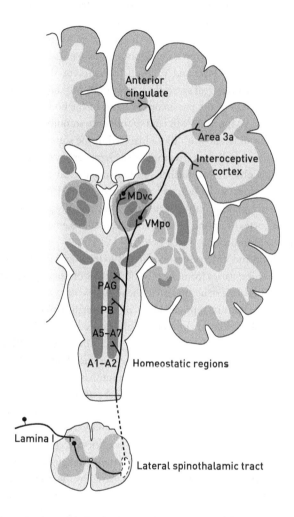

FIGURE 5.2

Summary of the projections of the lamina I system in primates. Modality-specific lamina I neurons project first to autonomic sites in the spinal cord (not shown) and to homeostatic sites in the brainstem (including the noradrenergic cell groups A1–A2 and A5–A7, the parabrachial nucleus [PB] and the periaqueductal gray matter [PAG]). In primates, lamina I neurons also project by way of the crossed lateral spinothalamic tract to two sites in the thalamus: the posterior part of the ventral medial nucleus (VMpo) and the ventral caudal part of the medial dorsal nucleus (MDvc). The VMpo provides a high-resolution, modality-specific sensory representation of the physiological condition of the body in interoceptive cortex at the dorsal margin of the insula, and it sends a corollary projection to area 3a in the sensorimotor cortex. The MDvc integrates lamina I input with brainstem homeostatic activity (from PB and PAG) and produces behavioral drive in limbic motor cortex (anterior cingulate). These generate the feeling and the motivation, respectively, that constitute the homeostatic emotion of pain. From Craig AD. A new view of pain as a homeostatic emotion. *Trends Neurosci.* 2003;26(6):303–307. Reprinted with permission.

and (d) influence somatic motor control, Craig considers them to form a cohesive homeostatic afferent system.

Sophisticated tract-tracing experiments in primates have demonstrated that lamina I neurons project to the contralateral thalamus by way of the lateral spinothalamic tract. Other studies have shown that precise lesions in these ascending pathways within the spinal cord can interrupt feelings from the body, such as pain, temperature, itch, and sensual touch. Lamina 1 neurons project to the posterior part of the ventromedial nucleus of the thalamus (VMpo), which is small in the monkey but proportionately very large in the human thalamus, and to the ventral caudal portion of the medial dorsal nucleus (MDvc). The VMpo is contiguous to the basal aspect of the ventrome-dial nucleus (VMb). The VMpo and VMb nuclei represent all homeostatic afferent flow from the body. In a very real sense, the VMpo and VMb can be viewed as forming an *internal representation* of the physiological status of the body. The small-diameter fiber pathways to the VMpo and VMb tend to influence smooth muscle activity. They develop in a fashion different from those involved in the somatosensory representa-tion of mechanical and proprioceptive input that characterizes skeletal muscle activity. Craig feels that this observation further substantiates the existence of two distinctly different representations in the human brain. Furthermore, these direct pathways to VMpo and VMb are present only in primates. Thus, the VMpo and IC (considered the interoceptive cortex) respond to virtually all sensations emerging from within the body that are related to the body's well-being.

The fact of VMpo and VMb projecting directly to the dorsal insular cortex (dIns) in a topographical fashion varies from the traditional view of nociceptive activity simply "passing through" thalamic structures on to the somatosensory cortex. The dIns would appear to contain a sensory representation of the small-diameter afferent activity that transmits the physiological condition of the entire body (primary interoceptive image of homeostatic afferents). The absence of a direct interoceptive representa-tion in subprimates implies that they cannot experience bodily feelings as humans do. Furthermore, the relative size of the thoracolumbar tracts and the development of sequential re-representation of the physiological state of the organism in the right insula cortex differ substantially from that of the monkey. Humans, therefore, pos-sess a neuroanatomical system that enhances our ability to experience the feelings we perceive, which, for Craig, ultimately makes up our self-perception, or consciousness.

Craig notes that research findings from functional imaging, lesion, and stimula-tion studies in humans confirm the critical role played by the dIns. Lamina I input to VMpo, as well as the cortical projections from VMpo and VMb to dIns, are topograph-ically organized in the anterior-to-posterior direction. The evidence also indicates that the dIns is activated in a graded fashion by pain, temperature, itch, dynamic or painful muscle sensation, sensual touch, hunger, thirst, gestation, cardiorespiratory activity, and "air hunger" (for references see Craig, 2002, 2003a,b). The dIns appears to serve as the primary sensory cortex for each of these distinct interoceptive "feelings" from the body. In addition to being activated in a graded fashion by these sensations, stimu-lation in the dIns region or VMpo and VMb can produce these sensations whereas lesions in these areas selectively disrupt such sensations.

Data provided by Craig also show that both the size and activation of the ante-rior insula cortex (AIC) are highly correlated with the subjective awareness of internal feelings. The conditions of pain asymbolia (pain is perceived but there is no sense of unpleasantness, suffering, or emotional response), amusia (disruption in one's ability to appreciate the emotional content of music), anosognosia (the lack of emotional awareness of one's self), or anergia (complete listlessness) have each been associated with damage to the insula cortex. Individual differences in the size of the AIC and the anterior cingulate cortex (ACC) have also been found to correlate with one's ability to be empathic. It is easy to forget that the structure and size of the brain, like many other aspects of the human anatomy, are highly individualized. Taken together, these findings provide evidence for a neural basis for subjective feelings. Therefore, individual differences in subjective interoceptive awareness, and thus emotional depth and complexity, may well be expressed by the size of the AIC and adjacent orbitofrontal cortices.

The limbic system includes the ACC (limbic motor cortex) and insula (limbic sensory cortex). Both of these structures are interconnected with the amygdala, hypothalamus, and orbitofrontal, and brainstem homeostatic regions. Joint activation of dorsal posterior insula (dpIns) and the ACC by the distinct homeostatic modalities seems to correspond well with the idea that the feelings from the body constitute homeostatic emotions that simultaneously generate both a sensation and a motivation. Craig concludes that activation of the ACC is associated with motivation and that of the insula with feeling; together they form an emotion. ACC activity has been directly associated with the affective-motivational component of pain (unpleasantness), suggesting that this pathway engenders the affect and motivation that renders *pain a homeostatic emotional drive*. That is, temperature, pain, itch, and muscle ache are, in fact, homeostatic emotions that drive behavior in a fashion similar to hunger and thirst. Furthermore, the condition of our bodies directly affects our feelings and our motivations on an ongoing basis. The motivational component appears to reside in the ACC. Interestingly, studies of placebo analgesia reveal coordinated activation of the ACC and rostral anterior insula (rAI), suggesting that the integration in rAI of the activity in the ACC (the behavioral agent) not only produces a representation of motivation within subjective emotional awareness but also enables motivation to directly modulate subjective feelings.

In summary, for Craig, pain is not a binary modality, either existing or not. Furthermore, the sensation of pain involves specific sensory channels (labeled lines) from lamina I and convergent pathways from lamina V. Therefore,

pain in humans is a homeostatic emotion reflecting an adverse condition in the body that requires a behavioral response. It involves a distinct sensation, engendered in interoceptive and anterior insula cortex (the feeling self), and an affective motivation, engendered in the ACC (the behavioral agent). It generates reflexive autonomic responses and motor responses that are under cortical control. (Craig, 2003a, p. 306)

Craig acknowledges that his view of pain is fundamentally different from the more conventional approaches, in a number or respects. First, it incorporates specific sensory channels or labeled lines for different kinds of pain and for pain of different tissue origins. Second, it provides a fast (sharp) pain channel that can elicit fight-or-flight behavior and a slow (burning) pain channel that can engage long-term responses, sickness behavior, and immune function. And third, the discriminative, topographic representations in the interoceptive cortex obviate the involvement of S1 in feelings from the body.

CONCLUSION

There are, of course, many other theories of pain. Most notably, there is the model outlined by Apkarian et al. (2009), which emphasizes chronic pain and the mechanism of chronification. Ray et al. (2013) suggest that the pain is akin to a holographic image, with its various components functioning like laser beams to create a particular representation. The pain image or representation is altered by modifying the intensity or nature of the laser beam(s).

Although the various theories seem able to account for experimental and clinical observations, they struggle to capture the dynamic and complex interactions among the individual's genetics and experiences and the ongoing external and internal stimulation. Craig's model of pain as a homeostatic emotion perhaps provides the closest approximation, as he describes homeostasis to be a dynamic process. Furthermore, Craig has pointed out neuroanatomical differences between primates and subprimates, as well as between primates and humans, suggesting that each experiences pain differently. Thus we the need to be cautious when making generalizations from one species to another (Lascelles and Flecknell, 2010). There can be little doubt that the concept of pain and the manner in which it is understood has evolved and must continue to do so.

In Chapter 9, we explore whether or not the fetus or neonate actually feels pain, in the ordinary sense of the word. If Melzack's neuromatrix theory is correct, then the fetus, neonate, and infant, assuming an intact central nervous system and brain, experiences pain of a type. It is not the same pain experienced by an adult, in whom the neurosignature has been modified by years of cyclical processing and synthesis. Derbyshire (1999) would appear to be correct in asserting that the pain experienced by the fetus and neonate is different from that of the adult. This begs the question regarding the definition of pain, of which there are many, as noted in Chapter 1. Indeed, a 2008 conference held in Kyoto, Japan was convened for the very purpose of examining the current notions of pain, related terminology, and definitions, confirming this as an ongoing etymological process (Loeser and Treede, 2008).

Despite being a common experience across recorded time, our understanding of pain is still in its scientific infancy. Therefore, pain-related definitions and terminology should be subjected to ongoing scrutiny. Definitions exist to facilitate communication, not to restrict it. By their very nature, theories go beyond the existing data. Strict adherence to materialism may limit progress and imagination. Indeed, in his discussion of quarks and gluons in quantum theory, Polkinghorne (2007) pointed out that there are many "unseen realities." We may be best served to view terms and their definitions as "hypothetical constructs" and not "intervening variables," à la MacCorquodale and Meehl (1948). As hypothetical constructs, terms are understood to be a shorthand way of labeling, categorizing, or expressing a phenomenon. Hypothetical constructs remain open to testing, verification, and modifications. Intervening variables, by contrast, tend to be treated as nouns representing some existing entity and, therefore, often assume facts not in evidence. As a hypothetical construct, pain might very well be viewed as a shorthand way of referring to the outcome of a highly integrated network of systems and subsystems—an emergent phenomenon. This approach has significant implications for pain treatments that will be discussed later in the book (see Chapter 14).

Apkarian AV, Baliki MH, Geha PY. Towards a theory of chronic pain. *Prog Neurobiol.* 2009;87:81–97.

Beecher H. *Measurement of Subjective Responses.* New York: Oxford University Press; 1959.

Craig AD. How do you feel? Interoception: the sense of the physiological condition of the body. *Nat Rev Neurosci.* 2002;3:655–666.

Craig AD. A new view of pain as a homeostatic emotion. *Trends Neurosci.* 2003a;26(6):303–307.

Craig AD. Pain mechanisms: labeled lines versus convergence in central processing. *Annu Rev Neurosci.* 2003b;26:1–30.

Craig AD. Interoception and emotion: a neuroanatomical perspective. In Lewis M, Haviland-Jones JM, Barrett LF, eds. *Handbook of Emotions,* 3rd ed. New York: Guilford; 2008:272–288.

Craig AD. A rat is not a monkey is not a human: comment on Mogil. *Nat Rev Neurosci.* 2009;10:466.

Derbyshire SWG. Locating the beginnings of pain. *Bioethics.* 1999;13(1):1–31.

Doleys DM, Davidson RS. Effects of pairing electric shock with reinforcement delivered on a VI schedule. *Psychol Rep.* 1976;39:483–489.

Hebb DO. Drives and the C.N.S. (conceptual nervous system). *Psychol Rev.* 1955;62:243–254.

Honore P, Rogers SD, Schwell MJ, et al. Murine models of inflammatory, neuropathic and cancer pain each generates a unique set of neurochemical changes in the spinal cord and sensory neurons. *Neuroscience.* 2000;98(3):585–598.

Jensen TS, Krebs B, Nielsen J, Rasmussen P. Phantom limb, phantom pain and stump pain in amputees during the first six months following limb amputation. *Pain.* 1983;17(3):243–256.

Jensen TS, Krebs B, Nielsen J, Rasmussen P. Immediate and long-term phantom limb pain in amputees: incidence, clinical characteristics and relationship to pre-amputation limb pain. *Pain.* 1985;21(3):267–278.

Katz J, Melzack R. Pain "memories" in phantom limbs: review and clinical observations. *Pain.* 1990;43:319–336.

Lascelles BD, Flecknell PA. Do animal models tell us about human pain? *Pain Clinical Updates.* 2010;18(5):1–6.

Leknes S, Tracey I. A common neurobiology for pain and pleasure. *Nat Rev Neurosci.* 2008;9:314–320.

Loeser JD, Treede RD. The Kyoto protocol of IASP basic pain terminology. *Pain.* 2008;137:473–477.

MacCorquodale K, Meehl PE. On the distinction between hypothetical constructs and intervening variables. *Psychol Rev.* 1948;55:95–107.

Mannion RJ, Woolf CJ. Pain mechanisms and management: a central perspective. *Clin J Pain.* 2000;16:S144–S156.

Melzack R. Phantom limbs, the self and the brain (The D.O. Hebb Memorial Lecture). *Can Psychol.* 1989;30:1–16.

Melzack R. From the gate to the neuromatrix. *Pain.* 1999;6:S121–S126.

Melzack R. Pain and the neuromatrix in the brain. *J Dent Educ.* 2001;65(12):1378–1382.

Melzack R, Casey K. Sensory, motivational and central control determinants of pain: a new conceptual model. In Kenshalo D, ed. *The Skin Senses.* Springfield, IL: Thomas; 1968:423–443.

Melzack R, Israel R, Lacroix R, Schultz G. Phantom limbs in people with congenital limb deficiency or amputation in early childhood. *Brain.* 1997;120:1603–1620.

Melzack R, Loeser JD. Phantom body pain in paraplegics: evidence for a central "pattern generating mechanism" for pain. *Pain*. 1978;4:195–210.

Melzack R, Wall P. Pain mechanisms: a new theory. *Science*. 1965;150:971–979.

Mitchell SW. *Injuries of Nerves and Their Consequences*. Philadelphia: J.P. Lippincott; 1872.

Murphy JP. Frontal lobe surgery in treatment of intractable pain: a critique. *Yale J Biol Med*. 1951;23(6):493–500.

Pavlov IP. *Conditional Reflexes*. New York: Dover; 1927.

Polkinghorne J. *Quantum Physics and Theology: An Unexpected Kinship*. New Haven: Yale University Press; 2007.

Price DD. *Psychological Mechanisms of Pain and Analgesia*. Seattle: IASP Press; 1999.

Price DD. Psychological and neural mechanisms of the affective dimension of pain. *Science*. 2000;288(5472):1769–1772.

Ray AL, Ullmann R, Francis MC. Pain as a perceptual experience. In Deer T, et al, eds. *Comprehensive Treatment of Chronic Pain by Medical, Interventional, and Integrative Approaches*. New York: Springer; 2013:745–757.

Sherrington CS. *Textbook of Physiology*. Schaffer EA, ed. Edinburgh: Pentland; 1900:920–1001.

Wall PD, McMahon SB. The relationship of perceived pain to afferent nerve impulses. *Trends Neurosci*. 1986;9(6):254–255.

Woolf CJ. Pain: moving from symptom control toward mechanism-specific pharmacologic management. *Ann Intern Med*. 2004;140:441–451.

Woolf CJ, Max, MB. Mechanism-based pain diagnosis: issues for analgesic drug development. *Anesthesiology*. 2001;95:241–249.

6 The Complexities of Measuring Pain

If only my anguish could be weighed and all my misery be placed on the scale
It would surely outweigh the sand of the seas...
My suffering is too great for words
–Job 6:1–3

INTRODUCTION

In recent years, pain has been dubbed the "fifth vital sign," along with blood pressure, heart rate, respiration, and temperature. Measuring pain, however, is fraught with difficulties. Pain is viewed by many to be a subjective experience and phenomenon without any objective signs or symptoms. This would imply that the only measure of pain is the individual's self-report. This view leaves the patient open to much scrutiny as to the reliability and validity of their report. Determination of the validity of the report would rest entirely in the hands of the person receiving the report. If a patient reporting a pain level of 8 does not look or act like what the observer might believe should be an 8, the patient might be judged to be faking, malingering, or at the very least exaggerating. Approached in this manner, the measurement of pain would be very unlike measuring other medical condition. Regardless of whether a patient appears to have a temperature or not, if the thermometer registers 102°F, no one would question the fact. If a person's blood pressure is 190/120, no one is likely to argue, despite how comfortable or relaxed the person appears, that the individual is experiencing hypertension that needs to be addressed. Unquestionably, the absence of any litmus test for determining legitimate or "real" pain poses a significant diagnostic and therapeutic dilemma.

Although pain is generally considered to be a multidimensional and multifactorial subjective experience, there are a variety of approaches to its assessment. Pain can be assessed at the micro level or at the macro level. In the research setting it is not uncommon to focus on a single dimension, such as the sensory or intensity aspects of pain (micro level) in response to an acute stimulus or a procedure (venipuncture). In the clinical and especially chronic-pain situation, the use of such a simplistic measure, albeit reflective of the individual's experience, is rejected in favor of a much more comprehensive assessment (macro level). This may include assessing the qualitative and quantitative aspects of pain, the patient's mood states and personality, the coping style, and the impact of the pain experience (disability and quality of life), using instruments such as the SF-36 (Ware et al, 1994; Ware and Sherbourne, 1992).

This chapter will review some of the more common tests and questionnaires used to assess pain. Recent and perhaps less well-known approaches such as narrative analysis and fractal analysis will also be discussed. In addition, specialized tools and approaches for assessing pain in specific and unique populations, such as cognitively impaired persons, infants, older adults, and developmentally delayed individuals, will be reviewed. The goal is to provide an illustration of the complexities encountered when measuring pain, especially chronic pain, as an experience, and to highlight the potential shortcomings of instruments and a philosophy that emphasize scientific materialism and linearity.

APPROACHES TO MEASURING PAIN

The measuring of pain has included both quantitative and qualitative approaches. The most basic quantitative approach to assessing pain is through the controlled application of mechanical, electrical, thermal, or chemical stimuli—experimentally induced pain (EIP: Edwards et al, 2005; Gracely, 1999). Through this method, inter- and intraindividual differences in pain threshold and tolerance can be established. Comparisons can be made across time or conditions. However, the relevance of EIP in the laboratory to pain experienced in the naturalistic setting, in animals compared to that humans, and in healthy individuals compared to that in the clinical population, remains questionable.

Perhaps the most common approach to assessing clinical pain is the patient's self report using a 0–10 numerical rating scale (NRS) or a visual analogue scale (VAS). A study by Myles et al. (1999) of patients with postoperative pain was able to demonstrate that the VAS had linear characteristics, at least in that setting. Although appearing very much alike, Lund and her associates (2005) reported a lack of interchangeability between visual analogue and verbal rating scales. Variations of NRS and VAS have been developed for use with children, developmentally disabled persons, and the cognitively impaired, and will be discussed later in the chapter.

For most patients, their pain level varies throughout the day, much like blood glucose or blood pressure levels. If a patient were asked to rate their pain on an hourly basis over an extended period of time, it would surely strain credulity if all the pain ratings were identical. Most commonly, chronic pain will wax and wane over time. There will be episodes of increased pain, which may be associated with some provocative stimulus or activity, or spontaneous bursts of pain. Many patients with neuropathic pain report spontaneous bursts or paroxysms of pain that can last for a few seconds to minutes.

The occurrence of a change in pain intensity over a background of chronic pain has been referred as *breakthrough pain* (BTP). There are many sources of BTP, including (a) the end of a dose of pain medication, (b) disease progression, (c) incident, (d) weather sensitivity, and (e) psychosocial factors (e.g., anger, depression, anxiety, conflict), to name a few. *Incident pain* can be conveniently divided into volitional and non-volitional. Svendsen et al (2005) describe these various kinds of pain as "stimulus-dependent" types of BTP. *Volitional* episodes are further divided into pain evoked by normally nonpainful stimuli (allodynia), such as walking, standing, mechanical pressure, moderate cold or heat, and increased pain response to normally painful events (hyperalgesia). *Non-volitional* BTP includes bladder or bowel distention, diurnal patterns, and hormone-related changes. In addition, the pattern of BTP may be anti-persistent or persistent (Foss et al, 2006). In an *anti-persistent* pattern, the occurrence of high-intensity BTP is followed by one of lower intensity, suggesting the activation of some type of physiological or psychological coping mechanism. By contrast, in the *persistent* pattern, high-intensity BTP is often followed by episodes of similar intensity, thus appearing more recalcitrant and self-perpetuating.

Psychologists have led the effort in evaluating patients' overt (observable) and covert (mental) behaviors. This type of semiological (from the Geek word *sēmeiōtikosics*, meaning "observant of signs") research was launched by Wilbert E. Fordyce's 1976 book, *Behavioral Methods for Chronic Pain and Illness*, which details the role of psychological factors, particularly those related to conditioning and learning theories. Several scales and questionnaires have been developed to measure behaviors thought to be associated with the experience of pain, such as posturing, bracing, grimacing, limping. Theoretically, these pain behaviors are seen as fairly natural in the presence of some type of injury and may have some protective utility. Other pain behaviors are designed to communicate one's pain to others. In the context of behavioral theory, however, there is evidence that if these pain behaviors lead to rewarding consequences, such as positive or negative reinforcement, they may well persist even when the injury that precipitated them has resolved. It is important to interpret these behaviors in the context of the patient's culture.

These pain behaviors are thus considered to be "nonorganic" signs. Such nonorganic signs are behaviors that no longer relate to any underlying physical pathology and thus are more psychological in nature. Pain behaviors are usually assessed by observers tabulating their individual frequency over a given period of time and in different situations, using scales such as the UAB Rating Scale, devolved by Richards and colleagues (1982), or the Pain Behavior Scale, by Keefe and Block (1982). A reduction in the frequency of these pain behaviors is a common goal of behavioral-based therapies and assumed to represent observable evidence of pain relief.

The McGill Pain Questionnaire (MPQ) (Melzack, 1975) is one of the most common of the qualitative approaches. The MPQ is used to detail the characteristics of the pain experience. Approximately 80 different words are grouped into 10 categories representing the "sensory" component of pain, and the other 10 categories the "non-sensory," or what is referred to as evaluative and affective, components of pain. Descriptors in the sensory category include "sharp," "shooting," and "aching." Those in the non-sensory categories include terms such as "aggravating," "agonizing," "exhausting," "cruel," and "wretched." The MPQ may, in fact, be one of the most frequently used instruments in clinical and research settings. It obviously requires a certain level of comprehension and understanding on the part of the patient. Assuming a thoughtful and deliberate patient, the MPQ has been shown to be able to differentiate among different painful conditions, such as arthritis, nerve-related pain, and musculoskeletal pain, and is useful in evaluating the outcomes of pain therapies.

The Brief Pain Inventory (BPI) (Cleeland, 1991; Daunt et al, 1983) was originally designed for use with patients having cancer pain, but it has been modified for assessing pain related to multiple other disorders, including spinal cord injury, amputation, diabetic peripheral neuropathy, cerebral palsy, and low back or non-cancer pain. The 1991 version of the BPI, developed by Cleeland, contained a mannequin on which the patient could indicate the areas of pain. Patients were asked to rate their "current pain, lowest, highest, and worst" pain over the last 24 hours and their pain "right now" on a 0 (no pain) to 10 (pain as bad as you can imagine) scale. They were also asked to report the degree of pain relief provided by medications in the last 24 hours on a 0–100% scale. The BPI, was then used to assess the degree to which the pain interfered with mood, relations with others, walking ability, general activity, normal work (including both work activity outside the home and housework), sleep, and enjoyment of life.

On the BPI and other similar instruments, numerical pain rating scores of 1–3(4)/10 have come to represent mild pain, 4–6/10 moderate pain, and 7–10/10 severe pain. This grouping also holds for the levels of "pain interference." That is, those patients in the severe range of pain report substantially more pain interference than those reporting moderate pain. In fact, there appears to be little variation among patients within a group. For example, the level of pain interference is very similar for patients reporting pain at the 7, 8, or 9 levels. Therefore, from a therapeutic perspective, shifting from one category to the next, for example, from severe to moderate, may be more clinically meaningful than a reduction in NRS within the same group, even if the latter is statistically significant. This observation appears to be supported by studies indicating a minimum of a 2- to 3-point change in NRS or an estimated 30% improvement by the patient for the outcome of a treatment to be considered "minimally" effective clinically (Farrar et al, 2001).

Von Korff and Dunn (2008) have taken a "prospective" vs. a "duration-based" approach to assessing and defining chronic pain. They state, "Chronic pain should be viewed as a condition whose future implications are uncertain and mutable, rather than as a fixed trait identifying patients with intractable pain" (p. 274). Thus they assess chronic pain in the context of the probability of the pain persisting in the future, by means of a risk score, which can be used to predict the probability of clinically significant pain continuing. Questions relating to pain intensity (average, worse, and current), pain interference (with usual activities, work or household activities, family and social activities), depression, number of pain sites, and number of days with the index (primary) pain in the previous 6 months are presented. Numerical values are assigned to response choices. When added together, a risk score ranging from 0 to 28 can be obtained.

Patients with headache, low back pain (LBP), and orofacial pain patients were studied by Von Korff and Dunn (2008) The cutoff scores for predicting continued chronicity with 50% accuracy ranged from 12 to 16, and for 80% accuracy from 20 to 25. Furthermore, the cutoff scores differed for the three groups of patients. The authors also concluded that chronic pain exists on a continuum, rather than constituting a distinct class of patients.

The manner in which a patient reacts to an injury or disease can influence the overall experience of pain. A number of questionnaires have emerged to evaluate a patient's coping strategies. The Coping Strategies Questionnaire (CSQ; Rosenstiel and Keefe, 1983) evaluates the use of coping strategies such as distraction, activity avoidance, seeking assistance, and praying. Some coping strategies have been deemed more adaptive than others, as they tend to be associated with higher levels of functioning and enhanced quality of life. Excessive and unnecessary worry can result in an unhealthy preoccupation with one's condition and symptoms leading to activity avoidance and social isolation. whereas distraction thorough physical and social activity can divert one's attention away from the pain. Patients' whose coping style is characterized by a general sense of optimism, or dispositional optimism (Scheier et al, 1994), tend to cope more effectively than those who are more pessimistic (Nes and Segerstom, 2006).

Sullivan et al (1995, 1998, 2001) have developed a questionnaire to assess the tendency of patients to catastrophize. Catastrophizers are often described as being hysterical in their reaction. Such statements as "I can't get it off my mind," "it will never get any better," and "I can't live like this," especially when accompanied by intense displays of emotion such as sobbing or crying that can almost be interpreted as self-induced, have been shown to be correlated with intensification of the experience of pain. Cognitive behavioral therapy (CBT) is designed to help the patient recognize the maladaptive and harmful nature of their catastrophic thinking and replace it with more appropriate statements. Imaging from successfully treated patients has demonstrated alterations in the activity of the brain's pain matrix (Ritchy et al, 2011).

A somewhat more recent area in the measurement of pain is that of acceptance. McCracken et al (2003, 2004) have defined *acceptance* as a realistic appraisal of pain and its consequences, as opposed to giving in or catastrophizing. Two main characteristics of the acceptance questionnaire include activity engagement and the willingness to disengage from attempts to control the situation. In the first instance, patients are evaluated on the degree to which they are willing to engage in activities that, although uncomfortable, do not pose any risk of harm or injury. The willingness to disengage from controlling the pain is highlighted by accepting that the pain will persist to one degree or another indefinitely. The patient "accepts" the pain, much like they would diabetes, and makes the decision to get on with life rather than devoting a disproportionate amount of physical, emotional, and financial resources in search for a cure. A companion concept is that of readiness to change (Kerns and Habib, 2004), which has grown out of the addiction literature and assesses how prepared and committed the patient is to making a change in his or her behavior.

MEDICAL TESTS

Various types of medical tests continue to be used in the assessment of pain. The use of imaging technology (CT scan, X-ray or MRI), electromyographic and nerve conduction studies, and discography are common. Discography involves the injection of a radiopaque dye into one or more intervertebral discs in an effort to determine disc morphology or damage to the annulus. Annular tears can be associated with the extravasation of chemicals potentially producing an inflammatory reaction and a neuropathic type pain. Although such tests are important for determining the existence of a structural abnormality which, if left uncorrected, might cause further harm to the patient, it is a mistake to assume a one-to-one correspondence between the type and degree of physical pathology and pain. Indeed, abnormal MRI findings of the lumbar spine are not uncommon among individuals asymptomatic for low back pain (Jensen et al, 1994).

Interpretation of the relationship between a structural abnormality and pain can be very complex, particularly in the setting of chronic pain. If pain is a product of a complicated interaction of different aspects of brain functioning, including sensory, affective, and evaluative aspects, it becomes important to differentiate between a nociceptive generator and a pain generator. A physical anomaly may or may not trigger the activation of a peripheral nociceptor. Depending on a multitude of variables, the sensory input may or may not be experienced as painful; that is, pain and physical damage are not the same thing.

A thoughtful and deliberate medical examination is a necessary component in the evaluation of a patient with pain, particularly following some type of injury or significant change in the location and type of pain. But caution must be exercised when interpreting the outcome. Unfortunately, the removal or destruction of an abnormal appearing structure is not always associated with long-term pain relief. The nociceptive generator represents the structure or stimuli causing activation of the nociceptive system. If there is a pain generator, it is likely to be the brain (see Chapters 4 and 7).

PSYCHOLOGICAL FACTORS

The role of psychological factors, including mood states and personality, in the patient's experience of pain is well established. In some instances, such as a genetically based depression, these factors will predate the pain and may affect its severity. In other cases, psychological issues will emerge in response to the pain. These mood and personality variables, as well as the patient's readiness for change (Kerns and Habib, 2004), can significantly impact the outcome of treatment.

The clinical interview is an indispensable source of information and gives the patient an opportunity to "tell his or her story" (see Narrative section later in this chapter). Information regarding the patient's fears, expectations, and perceptions can be obtained. Most important is the patient's concept of the cause(s) of the pain and what might be required for the situation to improve. Some people are so discouraged that they have become psychologically immobilized and display symptoms of demoralization characteristic of learned helplessness. The sense of being burdensome to others has been strongly associated with suicidal thoughts. The involvement of a significant other in the evaluation can yield another perspective and provide insight to the impact of the pain on the family as a whole (Monroe, 2003).

A variety of psychological tests are available to aid in assessment. Mood states such as depression and anxiety can be assessed using the Beck Depression Inventory (Beck et al, 1961) and the State-Trait Anxiety Inventory (STAI; Spielberger, 1970; van Knippenberg et al, 1990). Overall psychological functioning and personality style is commonly measured using the Minnesota Multiphasic Personality Inventory (MMPI: Keller and Butcher, 1991), Symptom Checklist 90-Revised (SCL 90-R; Derogotis, 1977), or Millon Behavioral Health Inventory, third edition (MBHI) (Labbe et al, 1989; Millon et al., 1982, 2006). Validated instruments should be used and results interpreted in the context of the patient interview. It is useful to obtain as comprehensive a picture as possible of the individual in pain, to facilitate an understanding of the various psychological components that may be contributing to the pain experience and develop a meaningful therapeutic algorithm (see Doleys and Doherty, 2003, for a more detailed discussion of specific instruments).

Evaluation of patients with cancer-related pain is somewhat more complex (Ahles et al, 1983; Turk and Fernendez, 1990; Turk et al, 2002; Zaza and Baine, 2002). The diagnosis of cancer and its associated pain can give rise to a variety of emotional reactions and fears. Among these are the fear of loss of bodily functions, disfigurement, loss of autonomy and independence, abandonment and isolation, becoming a burden, and financial impact. Few concerns generate more distress than the fear of uncontrolled pain and other related end-of-life issues. Caregiver reactions may inflame or moderate those of the patient. Patients may become very somatically vigilant in "searching" for any physical symptom, such as pain, that might herald the return of a previously eradicated cancer. Cancer-related pain is often interpreted as a sign of disease progression or part of the fatal consequences of the disease.

Pain is seen as inevitable and thus is frequently an undertreated aspect of cancer therapy (Kane et al, 1985). It also can vary with the context: Despite the presence of a physical abnormality, some women with metastatic breast cancer experience pain only after being informed of their diagnosis (Spiegel and Bloom, 1982). This emphasizes the importance of the meaning of the pain. In one study, an estimated 38% of women with breast cancer developed a comorbid psychological disorder after the diagnosis of cancer was made or at the time of a reoccurrence (Derogotis et al, 1983).

The rapid changing status of the disease and the impact of various treatments can affect the patient's emotional status and adjustment on an almost day-to-day basis (Massie and Holland, 1992). For this reason there are advantages to taking a *state-related* approach rather than the *trait-related* approach customarily used with non-cancer pain. A state-related approach emphasizes assessment of the psychological variables that tend to be sensitive to situational changes, including fear, anxiety, depressed mood, and acceptance (Doleys, 2011).

Depressed mood is often a natural reaction (Endicott, 1984; Kelsey et al, 1995) but needs to be distinguished from a pre-existing depressive illness, which may be exacerbated by the cancer and related pain. Some of the more distinctive features of depression in cancer patients include social withdrawal, failure to response to good news or humorous situations, persistent tearfulness, feeling like a burden to others, recalcitrance to pain-relieving therapies, and tendency to perceive the cancer as a personal punishment. Cancer pain has even been known to reactivate prior emotional trauma. Severe forms of depression can influence the patient's motivation and compliance and stimulate death wishes, suicidal behavior, and even the desire for euthanasia (Monroe, 2003).

Anxiety and stress can lower the pain threshold and interfere with patients' willingness to disclose their symptoms (Keogh and Cochran, 2002; Miller and Massie, 2006). They may harbor the fear that their reported pain will be interpreted as psychological. They may also hesitate to fully disclose their post-treatment residual pain, for fear of disappointing their physician. These and other fears are more common among older adults and less educated patients, as well as those of lower socioeconomic status. Anxiety may become generalized or take on the form of a phobic disorder, panic attack, or posttraumatic stress disorder (Gold et al, 2005). Some individuals will demonstrate a fear of even feeling the often innocuous physical manifestations of anxiety, as they tend to misinterpret these as threatening or as indicative of disease progression.

Anxiety tends to peak at specific points during the disease process, including at initial diagnosis and initiation of cancer treatment, and with cancer recurrence, failure of treatment, and perception of dying. The Hospital Anxiety and Depression Scales (HADS; Moorey et al, 1991), STAI (Spielberger, 1970), and Hamilton Rating Scale for Anxiety (Hamilton, 1959) are commonly used in this setting.

SPECIAL POPULATIONS

Pain in neonates and infants is a complex issue (see Chapter 9). Likewise, the measurement of pain in neonates, infants, and children requires some special consideration. By virtue of existing emotional, intellectual, and communicative barriers, measurement of pain in developmentally delayed individuals poses similar challenges. For the patient it may be like trying to communicate one's pain and suffering to someone who is blind, deaf, and unable to speak or comprehend their language.

Darwin (1872/2007) reported specific eye and mouth movements and positions in attempting to describe facial expressions of a person in pain. These facial features include a closely compressed mouth, lips retracted with the teeth clenched or ground together, eyes staring wildly "as in horrified astonishment," and heavily contracted eye brows (Schiavenato et al, 2008).

de Williams (2002) has reviewed the evidence for specific facial expressions of pain from infancy to old age and proposed that human expression of pain arises from evolved propensities. Facial expressions of pain, or at least the underlying propensities, appear to be hard-wired, although modifiable through learning. Indeed, she has suggested that such facial expressions are consistent across different types of stimulation, sex, and ethnicity.

Neonates, Infants, and Children

A number of ingenious scales have been developed that are amenable to use in special populations of patients. In general, behavioral rating scales and observations are recommended for measuring pain in neonates, infants, children under age 4 years, and the developmentally delayed. Observational scales reflect the occurrence, frequency, and magnitude of behaviors such as crying, reflex withdrawal, and facial grimacing and associated physiological responses, for example, heart rate. One example is the COMFORT-Behavior (COMFORT-B) scale, developed by Carnevale and Razack (2002), which notes the presence of grimacing, crying, body movements, and muscle tension. It has been validated in the pediatric intensive care setting and found to be applicable to children with Down syndrome (Valkenburg et al, 2011).

Hummel and Van Dijk (2006) reviewed some 16 scales designed for use with neonates and infants. Commonly assessed behaviors included facial action, body movement and tone, cry, sleep, and consolability. Some also examined presumed physiological indicators of pain, such as increased heart rate, respiratory rate, blood pressure, decreased heart rate variability, and oxygen desaturation. Others were more oriented toward assessing procedural pain, such as venipuncture (Benini et al, 2004), or postoperative pain, such as the Neonatal Infant Pain Scale (NIPS), designed for premature newborns during painful procedures. The Faces, Legs, Activity, Cry,

Consolability (FLACC) pain assessment tool can be used in preverbal children aged between 2 months and 7 years who cannot report pain, to assess postsurgical pain.

Pain in infants as young as 27 weeks can be assessed using the Premature Infant Pain Profile (PIPP), developed by Stevens and colleagues (Ballantyne et al, 1999; Stevens et al, 1996). The PIPP was validated to measure pain during invasive care in premature newborns and takes into account the newborn's age when comparing behaviors before and after painful stimulation. Physiological responses, including heart rate and oxygen saturation, along with behavioral observations of brow bulge, eye squeeze, and nasolabial furrow, are used. Observations over a 30-second interval after an event are scored, tabulated, and compared to a 15-second baseline. Different pain management strategies are recommended on the basis of the total score.

Although potentially useful, such physiological measures rely heavily on unconscious reflexes, which may or may not reliably correlate with the sensory processing activity in the brain. For example, skin conductance activity does not reliably discriminate between painful and nonpainful stimulation (Harrison et al, 2006; Hellerud and Storm, 2002). Therefore, Fabrizi et al (2011) expanded the assessment of infant pain by combining analysis of the electrical activity in skeletal muscles via electromyography (EMG) and electroencephalography (EEG) to detect activity in the areas of the brain where unpleasant sensations are processed with behavioral observations. They recorded a distinctive response pattern when comparing non-noxious touch with noxious heel-lance.

Perhaps one of the most recognizable tools is the FACS (Facial Action Coding System; Ekman and Friesen, 1978) scale. It is composed of nine different faces, each with a separate expression, ranging from jubilation to neutral to tearfully horrific. For more impaired or younger individuals there is the Modified FACS scale, which has four faces that are larger and more exaggerated. Rather than selecting a number representing the pain, the child selects a representative facial expression.

The Cube Test makes use of four wood cubes ranging in size from 1 to 5 centimeters. The larger the cube selected, the greater the pain.

In the Eland Color Scale, the child uses different colors drawn on a mannequin to depict the location and severity of the pain. The Modified Eland scale uses colored cubes and a larger mannequin.

The FACS or color-analogue scales are recommended for children ages 3 to 8 years. Children aged 8 years or older can effectively use a VAS or NRS.

Older Adults

Measurement of pain in older adults is beset with its own unique problems (Upshur and Wootton, 2003), not the least of which is the tendency of the patient to view pain as a normal part of aging. Even in the midst of advanced treatment for pain, older adults are often hesitant to speak up. The reasons are many and varied. Some fear being labeled as a bad patient. Far too many already anticipate being "placed in a facility" if they become burdensome to their family or caregivers. Pain is often seen as a major sign of the beginning of the loss of independence. The unfounded fear of addiction to pain medicine and that such medicine should be saved for "the end" is a testimony to these individuals' lifelong self-reliance. Many interpret pain as a sign of a serious illness. They develop anxiety and dread over the prospect of undergoing medical tests and the cost of such tests.

Changes in cortical structure and functioning as a result of aging, illness, or compromised health can have an impact on how incoming information is perceived and expressed. Indeed, Buckalew et al (2010) reported the presence of altered brain structure and function in a group of elderly pain patients with a history of disabling low back pain compared to that of individuals with non-disabling low back pain. Benedetti and his colleagues (2006) and Cole et al (2011) have demonstrated diminished response to opioids and increased connectivity resulting in enhanced activity in parts of the pain matrix in patients with cognitive dysfunction secondary to Alzheimer's disease. Diminished cognitive capacity can make the describing of pain frustrating for the patient and practitioner alike. In feeling despair and desperation, the elderly patient's situation becomes complicated by a sense of learned helplessness and depression.

Altered central processing, pain perception, and expression of pain, and fear or other affective responses may plague older adults who have compromised cognitive functioning. Thus, often it is important to assess their level of cognitive impairment. Performing a standard Mental Status Exam (Haddox and Kerner, 2013) may suffice. More comprehensive evaluations might include the Wechsler Intelligence Scale, Trail Making Tests A and B, or a full neuropsychological battery, although these can be rather expensive and are rarely necessary.

Patients with Brain Damage or Coma

For patients who have suffered head injuries, concussions, or brain insults, especially those associated with loss of consciousness, a comprehensive neuropsychological evaluation is appropriate. All too often the presence of a normal brain MRI is taken as evidence of the absence of any damage. As the brain is suspended in fluid, the forces exerted by blasts, auto accidents, or whiplash-type motion can have a sheering effect on neuronal structures. This can affect cognitive, behavioral, and emotional function but go undetected by standard brain MRI.

The use of a one-dimensional assessment, for example, an NRS, or assessment of coping skills, acceptance, catastrophizing, or pain-related disability. in patients with a traumatic brain injury (TBI) is generally inadequate. Even multidimensional approaches exploring the affective and sensory components of pain fall short. Such cases require an understanding of the impact of the TBI on the patient's behavioral, psychological, and cognitive functioning. Some will demonstrate a good deal of poor judgment and impulse control, leaving them to appear noncompliant, a feature of frontal lobe syndrome. Altered recall, short-term memory, and comprehension will compromise learning efficiency.

Severely brain-damaged and noncommunicative patients are challenging to assess regarding pain. Patients in a persistent (at least 3 months) or permanent (lasting 1 year or longer) vegetative state (VS) give no evidence of any conscious awareness of themselves or their environment. They do not respond to sensory stimuli, nor is there any suggestion of volition or conscious purpose. Evidence of language comprehension or meaningful expression is lacking. Behaviors such as inappropriate smiling, crying, or grimacing occur occasionally, but do not appear to be voluntary or goal directed.

Those in a minimally conscious state (MCS) demonstrate inconsistent signs of consciousness, such as responding to a verbal order, localization to noxious stimuli, and automatic movements (e.g., scratching); environmentally contingent emotional responses; object localization and manipulation; sustained visual fixation and pursuit; verbalizations; and intentional but unreliable communication. Although inconsistent, such signs are reproducible during examination. Neuroimaging and EEG studies have suggested the maintenance of functional connectivity among various cortical and sub-cortical networks, especially the default mode network (DMN, see Chapter 4), in MCS patients, thus the experience of pain is a possibility (Baars et al, 2003; Laureys and Schiff, 2012; Owen et al, 2006).

The Nociceptive Coma Scale (NCS) was developed by Schnakers and colleagues (2010) for patients emerging from coma and was validated on VS and MCS patients. Motor, verbal, and visual responses as well as facial expression are recorded in response to painful stimulation. The NCS proved capable of assessing nociception but also response to analgesics.

Schnakers et al. reviewed a number of other scales as well. The DOLOPLUS2, Pain Assessment Checklist for Seniors with Limited Ability to Communicate (PACSLAC), Echelle Comportementale pour Personnes Agées (ECPA), and the Pain Assessment in Advanced Dementia scale (PAINAD) demonstrated higher psychometric qualities. The COMFORT scale, the Behavioral Pain Scale (BPS), and a DOLOUSI have been used with sedated and intubated patients. The DOLOUSI measures mechanical ventilation, facial expression, tears, and motoricity.

Assessment and interpretation of pain in the noncommunicative population has raised many questions regarding the nature of consciousness and its role in pain (see Chapter 13). The degree to which these measures represent an adequate proxy for both the sensory and affective awareness thought to be necessary for the experience of pain continues to be investigated.

NARRATIVES

Analysis of a patient's narrative as a qualitative approach to measuring pain is receiving greater attention (Carr et al, 2005). Narratives written or told can provide information unique to a given patient. Narratives are viewed as a type of "script" that records the particular goals, beliefs, and activities that occur at a specific time and place. Patients often find it difficult to describe their pain other than through analogies, for example "It is like a knife in my back" or "It feels like hot icy water running down my leg." Sometimes, they will admit that their descriptions do not makes sense. even to them: "It is like it's numb and painful at the same time." Patients often have "a story" which they deem very relevant and important but which frequently goes unheard or ignored because of the tendency of clinicians to use objective tests or structured questionnaires. Patients may claim that "no one is listening to me." With narrative analysis of pain patients can communicate their problems, symptoms, conditions, and diseases in many diverse fashions.

Narratives offer a means of understanding the essential qualities and complexities of the patient's pain experience, including inner hurt, despair, grief, and moral pain, that frequently accompany and may even constitute the person's illness (Greenhalgh and Hurwitz, 1999). Narratives can provide the clinician with the meaning of pain to the patient and a contextual perspective. *Narrative competence* (NC) is a set of skills required to recognize, absorb, interpret, and be moved by the story one hears. NC gives the clinician the ability to understand not only the patient but also the disease itself.

There are myriad reasons to study narratives. Within the diagnostic encounter, narratives are the phenomenal form in which patients experience poor health. They can be a means of encouraging empathy and promoting understanding between the clinician and patient, and they enable the construction of meaning and provide analytic clues. From a therapeutic perspective, the use of narratives encourages a more holistic approach to pain management. They may possess some therapeutic or palliative value in and of themselves, not unlike a patient interacting with a psychologist.

Narratives have been found to aid in determining therapeutic options. Learning what a patient really believes about a specific therapy is not insignificant. One might be disinclined to pursue a treatment knowing the patient has no confidence or faith in it or, worse, anticipates negative consequences. In the realm of education, narratives are often memorable, grounded in experiences, and encourage reflection.

Finally, narratives can serve as a catalyst for new ways of conceptualizing a problem and challenging conventional wisdom. For example, Melzack's neuromatrix theory appears to have grown out of listening to the narratives of patients with phantom limb pain, especially those in whom the limb was congenitally absent.

Björkman et al (2008) investigated the experience of female patients following mastectomy for breast cancer who were reporting phantom breast(s) sensation or pain. A semi-structured interview with open-ended questions allowing the patients to elaborate on their response was used. For example, rather than asking, "Do you feel any burning pain in your phantom breast?" they were asked, "Tell me how your phantom breast feels to you?" The eight women interviewed tended to have a difficult time describing and spatially positioning the phantom breast(s). The experience of a phantom breast differed from that of a phantom extremity. The phantom breast did not appear to cause much distress. Finally, the phantom would appear, disappear, and reappear over time.

A study by Cedraschi et al (2012) examined the narratives of women with fibromyalgia and compared them to those of women with LBP. The women with fibromyalgia highlighted issues related to medical and social legitimacy and significant psychological factors associated with symptom onset, and they tended to dramatize their feelings of loss of control. By contrast, those with LBP emphasized issues of wear and tear, noting that the body "wore out" but was still a potentially reparable machine.

Pennebaker and Seagal (1999) evaluated the potential health benefits of narrative writing. A group of patients spent 15 minutes a day on four consecutive days writing about their situation without stopping or giving any regard to spelling, grammar, or sentence structure. The narratives were analyzed for the number of (a) emotional categories (positive vs. negative words) and (b) cognitive categories, that is, causal expressions (e.g., "because," "reason") vs. insight (e.g., "understand," "realize"). The results of this and similar studies showed that those patients using many positive words and only a moderate amount of negative words had the greatest health improvements. Immune system activity increased, including T-cell activity and antibody response to Epstein-Barr virus and hepatitis B vaccinations. Hostile and suspicious patients writing about someone else's trauma as though the writer had experienced it had similar benefits to those writing about their own trauma. Reduced pain, fewer physician visits, and decreased medication use were noted.

Several mechanisms have been proposed to explain these benefits: (1) individuals become more health conscious and change their behaviors accordingly; (2) writing allows for self-expression; and (3) emotions and images are converted into words, changing the way a person organizes and thinks about the trauma; the integration of thoughts and feelings provides a more coherent narrative of the experience. Indeed, through the use of neuroimaging techniques, Gallagher and Frith (2003) and Northoff and colleagues (2006) have begun to unravel changes at the cortical level that occur in response to such self-reflection.

NONLINEARITY AND PAIN

Is pain of intensity 6/10 twice as great as 3/10? Is pain rated 4/10 only half as severe as that of 8/10? Is an acute pain of 7/10 the same as a 7/10 chronic pain? Is pain provoked by a 4-volt stimulus exactly twice as severe as that from 2 volts? Is a nociceptive pain of 7/10 the same as a neuropathic pain of 7/10? Do all patients with a pain level of 8/10 have the same level of functioning? Is a pain rating of 6/10 accompanied by depression the same as pain rated 6/10 without depression? These are very transparent, yet important, questions. Hardly anyone would answer the above in the affirmative. It seems intuitive that pain is a *nonlinear* phenomenon, though it may be more parsimonious to think of it as linear.

The concept of linearity relates to the study of linear systems that are described as "well-behaved:" The magnitude of the response is proportionate to the strength of the stimulus (proportionality). Linear systems can be fully understood and predicted by dissecting out the components (reductionism)—the subunits of a linear system add up; the whole is equal to the sum of its parts.

Nonlinear dynamics is the study of systems that respond disproportionately. Nonlinear systems have the appearance of randomness (chaos). Furthermore, the components of nonlinear systems interact in complex fashions. Plotting data points over time does not yield a predictable sinusoidal pattern. Erratic variations give the appearance of randomness. Because of this, reductionistic analysis (i.e., attempts to find the least common denominator, as it were) often fails.

Loggia et al (2012) illustrated the coexistence of linear and nonlinear brain response patterns to deep tissue pain in non-pain subjects. Using classical psychophysiological methodology, cuff-pressure algometry, and fMRI, the authors were able to identify three types of cortical response patterns: (a) constant (uniform response to the presence of pain independent of it intensity), (b) linear (response pattern demonstrating a linear relationship with pain intensity), and (c) quadratic (response pattern characterized by a quadratic or U-shaped relationship). The constant pattern was characterized by bilateral activation in anterior insula/frontal operculum and medial frontal gyrus, a contralateral activation pattern in posterior insula and dorsolateral prefrontal cortex, and a deactivation pattern in a widespread network of structures including core areas of the bilateral DMN. Linear patterns included contralateral activation of the postcentral, precentral, and medial frontal gyri, and deactivation patterns in temporal and occipital cortices were noted. Bilateral quadratic patterns were seen in dorsal and medial prefrontal cortices and hypothalamus and left nucleus accumbens, among other regions. These data highlight the enormous complexity of the cortical response to nociception, involving broadly distributed networks rather than a fixed group of cortical structures responding in a deterministic fashion (Schriff et al, 1994; Tsuda, 2001).

Chaos theory describes systems that appear disordered, displaying a random type of variability but manifesting an underlying order (Gleck, 2008). *Nonlinear chaos* defines a constrained kind of randomness, which may be associated with fractal geometry. *Fractals* consist of geometric fragments of varying size and orientation but similar in shape. All fractals have an internal, look-alike property or self-similarity. In nature, for example, complicated structures such as branching trees, clouds, and irregular coast lines reveal fractals. That is, the shape or design of a part of the whole mimics the whole. If one examines arterial or venous trees, the secondary branches show self-similarity (are geometrically similar) to the primary branch. This can also be seen in the dendritic branches of neurons. Nonlinearity, chaos theory, and fractal analysis have been applied to the study of human physiology for decades (Goldberger, 1996; Goldberger et al, 1990; Huokuri et al, 2000) but only recently to the study of pain (Foss et al, 2006; Martinez-Lavin et al, 2008).

The concept of fractal geometry can be applied to examining complex times series wherein there is no standard length of time (a common denominator). The times series within which an event or events occur seem random. Thus, instead of looking at fractal objects one is looking at fractal time-series. Both fractal objects and fractal time-series can be characterized by their fractal dimension. One such example of a fractal time-series might be the occurrence of spontaneous pain in postherpetic neuralgia (PHN) (Foss et al, 2006). These episodes are often described by patients as variable and unpredictable in intensity and frequency. PHN may be an example of an intrinsically chaotic system. A system is considered intrinsically chaotic if much fluctuation is found even in the absence of any fluctuating external stimuli, rather than the system relaxing to a homeostatic or steady state.

Foss, Apkarian, and Chialvo (2006) conducted an experiment using a group of LBP patients, PHN patients, and normal adults without pain to examine the fractal dimension of spontaneous pain. In one phase of the study, all subjects were asked to rate their ongoing pain for 6 to 12 minutes. One subgroup of normal subjects was asked to imagine having LBP and rate its fluctuations. Another subgroup of normal subjects and LBP patients rated the intensity of various thermal stimuli, some quite intense, presented in a random fashion. The authors used a power spectrum analysis and rescaled range analysis to determine the fractal dimension. (The interested reader is referred to the original article.)

A graphic display of the ongoing numerical pain ratings for the two pain groups showed them to be much more erratic with multiple noncyclical fluctuations, that is, they appeared noisier than that of the imagined or thermal-stimulation group of normal individuals (see Figure 6.1). Upon examining a segment of the pain ratings, for example, from seconds 550 to 650 of the ongoing pain rating period, at different levels of magnification, self-similarity was noted. This pattern was not identified in the normal group. Statistical self-similarity was noted within a given patient. A subgroup of LBP patients also underwent brain scanning with fMRI. The medial prefrontal cortex and cingulate at the level of genu, which have been shown to be activated by spontaneous pain, correlated with the pain rating fractal dimension, whereas activity in the temporal brain regions did not.

This study makes several points. First, the temporal properties of spontaneous pain in LBP and PHN patients are different and nonlinear, and can be described in terms of their fractal dimension. Second, these conditions cannot be approximated by non-pain subjects imagining the pain or by use of random noxious thermal stimulation with

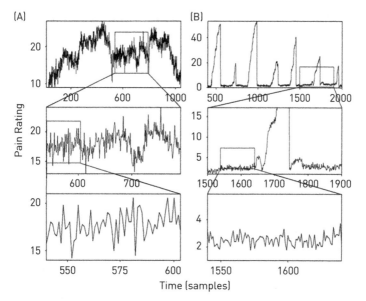

FIGURE 6.1

Properties of fractal pain ratings. (A) Statistical self-similarity of a fractal pain rating. A back pain patient's pain rating as a function of time in samples (1 sample = 400 ms) is shown at three different scales. The general time variability pattern is self-similar at all three magnifications. The boxes on each plot indicate the ranges in the plot below. (B) Pain rating from thermal stimulation. Magnifying a rating that is minimally fractal fails to show self-similarity. Note that vertical range is extremely dependent on exact horizontal location. From Foss JM, Apkarian AV, Chialvo DR. Dynamics of pain: fractal dimension of temporal variability of spontaneous pain differentiates between pain states. *J Neurophysiol.* 2006;95:733. Reprinted with permission.

non-pain subjects. Third, patients with LBP showed an anti-persistent pattern of fluctuating pain in which more intense pain was followed by less intense pain. Patients with PHN, however, showed both anti-persistent and persistent time series patterns. The anti-persistent and persistent patterns may reflect activation of the descending inhibitory system or facilitatory pathways. The presence of the persistent pattern suggests a relatively reduced ability to control spontaneous pain. And fourth, fluctuations in pain are likely to be a product of a complex interaction of the peripheral and central nervous systems.

Harnessing the ability to determine fractal time series and dimensions could be useful in identifying malingerers and in determining therapeutic algorithms and treatment efficacy. These data also raise the question of the relevance of studying pain responses in non-pain subjects to clinical pain conditions and the potential disconnect between experimentally induced pain and clinical pain.

SYSTEMS APPROACH

Chapman, Tuckett, and Song (2008) have illustrated a systems approach to evaluating and understanding pain (also see Chapter 8). They describe a "pain and stress supersystem" model which highlights the interaction among the nervous, endocrine, and immune systems. Nested within the supersystem are many subsystems, such as the immune-nervous, immune-endocrine, and endocrine-nervous systems. Furthermore, each individual system operates in accordance with its own set of "programmed" responses. The supersystem and subsystems function to regulate the adaptive actions to any perturbation (complex adaptive system). Some aspects of the systems are sensitive to even the slightest changes, for example, a mosquito bite; others have a higher threshold, for example, multiple anatomical damages following a motor vehicle accident, or metastatic cancer involving multiple structures.

One example of a systems analysis is the dynamic relationship that exists between the sympathetic and parasympathetic systems in the autonomic nervous system (ANS) which can influence baroreceptor activity. Baroreceptors are sensory nerve endings in blood vessels able to detect the pressure of blood flow and transmit information to the central nervous system to increase or decrease peripheral resistance and cardiac output. Heart rate is one measure of this interaction. Studies using electrocardiograms (ECG) have revealed cyclic changes in sinus rate over time, or heart rate variability (HRV). The absence of this HRV has been linked to a number of illnesses and disease states (Lombardi, 2000; Vaschillo et al, 2002). Martinez-Lavin and his colleagues (2008) have implicated this reduced HRV as one sign of decomplexification of the ANS in patients with fibromyalgia.

Decomplexification of the ANS results in a persistent inflexibility of circadian sympathetic response (Lipsitz and Goldberger, 1992). This unyielding sympathetic hyperactivity leads to neuroplasticity in the form of the development of abnormal connections between the sensory and sympathetic nervous systems. For instance, some women may manifest a defect in the catecholamine clearing enzymes, a type of gene polymorphism, rendering them more susceptible to fibromyalgia. Indeed, ECGs of patients with fibromyalgia have demonstrated a significant reduction in HRV, sympathetic hyperactivity with reduced parasympathetic activity at rest, and decreased sympathetic response to stress (decomplexification). Light et al (2009) provided additional evidence supporting the role of adrenergic dysregulation in fibromyalgia.

In general, patients with fibromyalgia tend to demonstrate an autonomic dysregulation, expressed as increased sympathetic tone, with concomitant decreased vagal tone at rest reflecting a dysfunction of autonomic neuroregulation (Cohen et al, 2000). Abnormal autonomic response to sympathetic challenge including physical and emotional stresses culminates in low muscle tissue oxygen (hypoperfusion), abnormal muscle phosphate metabolism, decreased pain threshold, and increased fatigue. Fatigue, sleep disturbance, irritable bowel syndrome, and paresthesias can result from this overactivity at rest. Conceptualized within this framework, fibromyalgia is the consequence of a degraded complex adaptive system requiring the use of nonlinear methodology and instruments in its assessment, viewed though a holistic (biopsychosocial) instead of a reductionistic model, and requiring treatment within a multidisciplinary context (Martinez-Lavin et al, 2008).

CONCLUSION

The continued use of the NRS and VAS is supported by convention and reinforced by pain being designated as the fifth vital sign. However, such quantitative measures often do not reflect the complex or dynamic nature of a phenomenon such as pain, especially chronic pain (Malterud, 2001a,b). As the definition of pain continues to evolve, what constitutes an adequate, useful, and meaningful measurement will change as well. Indeed, attempts to identify a neurologically or brain-based signature of pain through the use of fMRI and machine-learning analysis are being explored (Brown et al, 2011; Wager et al, 2013; see Chapter 14).

The manner in which the experience of pain is measured may have to vary, based on the clinical condition and the individual patient. Allowing patients the flexibility of determining the main features of their individual pain experience (cognitive, sensory, behavioral, emotional, activity engagement, quality of life) may be more meaningful than an NRS and scores on tests and questionnaires. Rigid adherence to a statistically oriented measurement may detract from uncovering some of the nuances of the individual experience. In some cases, the assessment may need to become less structured and outcomes conceptualized in terms of number of individual goals achieved or a more global assessment of improvement.

Here I have to acknowledge two biases related to the assessment of chronic pain: (a) descriptors, not predictors, and (b) "pain" generators over nociceptive generators. Briefly, the preference for descriptors refers to a bias toward an assessment or measurement process focused on elucidating the salient features (descriptors) of the pain condition and the patient for the purposes of developing a therapeutic algorithm and assessing the efficacy of treatment. Our reductionistic and materialistic heritage encourages the pursuit of some mystical formula that will, through the magic of statistics, predict the patient's immediate and future response. This approach betrays the complexity of the situation, often making the patient too accountable if they do not respond in the predicted fashion.

The second bias, of pain generators over nociceptive generators, highlights the distinction between the activation of the nociceptive system (nociceptive generator) and the experience of pain (pain generator). In a sense, this entire book is about the latter—that is, coming to understand what is known, what is not known, and what is yet to be learned about how a seemingly simple event like bruising one's hand could trigger a cascade of events that would leave one person with a severe complex regional pain syndrome (CRPS) that disables the person enough to prevent basic enjoyment of life, and leave another person to recover unscathed by the event.

William Osler (1909, 1925) is credited with stating that it is more important to know what sort of patient has the disease than what sort of disease the patient has. Less widely known is his comment: listen to your patient, he or she is telling you the diagnosis. Technological advances such as the electronic medical record tend to impose a computer-friendly rather than patient-relevant structure on the area of pain assessment and the patient–doctor relationship. Computerized templates for the patient's history and physical and office visits offer a fill-in-the-blank approach to assessment and are likely to dominate over more time-consuming approaches like narrative analysis. As the conception of pain continues to evolve, so will its measurement. At this point, it is difficult to know what critical bits of information are sacrificed for efficiency. It may be difficult to reconcile a nonlinear and systems-based orientation with the current philosophical approach to the measurement of pain.

Clinical pain is a complex interaction among genetic, physiological, neurochemical, and psychosocial variables. The ever-changing interactions among this host of variables constitutes a dancing landscape in systems theory and encourages an appreciation for the fluidity of the situation. The system's continual adaptation to changes in exogenous and endogenous stimuli may produce physiological changes that may appear random and chaotic but manifest an underlying order. Complexity theory may provide a framework and terminology within which to describe and understand these changes. For example, *decomplexification* refers to the loss of this dynamic relation among different systems and the relative inability to adapt, and *dysregulation* to a prolonged dysfunction in the ability of the system to recover its normal function and adaptive ability. Both can be very detrimental to the organism.

It seems clear that the assessment of pain must consider this complex interaction among systems. Viable and sustainable biological systems are often characterized by adaptability and flexibility. Indeed, some of the definitions of pain reviewed in the Introduction (Chapter 1) refer to pain in the context of a homeostatic (homeodynamic) regulatory system. This feature manifests itself through a very complex relationship between the internal and external environment and subsystems. Likewise, the patient's ability to cope with and manage pain rests on the various systems ability, individually and collectively, to adapt. Therefore, developing a means of assessing the individual's (system) degree of complexity and adaptability seems logical, if not a necessity. Finally, we must acknowledge that although through the process of measurement much can be known, little is understood.

REFERENCES

Ahles TA, Blanchard EB, Ruckdeschel JC. The multidimensional nature of cancer-related pain. *Pain.* 1983;17:277–288.

Baars BJ, Ramsey TZ, Laureys S. Brain, conscious experience and the observing self. *Trends Neurosci.* 2003;26(12):671–675.

Ballantyne M, Stevens B, McAllister M, Dionne KR, Jack A. Validation of the Premature Infant Pain Profile in the clinical setting. *Clin J Pain.* 1999;15(4):297–303.

Beck AT, Ward CH, Mendelson MM, Mock J, Erbaugh J. An inventory for measuring depression. *Arch Gen Psychiatry.* 1961;4:561–571.

Benedetti F, Arduino C, Costa S, et al. Loss of expectation-related mechanisms in Alzheimer's disease makes analgesic therapies less effective. *Pain.* 2006;121:133–144.

Benini F, Trapanotto M, Gobber D, et al. Evaluating pain induced by venipuncture in pediatric patients with developmental delay. *Clin J Pain.* 2004;20:156–163.

Björkman B, Arnér S, Hydén L-C. Phantom breast and other syndromes after mastectomy: eight breast cancer patients describe their experiences over time: 2-year follow-up study. *J Pain.* 2008;9(11):1018–1025.

Brown JE, Chatterjee N, Younger J, Mackey S. Towards a physiology-based measure of pain: patterns of human brain activity distinguish painful from non-painful thermal stimulation. *PLoS One.* 2011;6(9):e24124, 1–8.

Buckalew N, Haut MW, Alzenstei H, et al. Differences in brain structure and function in older adults with self-reported disabling and nondisabling chronic low back pain. *Pain Med.* 2010;11(8):1183–1197.

Carnevale FA, Razack S. An item analysis of the COMFORT scale in pediatric intensive care unit. *Pediatr Crit Care Med.* 2002;3:77–180.

Carr D, Loeser J, Morris D. *Narrative, Pain and Suffering.* Seattle: IASP Press; 2005.

Cedraschi C, Luthy C, Girard E, Piguet V, Desmeules J, Aliaz AF. Representations of symptom history in women with fibromyalgia vs. chronic low back pain: a qualitative study. *Pain Med.* 2012;13:1562–1570.

Chapman CR, Tuckett RP, Song CW. Pain and stress in a system perspective: reciprocal neural, endocrine, and immune interactions. *J Pain.* 2008;9(2):122–145.

Cleeland C. *Brief Pain Inventory; User Guide.* 1991. www.mdanderson.org/education-and-research/departments-program.

Cohen H, Neumann L, Shore M, Amir M, Cassuto Y, Buskila D. Autonomic dysfunction in patients with fibromyalgia: application of power spectral analysis of heart rate variability [see comments]. *Semin Arthritis Rheum* 2000;29(4):217–227.

Cole L, Gavrilescul M, Johnston LA, Gibson SJ, Farrekk MJ, Eagan GF. The impact of Alzheimer's disease on the functional connectivity between brain regions underlying pain perception. *Eur J Pain.* 2011;15(6):568.e1–568.e11.

Darwin C. *The Expression of Emotion in Man and Animals.* New York: Filiquarian; 1872/2007.

Daunt RJ, Cleeland CS, Flannery RC. Development of the Wisconsin Brief Pain Questionnaire to assess pain in cancer and other diseases. *Pain.* 1983;17:197–210.

Derogatis LR. *Symptom-Checklist-90-R: Scoring and Procedures Manual I for the Revised Version.* Eagan MN: Pearson Assessments; 1977.

Derogatis LR, Morrow GR, Fetting J. The prevalence of psychiatric disorders among cancer patients. *JAMA.* 1983;249:751–757.

de Williams AC. Facial expression of pain: an evolutionary account. *Behav Brain Sci.* 2002;25:439–488.

Doleys, DM. Psychological considerations in intrathecal drug delivery. In Buvanendran A, Diwan S, Deer T, eds. *Intrathecal Drug Delivery for Pain and Spasticity.* Philadelphia: Saunders; 2011:48–55.

Doleys DM, Doherty DC. Psychological evaluation. In Raj PP, ed. *Pain Medicine: A Comprehensive Review*, 2nd ed. St. Louis: Mosby; 2003:152–160.

Edwards RR, Sarlani E, Wesselmann U, Fillingim RB. Quantitative assessment of experimental pain perception: multiple domains of clinical relevance. *Pain.* 2005;114:315–319.

Ekman P, Friesen WV. *Facial Action Coding System.* Palo Alto, CA: Consulting Psychology Press; 1978.

Endicott J. Measurement of depression in patients with cancer. *Cancer.* 1984;53(Suppl): 2243–2249.

Fabrizi L, Worley A, Patten D, et al. Electrophysiological measurements and analysis of nociception in human infants. *J Vis Exp.* 2011;58:e3118.

Farrar JT, Young JP, LaMoreaux L, et al. Clinical importance of changes in chronic pain intensity measured on an 11-point numerical pain rating scale. *Pain.* 2001;94:149–158.

Fordyce WE. *Behavioral Methods for Chronic Pain and Illness.* St. Louis: Mosby; 1976.

Foss JM, Apkarian AV, Chialvo DR. Dynamics of pain: fractal dimension of temporal variability of spontaneous pain differentiates between pain states. *J Neurophysiol.* 2006;95:730–736.

Gallagher HL, Frith CD. Functional imaging of theory of mind. *Trends Cogn Sci.* 2003;7(2):77–83.

Gleck J. *Chaos: Making a New Science.* New York: Penguin Books; 2008.

Gold J, Douglas M, Thomas M, Elliott J, Roa S, Miaskowski C. Pain and posttraumatic stress in adults treated for cancer. *J Pain.* 2005;6(3, Suppl):S78.

Goldberger AL. Non-linear dynamics for clinicians: chaos theory, fractals, and complexity at the bedside. *Lancet.* 1996;347:1312–1314.

Goldberger AL, Rigney DR, West BJ. Chaos and fractals in human physiology. *Sci Am.* 1990;(Feb):44–49.

Gracely RH. Studies of pain in normal man. In Wall PD, Melzack R, eds. *Textbook of Pain*, 4th ed. London: Churchill Livingstone; 1999:385–407.

Greenhalgh T, Hurwitz B. Why study narratives. *BMJ*, 1999;318:48–50.

Haddox JD, Kerner B. The "five-minute" mental status examination of persons with pain. In Deer T, et al, eds. *Comprehensive Treatment of Chronic Pain by Medical, Interventional, and Integrative Approaches.* New York: Springer; 2013:795–804.

Hamilton M. The assessment of anxiety states by rating. *Br J Med Psychol*, 1959;32:50–55.

Harrison D, Boyce S, Loughnan P, Dargaville P, Storm H, Johnston L. Skin conductance as a measure of pain and stress in hospitalised infants. *Early Hum Dev.* 2006;82:603–608.

Hellerud BC, Storm H. Skin conductance and behaviour during sensory stimulation of preterm and term infants. *Early Hum Dev.* 2002;70:35–46.

Hummel P, Van Dijk M. Pain assessment: current status and challenges. *Semin Fetal Neonatal Med.* 2006;11(4):237–245.

Huokuri HV, Makikallio TM, Peng C, Goldberg AL, Hintze U, Moller M. Fractal correlations properties of R-R interval dynamics and mortality in patients with depressed left ventricular function after an acute myocardial infarction. *Circulation.* 2000;101:47–53.

Jensen MC, Brant-Zawadzki MN, Obuchowski N, Modic MT, Malkasian D, Ross JS. Magnetic resonance imaging of the lumbar spine in people without back pain. *N Engl J Med.* 1994;331(2):69–73.

Kane RL, Bernstein L, Wales J, Rothenberg R. Hospice effectiveness in controlling pain. *JAMA.* 1985;253:2683–2686.

Keefe FJ, Block AR. Development of an observation method for assessing pain behavior in chronic low back pain patients. *Behav Ther.* 1982;13:363–375.

Keller LS, Butcher JN. *Use of the MMPI-2 with Chronic Pain Patients.* Minneapolis: University of Minnesota Press; 1991.

Kelsey DP, Portion RK, Thales HT, et al. Pain and depression in patients with newly diagnosed pancreas cancer. *J Clin Oncol.* 1995;13:748–755.

Keogh E, Cochrane M. Anxiety sensitivity, coping biases and the experience of pain. *J Pain.* 2002;3:320–329.

Kerns R, Habib S. A critical review of the readiness for change model. *J Pain.* 2004;7:357–367.

Labbe EE, Goldberg M, Fishbain D, Rosomoff H, Steele-Rosomoff R. Millon Behavioral Health Inventory norms for chronic pain patients. *J Clin Psychol.* 1989;45(3):383–390.

Laureys S, Schiff ND. Coma and consciousness: paradigms (re)framed by neuroimaging. *Neuroimage.* 2012;61(2):478–491.

Light, KC, Bragdom EE, Grewen, KM, Brownley KA, Gridler SS, Maixner W. Adrenergic dysregulation and pain with and without acute beta-blockade in women with fibromyalgia and temporomandibular disorder. *J Pain.* 2009;10(5):542–552.

Lipsitz LA, Goldberger AL. Loss of complexity and aging. *JAMA.* 1992;267:1806–1809.

Loggia ML, Edwards RR, Kim J, et al. Disentangling linear and nonlinear brain responses to evoked deep tissue pain. *Pain.* 2012;153:2140–2151.

Lombardi F. Chaos theory, heart rate variability, and arrhythmic mortality. *Circulation.* 2000;101:8–10.

Lund I, Lundeberg T, Sandberg L, Budh CN, Kowalski J, Svensson E. Lack of interchangeability between visual analogue and verbal pain scales: a cross-sectional description of pain etiology groups. *BMC Med Res Methodol.* 2005;5:31.

Malterud K. Qualitative research: standards, challenges, and guidelines. *Lancet.* 2001a;358:483–488.

Malterud K. The art and science of clinical knowledge: evidence beyond measures and numbers. *Lancet.* 2001b;358:397–400.

Martinez-Lavin M, Infante O, Lerma C. Hypothesis: the chaos and complexity theory may help our understanding of fibromyalgia and similar maladies. *Semin Arthritis Rheum.* 2008;37(4):260–264.

Massie MJ, Holland JC. The cancer patient with pain: psychiatric complications and their management. *J Pain Symptom Manage.* 1992;7:99–109.

McCracken LM, Eccleston C. Coping or acceptance: what to do about chronic pain? *Pain.* 2003;105:197–204.

McCracken LM, Vowles KE, Eccleston C. Acceptance of chronic pain: component analysis and a revised assessment method. *Pain.* 2004;107:159–166.

Melzack R. The McGill Pain Questionnaire: major properties and scoring methods. *Pain.* 1975;1(3):277–299.

Miller K, Massie MJ. Depression and anxiety. *Cancer J.* 2006;12(5):388–397.

Millon T, Green CJ, Meagher RB Jr. The Millon Behavioral Health Inventory (MBHI™). 2006. http://www.millon.net/instruments/MBHI.htm.

Millon T, Green CJ, Meagher RB. The Millon Behavioral Health Inventory, 3rd ed. Minneapolis: Interpretive Scoring Systems; 1982.

Monroe B. Psychological evaluation of patient and family. In Sykes N, Fallon MT, Patt RB, eds. *Clinical Pain Management: Cancer Pain.* New York: Oxford University Press; 2003:73–85.

Moorey S, Greer S, Watson M, et al. The factor structure and factor stability of the Hospital Anxiety and Depression Scale with cancer. *Br J Psychiatry.* 1991;158:255–259.

Myles PS, Troedel S, Boquest M, Reeves M. The Pain Visual Analog Scale: is it linear or nonlinear? *Anesth Analg.* 1999;89:1517–1520.

Nes LS, Segerstrom SC. Dispositional optimism and coping: a meta-analytic review. *Pers Social Psychol Rev.* 2006;10:235–251.

Northoff G, Heinzel A, de Greck M, Bermpohl F, Dobrowolny H, Panksepp J. Self-referential processing in our brain—a meta-analysis of imaging studies on the self *Neuroimage.* 2006;31:440–457.

Osler W. The treatment of disease. *Can Lancet.* 1909;42:899–912.

Osler W. *Aequanimitas: With Other Addresses to Medical Students, Nurses and Practitioners of Medicine.* Philadelphia: P. Blakiston's Son and Co; 1925.

Owen AM, Coleman MR, Boly M, Davis MH, Laureys S, Pickard JD. Detecting awareness in the vegetative state. *Science.* 2006;313(5792):1402.

Pennebaker JW, Seagal JD. Forming a story: the health benefits of narrative. *J Clin Psychiatry.* 1999;55:1243–1254.

Richards JS, Nepomuceno C, Riles, M, Suer Z. Assessing pain behavior: the UAB Pain Behavior Scale. *Pain.* 1982;14:393–398.

Ritchy M, Dolcos F, Eddington K, et al. Neural correlates of emotion processing in depression: changes with cognitive behavioral therapy and predictors of treatment response. *J Psychiatric Res.* 2011;45(5):577–587.

Rosenstiel AK, Keefe FJ. The use of coping strategies in chronic low back pain patients: relationship to patient characteristics and current adjustment. *Pain.* 1983;17:33–44.

Scheier MF, Carver CS, Bridges MW. Distinguishing optimism from neuroticism (and trait anxiety, self-mastery, and self-esteem): a reevaluation of the Life Orientation Test. *J Pers Soc Psychol.* 1994;67:1063–1078.

Schiavenato M, Byers JF, Scovanner P, et al. Neonatal pain facial expression: evaluating the primal face of pain. *Pain.* 2008;138:460–471.

Schnakers C, Chatelle C, Majerus S, Gosseries O, De Val M, Laureys S. Assessment and detection of pain in noncommunicative severely brain-injured patients. *Expert Rev Neurother.* 2010;10(11):1725–1731.

Schriff SJ, Jerger K, Duong DH, Chang T, Spano ML, Ditto WL. Controlling chaos in the brain. *Nature.* 1994;370:615–620.

Spielberger C. The State-Trait Anxiety Inventory. New York: Academic Press; 1970.

Spiegal D, Bloom JR. Group therapy and hypnosis reduced metastatic breast carcinoma pain. *Psychosom Med.* 1982;45:333–339.

Stevens B, Johnston C, Petryshen P, Taddio A. Premature Infant Pain Profile: development and initial validation. *Clin J Pain.* 1996;12(1):13–22.

Sullivan MJL, Bishop SR, Pivik J. The Pain Catastrophizing Scale: development and validation. *Psychological Assessment.* 1995;7(4):524–532.

Sullivan MJL, Stanish W, Waite H, Sullivan ME, Tripp D. Catastrophizing, pain, and disability in patients with soft tissue injuries. *Pain.* 1998;77:253–260.

Sullivan MJL, Thorn B, Haythornthwaite JA, et al. Theoretical perspectives on the relation between catastrophizing and pain. *Clin J Pain.* 2001;17:52–64.

Svendsen KB, Arnason S, et al. Breakthrough pain in malignant and non-malignant diseases: a review of prevalence, characteristics and mechanisms. *Eur J Pain.* 2005;9: 195–206.

Tsuda I. Toward an interpretation of dynamic neural activity in terms of chaotic dynamical systems. *Behav Brain Sci.* 2001;24:793–847.

Turk DC, Fernandez. On the putative uniqueness of cancer pain: do psychological principles apply? *Behav Res Ther.* 1990;28:1–13.

Turk DC, Monarch ES, Williams AD. Cancer patients with pain: considerations for assessing the whole person. *Hematol Oncol Clin North Am.* 2002;16:511–525.

Upshur C, Wootton J. Depression and chronic pain in the elderly: dual challenges. *Clin Geriatrics.* 2003;11:30–36.

van Knippenberg FC, Duivenvoorden HJ, Bonke B, Passchier J. Shortening the State-Trait Anxiety Inventory. *J Clin Epidemiol.* 1990;43:995–1000.

Valkenburg AJ, Boerlage AA, Ista E, Duivenvoorden HJ, Tibboel D, van Dijk M. The COMFORT-behavior scale is useful to assess pain and distress in 0- to 3-year-old children with Down syndrome. *Pain.* 2011;152:2059–2064.

Vaschillo E, Lehrer P, Rishe N, Konstantinov M. Heart rate variability biofeedback as a method for assessing baroreflex function: a preliminary study of resonance in the cardiovascular system. *Appl Psychophysiol Biofeedback.* 2002;27:1–27.

Von Korff M, Dunn K. Chronic pain reconsidered. *Pain.* 2008;138:267–276.

Wager TD, Atlas LY, Lindquist MA, Roy M, Woo C, Kross E. An fMRI-based neurologic signature of physical pain. *N Engl J Med.* 2013;368(15):1388–1397.

Ware JE, Kosinki M, Keller SD. *SF-36 Physical and Mental Health Summary Scales: A User's Manual.* Boston: The Health Institute; 1994.

Ware JE, Sherbourne CD, The MOS 36-Item Short-Form Survey (SF-36). *Med Care.* 1992;30:473–481.

Zaza C, Baine N. Cancer pain and psychological factors: a critical review of the literature. *J Pain Symptom Manage.* 2002;24:526–542.

7 Psychogenic Pain: Is It a Useful Concept?

[P]ain can also be fully internally generated instead of driven by afferent input.
–H. Grunel and T.R. Tolle (2005, pp. 91–92)

I'm suffering in my mind because I can't suffer in my body.
–Namo, *a leprosy patient. Quoted in Brand and Yancy* (1997, p. 125)

INTRODUCTION

Broggi (2008) noted that human pain could be divided into two main categories: physical pain and psychological (psychogenic) pain. *Psychogenic* or *psychogenesis* is defined Webster's dictionary as "an event that originates or develops within the psyche/mind; the development of a physical disorder resulting from mental conflict versus organic cause." The mysteriousness of this term is enhanced by the psyche being declared as an entity beyond natural or known physical processes, apparently sensitive to forces beyond the physical world.

The Freudian era (Sigmund Freud, 1856–1939) saw an alteration in the conceptualization of the brain and the mind. The psyche became the mediator between the brain and the mind and in a sense disembodied from the body and brain. It appeared to function independently and, from a mechanistic perspective, evaluated and interpreted early events to which the individual was exposed. For Freud, the underlying motivational force in life was the gratification of biologically instinctual drives. Chronic, unexplained pain was thought to be a result of a drive the individual was unable to gratify in a socially acceptable manner. The unconscious "used" a physical insult to stabilize a dynamic conflict created by the awareness of repressed urges and to partially gratify this drive and conflict via subjective pain, disability, and emotional responses.

Thus, the superego, ego, and id were seen as the psychiatric triumphant which ultimately determined the manner in which the individual responded to life events. As the individual was not always aware of this activity, the unconscious became the arena in which these forces interacted. Importantly, the patient's personality and manner in which he or she would deal with life was established by adolescence. Although widely questioned, and in some circles thought to be discredited, the philosophical underpinnings of the Freudian dynamic approach have survived.

The history of low back pain (LBP) has been one of attempts to attribute the complaints to identifiable causes. The philosophy of materialism, reductionism, and linearity dominated. Indeed, a 1917 article noted, "If there's a functional problem, there must be, in any case, an anatomic abnormality. We just can't find them with our current devices" (from Raether, 1917; cited in Lutz et al, 2003, p. 1902). This underlying view of the human being and the role of anatomical abnormalities led to the use of various surgical procedures: "Surgical therapy has to be conducted at the anatomic abnormality" (Lutz et al, 2003, p. 1904). The emphasis on identifying a physical substrate (materialism) for pain is obvious. If the data from the physical examination and diagnostic testing did not add up (nonlinear), the problem was declared to be "psychogenic" (diagnosis by exclusion) and thus beyond the reach of acceptable medical therapies, but only after any structural abnormality was corrected. Any residual pain was relegated to the status of an epiphenomenon, and one in which only the patient, individually or with psychiatric or psychological guidance, was in a position to remediate.

Lutz et al (2003) note that throughout the history of treating LBP, the disconnect between anatomical abnormalities and pain has plagued the medical profession. Discussion of psychogenic causes appeared in nearly 60% of articles published from 1900 to 1950 and gradually declined to zero in the 1970s, followed by a resurgence in 1980–2000. As early as 1917 M. Raether observed, "Even non-specialists know from experience during the war and the numerous publications about 'war-neurotics,' that the psychogenic component is far more important than anyone would have expected" (Lutz et al, 2003, p. 1902). The proposed psychogenic explanations for chronic pain included sexual neurasthenia, excessive masturbation, abnormal and exaggerated sexuality, and fears and unfulfilled wishes (note the Freudian influence). This pattern seemed to parallel the advent of more sophisticated imaging technology and the degree of satisfaction with surgical outcomes. That is, the more that could be seen and the better the surgical outcomes were thought to be, the less emphasis was placed on psychogenic causes. More recently, this group of patients has been referred as manifesting "medically unexplained symptoms" (MUS).

PSYCHOGENIC PAIN

The contemporary use of the term *psychogenic pain* began with Engel (1959, 1980) and emerged in an era of psychodynamically dominated theory. Pain was thought to take on a central position in psychic development and function. Engle felt that pain was intricately involved in human relationships and punishment occurring early in the person's developmental history. Pain came to be associated with aggression and power in childhood, the actual or imagined loss of a loved one, as well as feelings of a sexual nature. The emphasis was on primary over secondary gain—that is to say, on the underlying psychic issues. Given these various meanings and functions, psychogenic pain was most likely to occur (a) when external circumstances failed to satisfy the unconscious need to suffer, (b) as a response to real, imagined, or fantasized loss, or (c) in response to guilt evoked by intense aggressive or forbidden sexual feelings.

The *Diagnostic and Statistical Manual, Fourth Edition (DSM-IV)*, published by the American Psychiatric Association 1994, does not contain the term *psychogenic pain*. It was replaced by Pain Disorder. The diagnosis of Pain Disorder was considered appropriate when psychological factors were judged to play a significant role in the onset, severity, exacerbation, or maintenance of pain. This seems to represent a shift away from appealing to the unconscious processes proposed by Freud to the more conventional and observable psychological factors. The DSM-IV, however, does not explain the mechanism(s) by which these psychological factors come to influence pain. Properly applied, this diagnosis requires the clinician to identify which psychological factors are related to the onset and maintenance of pain, effectively eliminating the process of diagnosis by exclusion.

The International Association for the Study of Pain (IASP) has been endowed with the responsibility of developing a nomenclature and classification system for pain. The second edition of the *Classification of Chronic Pain* (Merskey and Bogduk, 1994) uses the phrase "pain of psychological origin." There are three main categories: (1) delusional/hallucinatory, (2) hysterical, conversion, or hypochondriacal, and (3) associated with depression. For the diagnosis of pain of psychological origin to be applied properly, there needs to be evidence of pain without an adequate pathophysiological explanation (diagnosis by exclusion). However, there must also be separate evidence to support the view that a psychiatric illness is present. Proof of the presence of psychological factors by (1) relationship in time or (2) the patient avoiding undesirable activity or obtaining support from the environment otherwise not forthcoming (Merskey and Bogduk, 1994, p. 55) is required.

The IASP definition of pain as an unpleasant sensory and emotional experience associated with actual or potential tissue damage, or described in terms of such damage, allows for the experience of pain to occur in the absence of any external noxious stimulation or activation of the nociceptive system by a peripheral stimulus.

However, the search for the presumed pain generator continues. Physicians often seek to discover this illusive pain generator through several means. One is by injecting a nerve suspected to be carrying the pain signals with a local anesthetic. If the pain is substantially reduced or abolished for the time period of the anesthetic, that nerve or the structure it innervates is declared to be the pain generator. Another is via the use of a somatic block, which essentially suppresses the pain signals from reaching the brain. Presumably, if the patient continues to report pain during the procedure, this is taken as further evidence that the problem is supratentorial.

Discography represents another approach. Sterile needles are placed into several intervertebral discs. At least one of these discs is thought to be casing the pain (painful disc) and one not (a control disc). A solution containing a radiopaque dye is systematically injected into each disc. The patient's response to each injection is then recorded. The disc that the patient reports as reproducing the usual (concordant) pain is considered the pain generator. Confidence that the offending structure has been identified is heightened if the radiographs reveal some morphological changes, such as internal disc disruption (the injected solution forms an abnormal pattern inside the disc) or extravasations (leakage of dye from the inside of the disc through tears in the outer lining or annulus). Further convincing evidence is the presence of a nonpainful and morphologically normal control disc.

ALTERNATIVE EXPLANATIONS OF PSYCHOGENIC PAIN

Several lines of evidence call into question this notion of a pain generator. For example, it is well known that 30–40% of individuals with abnormal imaging studies have no complaints of pain (Jensen et al, 1994). Positive discograms have been found in asymptomatic patients (Carragee et al, 1999, 2000). Epidural scarring, frequently found after spine surgery and thought to be the cause of continuing pain, is not always associated with pain. Finally, there are multiple chemical mediators (substance P and glutamate) and nociceptive processing changes (central sensitization) that are associated with pain and can be independent of any identified structural abnormality. Taken together, these observations suggest that physical damage and pain are not the same. Indeed, Merskey and Bogduk (1994) stated that "activity induced in the nociceptor and the nociceptive pathways by a noxious stimulus is not pain, which is always a psychological state even though we may well appreciate that pain most often has a proximate physical cause" (p. 210).

Models of Pain Processing

In the absence of what Tracey (2005) refers to as a "nociceptive drive," and when pain is not improved by pharmacological or surgical therapy or altered by natural disease progression, she speculated that the pain was generated by (a) unidentified remnants of the nociceptive drive or tissue damage, (b) emotional or cognitive elements within the brain, (c) amplification or alteration of nociceptive or non-nociceptive input due to sensitization within the nervous system, or (d) the patient's imagination.

Melzack and Casey (1968) described pain processing as involving three major components. The sensory/discriminative component informs the person of the precise location and quality of their pain. The affective/motivational component reflects the impact of emotional states such as depression, anxiety, and fear. The parts of the brain associated with this component also serve as a repository for many repressed and past emotional traumas, the emotional aspect of which can be activated by new physical or emotional trauma and thus impact the degree of pain and suffering experienced by the patient. Finally, the cognitive/evaluative component is the harbinger of our knowledge, expectations, and meaning as it relates to the injury and subsequent pain. The effect of self-fulfilling prophecies such as "You just have to live with it"; "You'll never get any better"; "You will be in a wheelchair in 10 years" in a sense reside here and become manifest in the presence of physical harm by enhancing or turning up the volume, as it were, on the output of the interactive effects of the sensory and affective components.

Price (1999, 2000) outlined a pain processing system containing four components: nociception, primary pain affect, secondary pain affect, and the behavioral response. In his model, nociceptive activity triggered by some event is transmitted to the sensory component of the brain. If this event is perceived by the person as intrusive or threatening in some way, it is immediately followed by "pain unpleasantness" (distress, fear, annoyance). This pain unpleasantness gives way to second-order appraisals such as interruption in activities, difficulty enduring pain, or concern for the future.

Extended pain affect (depression, frustration, anxiety, anger) then follows. Finally, there is a behavioral response (avoidance, withdrawal, relief seeking). The models proposed by Melzack and Casey (1968) and Price (1999, 2000) clearly state that what is ultimately felt as pain is the product of a complex and dynamic interaction of multiple components and systems and may well be disproportionate to the inciting event.

If these models of pain processing are correct, then, by extension, any increase or decrease in negative emotions or maladaptive cognitive states should alter the pain (McCracken et al, 1998). This can be illustrated by examining the effect(s) of anticipation on pain. For example, parents carefully select their words when taking a toddler for immunization shots. Older siblings often enjoy taunting the younger ones with tales of woe about the experience. Parents frequently play games on the way to the doctor's office, use distraction while in the office, and promise a reward for being a "good boy." These maneuvers are all efforts to dissociate the anticipation and expectation of pain from the actual pain.

Neuroimaging

Sophisticated neuroimaging techniques have been used to study the reactions of healthy volunteers undergoing procedures designed to provoke acute pain. Expectation of pain was found by Ploghaus and his group (1999) to be associated with altered activity in several brain areas, including the medial frontal lobe, insular cortex (IC), and cerebellum. The study concluded that anticipation of pain can, in and of itself, cause mood changes and behavioral adaptations that exacerbate the suffering experienced by patients in pain.

Expectations regarding pain tend to emerge from some type of experience or learning. Sawamoto et al (2000) used nonpainful warm stimuli randomly intermixed with stimuli that produce shooting, neuropathic-like pain and demonstrated that uncertain expectations (uncertainty) are associated with an enhancement of the transient brain response to nonpainful warm stimulation. Expectations of a painful stimulus are known to amplify perceived unpleasantness of even innocuous stimulation, but they appear to have little effect on the reported pain intensity. In other words, when a person knows he or she will be exposed to a variety of events, some of which will be painful and others not, but without any means of knowing exactly when the painful ones will occur, even the previously nonpainful events will be experienced as painful. Yet, when asked to rate the degree of perceived unpleasantness and intensity of the event, the intensity rating remains unchanged, but the unpleasantness rating is higher. In essence, it is the brain's affective/emotional response to the stimuli that is influenced, not the intensity of the sensation. Likewise, a startle response is substantially altered when the event is predictable and expected compared to when it is not.

Kramer et al (2008) evaluated imagined allodynia (experiencing a nonpainful stimulus as painful). One group of subjects was chosen from among those who had participated in an earlier study in which they experienced experimentally induced allodynia. A stainless-steel needle was inserted under the skin of the right dorsal hand. A surface electrode was positioned directly above the needle. A constant electrical current was delivered for 50 minutes between the two. It was gradually increased over the first 20 minutes until the subject rated it at a level of 5/10 pain, after which it remained stable. Subjects were then asked to rate the intensity of a light brush stroke across that part of the hand. Ordinarily such a brush stroke would not be perceived as painful. However, after the electrical current, each subject found even lightly stroking or touching the dorsal right hand painful, rating it as 6/10 on a numerical pain scale (brush-evoke mechanical allodynia).

This group of subjects was then compared to another group without such an experience. Each of the two groups received tactile stimulation to both hands and then asked to imagine that it provoked a painful sensation (allodynia) to the right hand. Neuroimaging was then carried out. By virtue of their previous experience with tactile allodynia, this group, in fact, felt increased pain when asked to imagine it, whereas the other group did not. Furthermore, the cortical areas that were activated in the imagine group approximated those traditionally associated with real allodynia. This study suggests that following a previous experience with certain types of pain, simply imagining the pain experience can alter the manner in which the brain processes the information, thus turning a nonpainful light touch into a painful one.

Raij et al (2005) questioned whether the pain experienced in the absence of nociceptive stimulation would feel as real as that felt in response to an actual peripheral stimulus. Each of 14 "suggestion-prone" individuals was exposed to (a) suggestion of pain, (b) suggestion of pain relief, (c) low-intensity laser stimulus, and (d) painful laser stimulus. They were asked to rate the pain intensity, pain unpleasantness, and the reality of the pain experienced. The laser-induced pain was rated as 65 (0–100 scale) for intensity and 57 for unpleasantness. The suggestion-induced pain was rated 55 for intensity and 51 for unpleasantness. The reality score was 87 for the laser and 62 for the suggestion-induced pain. Neuroimaging studies using fMRI noted activation of the somatosensory cortex, anterior cingulated cortex (ACC), and insula in each condition. The researchers concluded that events often feel real or unreal rather than are known to be real or unreal. That is, pain stimulated by a mechanism other than peripheral noxious stimulation may well feel the same to the patient.

Derbyshire et al (2003, 2004) examined eight "highly hypnotizable" subjects exposed to a thermal stimulus while undergoing fMRI scanning. A single tap on the hand announced the arrival of the stimulus (noxious heat), two taps signified a rest period. There were a total of six trials, but the thermal stimulus was presented on only three of the six trials. Under hypnosis, the subjects were told to imagine the thermal stimulus (hypnotic-induced hallucination). Hallucinatory pain appeared to be mediated by structures similar to those mediating the stimulated pain but did not involve activation of subcortical structures.

In clinical practice, it is not uncommon to encounter patients reporting incessant ruminations regarding their pain. They worry that the pain will never get better and obsess over their feelings of helplessness. Descriptions of their pain and its effects on their life tend to be very exaggerated and dramatic, if not hysterical. This has been referred to as "pain catastrophizing." Such patients, and their complaints, are often dismissed and disregarded. They are frequently referred for psychological or psychiatric therapy, based on the doctor's belief that pain, if it exists at all, is imaged or psychogenic.

Gracely and his colleagues (2004) studied a group of such pain catastrophizers diagnosed with fibromyalgia using fMRI. They discovered increased activity in areas of the brain related to anticipation of pain (medial frontal cortex, cerebellum), attention to pain (dorsal ACC, dorsolateral prefrontal cortex), emotional aspects of pain (claustrum, closely related to the amygdala), and motor control. It seemed that catastrophizing influenced pain perception through altering attention and anticipation and through heightening the emotional response to pain. What was not apparent was whether this pattern of brain activity was somehow genetically determined, linked to certain types of personalities, a result of early childhood rearing practices, current patterns of reinforcement, or a combination of these factors.

Psychological Factors

The association of depression and pain has been well recognized. Indeed, it has been estimated that up to 65% of clinically depressed patients have unexplained pain, and 37% (range 5–85% depending on which study is quoted) of pain patients manifest clinically significant depression. The more the pain is allowed to interfere with daily functions, the greater the depressive symptoms. This may be a reflection of C. B. Ferster's (1973) reinforcement theory of depression. This theory hypothesized that depression is associated with the degree of rewarding events the person engages in and the amount of positive reinforcement from others. Therefore, as the individual with pain avoids engaging in desirable activities such as work, sporting events, family interactions, religious services, and sexual intimacy, depression begins and worsens. Therapies that emphasize a return to activity or the development of new reinforcing activities are more likely to affect depression. Treatments that reduce pain without improving the frequency of rewarding activity may not be as successful at improving mood.

Visceral pain involves internal organs, including the bowel, bladder, and stomach. Irritable bowel syndrome (IBS), chronic stomach upset (dyspepsia), and noncardiac chest pain have often been considered to be a result of anxiety, that is, psychogenic. Human (Myers and Greenwood-Van Meerveld, 2009) and animal (Larauche et al, 2011) studies have shown that early life stresses created by such events as maternal separation can result in an increased visceromotor response to colorectal distention. Colonic distension is created experimentally by temporarily inserting an inflatable balloon into the colon. Inflation of the balloon creates a sensation not unlike that of the need to defecate. The presence of a pain response to a level of distension generally perceived as innocuous is referred to as "visceral hyperalgesia." Unfortunately, such complaints of pain may lead to repeated invasive investigations and surgery, the outcome of which is to cause further irritation and the creation of adhesions. While it is clear that anxiety and stress play a role in the development of such disorders, there is also an underlying physiological mechanism that should discourage interpreting these as a purely psychological phenomenon.

The lack of any significant improvement in pain following spine surgery undertaken primarily as a treatment for chronic pain has been used as evidence that the pain is driven by psychological rather than physical variables. Upon closer examination, Schofferman et al. (1992) determined that many of the patients who fail to improve have certain developmental traumas in common, including physical or sexual abuse, evidence of alcohol and or drug abuse in a primary caregiver, being abandoned by a primary caregiver, or emotional neglect or abuse. In fact, the presence of three of more of these risk factors correlated with the lack of pain relief following spine surgery.

The term *limbically augmented pain syndrome* (LAPS) was introduced by Howard and Jeffery Rome (2000) describing the mechanism(s) by which these early childhood traumas could come to affect pain experienced many years after the fact. Kindling, corticolimbic sensitization, and the convergence of affective and sensory symptoms are put forth as possible mechanisms. Reduction in the size of the hippocampus (Bremner et al, 1997; Stein et al, 1997) and higher levels of cortisol (Weissbeckera et al, 2006) have been found in adult women with a history of childhood sexual abuse. Much less, but some, research has also been conducted with men and identified a similar relationship between childhood abuse and later experience of pain.

Surprisingly, an examination of the pre-pain lives of most of these abused individuals would lead one to conclude that they either did not perceive themselves as having been abused or they had successfully adjusted to the fact. It is unclear why some persons with histories of abuse respond like those without such a history. Taken as a whole, the data clearly suggest that childhood trauma can, indeed, influence the degree of the pain response in adult life, and that this heightened response has physiological correlates and thus should not be attributed to the hysterical ramblings of a patient with an unfortunate history.

Another means by which pain can be experienced without peripheral stimulation is through conditioning and learning. Classical conditioning principles were worked out by the Russian physiologist Ivan Pavlov (1927). Perhaps his most renowned demonstration is that of a dog salivating to the sound of a bell after the bell had been systematically paired (or associated) with food. The simplicity of this example betrays the complexity and elegance of classical conditioning theory and principles, but it is sufficient for our purposes. In a similar fashion, when olfactory cues have been paired with morphine-induced analgesia in animals, the odor itself induces the ability to elicit pain relief in the absence of morphine.

Classical conditioning is thought to be one of the mechanisms responsible for the well-recognized placebo response. Placebos, presumably, have little or no palliative qualities until they are paired, intentionally or not, with some type of analgesic. By extension, it seems logical that events that become associated with painful stimuli will come to elicit pain. This is precisely what Flor and her colleagues (1997) demonstrated when they recorded the same electrical brain-wave activity previously associated with a painful shock to the finger as that produced in response to a light that had been paired with the painful stimulus. If after being trapped in an elevator and experiencing an anxiety attack one can re-experience very similar physical sensations (increased heart rate, sweating, shortness of breath) upon coming in contact with an elevator, it should not be surprising that stimuli associated with events that activate the nociceptive system can come to elicit similar activation even in the absence of the original pain-producing event.

This type of conditioned nociception was recorded from the spinothalamic tract of monkeys by Duncan et al (1987). Spinothalamic tracts are known to be part of the nociceptive transmission system and conduct impulses from the periphery to the brain. In their study, monkeys were exposed to a variety of thermal stimuli presented via a thermistor attached to their lip. The monkey was to make a differential response according to whether or not a particular stimulus was perceived as painful. Once positioned in front of the console, a light cued the monkey that a trial was about to begin. Over time, activation of the spinothalamic tract was recorded in response to the light but before the presentation of any peripheral, painful or nonpainful, stimulus—conditioned nociception.

There is strong evidence that patients receiving a good deal of positive or negative reinforcement for their pain behavior may experience more pain and pain-related disability than those who do not. Indeed, when patients with chronic low back pain were given a mild electrical shock to their back in the presence of an overly sympathetic spouse, enhanced activity in the brain's pain matrix was noted compared to when the spouse was absent or if the patient's spouse tended to be more apathetic. Observations of this type have helped to form the basis for pain therapies that incorporate learning theory and conditioning principles.

Summary

Based on the findings discussed here, there appear to be several possible types of psychogenic pain. In one type, pain functions as a defense mechanism reflecting some unconscious process, à la Sigmund Freud's notion of a conversion reaction. A second type could be a psychophysiological response in which the pain is mediated by a physiological response, for example, an autonomic or muscular response, to an event. The classical tension headache in response to muscular tightness created in response to stress is an example. A third type of psychogenic pain could be a product of some psychological procedure or process, such as hypnosis or suggestion. Finally, the qualitative and quantitative aspect of pain can be influenced by psychosocial factors, including mood, attention, distraction, and developmental traumas.

There can be little doubt that a neural basis for psychogenic pain exists. Anticipation and expectation of pain activates the primary somatosensory cortex, ACC, periaqueductal gray matter, IC, prefrontal cortex (PFC), and cerebellum. The use of priming events is associated with increased EEG activity. Negative emotional states enhance pain perception through involvement of ACC and IC. Hypnotic suggestion altered pain-evoked activity that was region specific based on the nature of the suggestion.

MEDICALLY UNEXPLAINED SYMPTOMS (MUS) REVISITED

The term *medically unexplained* (or functional) *symptoms* (MUS) refers to "physical symptoms that prompt the sufferer to seek health care but remain unexplained after an appropriate medical evaluation" (Richardson and Engel, 2004). Such symptoms are often the basis for describing the problem as being psychogenic, somatoform, psychological, psychiatric, imaginary, or hysterical, essential declaring it to be in the mind of the patient rather than real. This is true even in the presence of physical manifestations such as swelling, fever, or muscular abnormalities. Common features of this group of patients with MUS include (a) being female, (b) early adverse experience, (c) sudden onset, often associated with some type of injury or infection, (d) multiple coexisting symptoms in the same patient with no set order of onset, (e) waxing and waning of symptoms, (f) heightened stress response involving altered adrenocortical and sympathetic nervous system functioning, and (g) recalcitrance to common treatments. The most unwavering criterion is whether or not the objective (medical) data and test results obtained by the clinician sufficiently account for the patient's symptoms.

The problems inherent in this situation are too obvious. First, what defines "medical"? This brings us back again to the issues of materialism and reductionism. Do genetic vulnerability and altered nociceptive processing constitute a medical explanations? Second, what defines an "appropriate workup"? Some rely on a physical exam; others, an interview; still others, imaging studies. All of these methods have been shown to be flawed when it comes to explaining pain. Third, there are broad discrepancies in the background, diagnostic sophistication, and training of physicians. No doubt, one can show the results of an exanimation and tests to three different clinicians and get three different interpretations. A further problem is the assumption that the degree of specificity and sensitivity of the present medical technology is sufficient to detect all related physical abnormalities. The advent of functional neuroimaging has significantly altered and expanded the conceptualization of pain. Perhaps MUS should be renamed as those disorders beyond the comprehension and sophistication of current medical science (BCSCMS), and place the burden of proof where it belongs.

Epigenetic, psychoneuroimmunological, and neurovisceral-integration models have been advocated as approaches to MUS. Each of these models emphasizes the biopsychological framework. Buffington (2009) has explored epigenetics as a contributing factor. *Epigenetics* (*epi* in Greek means "upon"; Zhang and Meaney, 2010) describes heritable changes in gene expression that do not involve DNA mutation. He outlines a model in which heightened sensitivity and vulnerability to stress and the development of such somatoform disorders as chronic pelvic pain, chronic fatigue syndrome, IBS, interstitial cystitis, and fibromyalgia can result from an epigenetic modulation of gene expression (EMGEX; McGowan et al, 2009).

Bruehl and Chung (2006) reported that offspring of parents with a history of chronic pain demonstrated enhanced pain sensitivity potentially attributable to alternation in endogenous opioid functions. There is evidence showing an alteration in gene expression in pregnant women genetically predisposed to being more sensitive to stress when exposed to certain types of stress (Buffington, 2009). The consequences of EMGEX, such as neuroendocrine abnormalities, are passed on to the offspring. For example, higher levels of cortisol and a greater likelihood of developing posttraumatic stress syndrome (PTSD) have been found in the offspring of Holocaust survivors and American women who were pregnant during the 9/11 World Trade Center attacks (Yehuda et al., 2002, 2005). Genetic polymorphisms that affect stress responsiveness include variations in COMT, serotonin transporter, and alpha 2-adrenergic receptor genes. Offspring of pregnant women carrying these polymorphisms may acquire an overly responsive stress-response system as a consequence of being exposed to the by-products of the mother's enhanced stress response.

This altered genetic pattern is passed on to the offspring, rendering them genetically vulnerable and predisposed to developing certain types of disorders or symptoms in response to what might otherwise be considered normal stresses. Buffington (2009) has reviewed a number of studies suggesting the presence of critical developmental periods when offspring are more vulnerable. However, it is also during this time period that high levels of physical contact and maternal responsiveness may mitigate a genetic predisposition toward a more extreme stress reaction (Anisman et al, 1998; de Kloet et al, 1996). These observations represent yet another example of the complex adaptive nature of the human organism (system).

Another approach to somatization or functional-pain disorders is described by Dantzer (2005) and referred to as the psychoneuroimmune perspective. Dantzer asserts that somatization "might be nothing else than the outward manifestation of sensitization of the brain cytokine system that is normally activated in response to activation of the innate immune system and mediates the subjective, behavioral and physiological components of sickness" (p. 948). Activation of the innate immune system by some pathogen-associated molecular pattern results in the synthesis and release of proinflammatory cytokines, including tumor necrosis factor alpha (TNF-α) and interleukins (IL). The brain cytokine system is then activated via various afferent and humoral systems, triggering a "sickness response" consisting of fever, neuroendo-crine responses, sickness behavior, and affective and cognitive alterations. Prolonged activation of this system can induce depression through modifications of tryptophan metabolism.

The role of IL-1, TNF, and nerve growth factor (NGF) in pain and being sick has been detailed by Watkins and Maier (2000). A study by Wallace and his col-leagues (2001) compared fibromyalgia (FM) patients with non-pain controls and found increased levels of IL-6 and IL-8 in the FM group. IL-6 is associated with hyperalgesia, fatigue, and depression; IL-8 is associated with sympathetic related pain. Dantzer also notes that the brain cytokine system can undergo sensitization as a result of stimulation during the early stages of development, repeated activa-tion by exposure to environmental stressors, and prior activations by exposure to environmental stressors.

Thayer and Brosschot (2005) have proposed a neurovisceral-integration model which involves the autonomic nervous system (ANS), central nervous system (CNS), and central autonomic network (CAN). The CAN is made up of PFC and limbic struc-tures and comprises the internal regulation system via which the brain controls vis-ceromotor, neuroendocrine, and behavioral responses related to goal-directed activity, adaptability, and health. Thayer and Brosschot also apply some of the concepts from complexity theory, such as "organized variability," which characterizes dynamic adap-tive systems, in contrast to "rigid regularity," which is associated with morbidity, ill health, and mortality.

In general, stress and alarm conditions precipitate the fight-or-flight response, including activation of the ANS. A prolonged state of alarm, action-readiness, uncer-tainty, threat (real or imagined), or negative emotions, places excessive demands on the system. An ANS imbalance highlighted by decreased parasympathetic tone emerges. The tonic inhibitory control usually exerted by the PFC is compromised, resulting in a state of disinhibition. The balance of sympathoexcitatory (vagal dominance) and inhibitory processes needed for preservation of the integrity of the system (health) is thus compromised. This common reciprocal inhibitory corticosubcortical neural circuit links psychological processes with health-related physiological processes. Sympathetic dominance alters CNS network activity that typically regulates auto-nomic balance via the CAN and thus influences social, attentional, affective executive, and motivated behavior. Deactivation of the PFC results in a loss of parasympathetic inhibitory controls (a state of relative disinhibition). The resulting sympathetic domi-nance leads to pathogenic outcomes, including psychological, somatic, and immune system dysfunction.

Low heart rate variability (HRV) is thought to be an index of this state of dis-inhibition and low parasympathetic activation. Hypervigilance, perseveration, and persistence of a sympathoexcitatory alarm state can exhaust the system, culminat-ing in various stress-related (functional) illnesses as well as depression and anxiety. This argument is bolstered by the work of Laederach-Hofmann et al (2008), who noted impaired autonomic regulation in 62% of patients diagnosed with a somati-zation disorder. They hypothesized that autonomic dysfunction could constitute an "independent somatic factor" in this group. A similar study by Reyes Del Paso et al (2010) reported a general lack of autonomic flexibility in patients with fibromyalgia compared to controls. Burton et al (2010) have also provided a compelling review regarding data supporting reduced complexity in patients with MUS.

Emotions tend to reflect the integrity of one's ongoing adjustment to ever-changing environmental demands, or "dancing landscapes" in systems theory. A properly functioning affective system results in flexible adaptation to shifting demands. Decreased parasympathetic activity may be the link between negative affective states and a disposition to disease and illness. Some of the studies summarized by Thayer and Brosschot (2005) noted anxiety, depression, PTSD, and schizophrenia to be among the disorders that have been associated with PFC hypoactivity and lack of neural inhibitory processes. HRV is an indication of CAN-ANS integration. ANS imbalance is indexed by low HRV and tends to be associated with a constellation of outcomes, including inactive lifestyle, substance abuse, hypervigilance, activation of defensive system to non-threatening stimuli, impaired attentional and cognitive resources, and negative health consequences. Indeed, a three-fold increase in mortality was found among persons with a resting HR greater than 90 beats per minute (bpm) compared to those with 60 bpm or less. A common mechanism could be excessive proinflammatory cytokines (TNF, IL-1 IL-6, C-reactive protein). Stress alone can lead to the release of cortisol, which is associated with increased proinflammatory cytokines and impaired cognitive function controlled by the PFC. Impaired cognitive control (memory, flexibility, attention, behavioral inhibition) in turn contributes to depression. This may also be a factor in the Macfarlane et al. (2001) study suggesting an increased death rate due to cancer in patients with widespread body pain (fibromyalgia) compared to those with regional pain or no pain.

The three models just discussed represent only a partial list of theories that have been proposed to account for MUS. van Ravenzwaaij et al (2010) identify no less than nine explanatory models: somatosensory amplification theory, sensitization theory, sensitivity theory, immune system sensitization theory, endocrine dysregulation theory, signal filter model theory, illness behavior model, autonomic nervous system dysfunction theory, and abnormal proprioception theory. Each of these theories differentially emphasizes somatic causes, perception, illness behavior, and predisposition. van Ravenzwaaij et al found the cognitive behavior therapy model proposed by Deary and colleagues (2007) to be inclusive of many domains. This model asserts that the cause of MUS is an autopoietic (self-created and self-perpetuated) multifactorial cycle involving a complex interaction among genetic, neurological, psychophysiological, immunological, personality, attentional, attributional, affective, behavioral, social, and interpersonal factors.

Lambert (2010) has taken on the task of attempting to explain migraine headache, a phenomenon that is occasionally seen as psychogenic because of the apparent absence of any peripheral pathology or activation of the peripheral trigeminal system. Relying on system theory concepts, he proposes "a noise model" consistent with viewing the CNS as the source of idiopathic migraine. In the noise model, nothing is required for a migraine to occur—it just happens. The CNS is seen as a stochastic system (one that changes randomly as time goes on). It manifests features of "self-organized criticality." Like many other dissipative systems, it operates near a state of minimal stability. This is not unlike mountains prone to landslides or avalanches.

Migraines, then, are a result of destabilization of a critical state by noise excursion. The cortex is described as the noisiest of the pain perception and modulatory systems because of its relatively greater network complexity. Lambert suggests there is ongoing "traffic" in the trigeminal nervous system and that the threshold for impulse firing varies. Random fluctuations in the system occasionally rise above the impulse firing threshold, and a migraine ensues absent any noxious stimulation. Therefore, normal subthreshold stimuli may ultimately cross over the pain threshold. This process is similar to a sensitive burglar alarm system set off by random environmental noises (a false alarm). Decreases in the descending control system can result in this CNS noise turning into pain.

If this is correct, this theory would support Living's 1873 hypothesis of migraines being a result of a "nerve- or brain-storm," which "just happens" as a result of random noise in an exquisitely sensitive and complex system. If indeed idiopathic migraine is a "false alarm," one would expect the rate to increase with heightened sensitivity and variability. Thus, it may not be a matter of coincidence that migraines occur at their highest rate in 25- to 35-years-olds, when the system displays its greatest sensitivity and dynamic flexibility. Lambert's approach to migraine headache is yet another example of how broadening the paradigm through which pain is viewed may provide for new research opportunities and explanations.

DSM-V

The fifth edition of the *Diagnostic and Statistical Manual of Mental Disorders*, DSM-V, was published in July 2013. Compared to DSM-IV, the diagnoses of Somatization, Hypochondriasis, and Pain Disorder, and Undifferentiated Somatoform Disorder, previously subsumed under Somatoform Disorders, have been eliminated in favor of Somatic Symptom Disorder. Furthermore, the phrase "medically unexplained symptom" as a diagnostic criteria was also abolished. The diagnosis is now be based on positive cognitive and behavioral features, as it became apparent that the DSM-IV disorders were overlapping with differing dimensions such as the number of somatic symptoms, health anxiety, and duration of disorder, among others. According to Dimsdale and Creed (2009), "The…classification identifies somatic symptoms as one aspect of complex somatic symptoms disorder; another aspect concerns misattributions, excessive concern or preoccupation with symptoms and illness. The third aspect is increased health care use" (p. 474).

The hope is that this new designation will help to eliminate the mind–body dualism fostered by terms such as somatoform and medically unexplained-symptoms. Rather, the emphasis will be on identifying common features, thus providing a substitute for diagnosis by exclusion. Somatic symptoms will now be viewed in the context of their severity and intensity as multiple or single, localized or nonspecific. Misattributions, excessive concern or preoccupation with symptoms and illness, and high levels of health-related anxiety are seen as common cognitive distortions. Behavioral manifestations proposed to characterize this group of patients include an increased pattern of health care utilization, being unresponsive to therapies, and new treatments tending to exacerbate symptoms or leading to new side effects or complications.

The debate as to whether patients who display behaviors such as excessive concern and anxiety about their pain can be said to have a mental illness continues. At the heart of this debate is who determines and how does one determine when the concern or anxiety is "excessive"? The DSM defines this by the presence of significant distress and impairment. One can easily counter that there are times when such a reaction to pain and its devastating consequences would be considered normal. Therefore, it is the pain and not the patient that is abnormal. Indeed, even within psychiatry, the definition and meaningfulness of the concept of mental illness (disease) remains unsettled (Schramme, 2013). A.J. Frances, chairperson of the committee that framed DSM-IV and a contributor to DSM-V, stated, "There could arguably not be a worse term than 'mental disorders' to describe the conditions classified in DSM-IV. Mental implies a mind–body dichotomy that is becoming increasingly outmoded" (Frances, 1994, p. VIII) Stein et al (2010) have also asserted that the term *mental* (psychogenic) promotes a Cartesian mind–body dualism that is inconsistent with contemporary philosophical and neuroscientific views.

CONCLUSION

Tracey (2008) has pointed out that recent neuroimaging data display activity of nearly the entire pain matrix without any nociceptive input, suggesting it is time to reconsider how central pain processing is defined with respect to the origin of the input and resultant perception and meaning. This is not to say that pain experienced without a nociceptive input (sometimes referred to as psychogenic pain) is any less real than physically defined pain. Indeed, neuroimaging studies have highlighted the physiological reality of such experiences as a result of the extensive neural activation that occurs. These studies illustrate how powerful the mind can be in terms of activating specific networks within the brain to subsequently produce a realistic and vivid experience.

Psychogenic, neurotic, nonorganic, functional, and *reactive* are often substituted for one another. This, however, is a superficial issue. At the heart of it is the mind–body problem (Bracken and Thomas, 2002) and the admitted uncertainty about the etiology of many pain experiences.

Because of the fundamental issues of causality, dualism, and normality, Lewis (1972) stated that "it would be as well at this stage to give it [the term *psychogenic*] a decent burial, along with some of the fruitless controversies whose fire it has stoked," including organic vs. functional, real vs. psychological, real vs. imagined. This sentiment was echoed some 30 years later by Katon et al (2001) when they declared that

disease and distress both produce physical symptoms. It is not productive to dichotomize symptoms as "somatogenic" and "psychogenic" because physiological and psychological processes are involved in all symptom production and perception. "Rule-out" diagnostic strategies that search for either a medical or a psychiatric cause of a physical symptom are not supported by epidemiological findings of a high rate of medical and psychiatric co-morbidity. (p. 922)

It appears that several conclusions can be drawn from this discussion. First, a person can experience pain in the absence of any stimulation of the peripheral nociceptive system. Second, stimulation of the nociceptive system by a non-noxious stimulus can be experienced as pain as a result of the impact of psychological factors. Third, painful stimuli can be made more unpleasant without influencing its perceived intensity. Fourth, to the extent that psychogenic pain means pain without stimulation of the peripheral nociceptive system, it does, in fact, exist. Finally, there is the intended or unintended consequence of applying a label indicative of a mental illness to a situation in which none may exist.

I would suggest here that the term *psychogenic pain* be abandoned because it continues to be applied as a diagnosis by exclusion, as evidenced by the oft-used criterion of medically unexplained symptoms. Also, the term continues to imply that the pain, especially chronic pain, can be something other than real pain, and the veracity of patients labeled as manifesting psychogenic pain is repeatedly questioned. Instead, the emphasis should be on identifying (a) historical and predisposing factors which, via epigenetic or other processes, alter the "system" in such a fashion as to make the emergence of chronic pain more likely, (b) current psychological and behavioral variables that mediate the severity of the chronic pain, and (c) factors that influence the homeostatic function of the human complex-adaptive system and, as such, would represent meaningful therapeutic targets. This approach eliminates the issue of "mental illness" and provides a more rational basis for the development of a treatment algorithm.

REFERENCES

American Psychiatric Association. *Diagnostic and Statistical Manual of Mental Disorders*, Fourth Edition (DSM-IV). Washington, DC: American Psychiatric Publishing; 1994.

American Psychiatric Association. *Diagnostic and Statistical Manual of Mental Disorders*, Fifth Edition (DSM-V). Washington, DC: American Psychiatric Publishing; 2013.

Anisman H, Zaharia MD, Meaney MJ, Merali Z. Do early-life events permanently alter behavioral and hormonal responses to stressors? *Int J Dev Neurosci*. 1998;16(3-4):149–164.

Bracken P, Thomas P. Time to move beyond the mind–body split. *BMJ*. 2002;325:1433–1434.

Brand P, Yancy P. *Pain: The Gift Nobody Wants*. Grand Rapids, MI: Vondervan; 1997.

Bremner LD, Randall P, Vermetten E, et al. Magnetic resonance imaging-based measurement of hippocampal volume in posttraumatic stress disorder related to childhood physical and sexual abuse: a preliminary report. *Biol Psychiatry*. 1997;41(1):23–32.

Broggi G. Pain and psychoaffective disorders. *Neurosurgery*. 2008;62(6 Suppl 3):1–19.

Bruehl S, Chung OY. Parental history of chronic pain may be associated with impairments in endogenous opioid analgesic systems. *Pain*. 2006;124:287–294.

Buffington CAT. Developmental influences on medically unexplained symptoms. *Psychother Psychosom*. 2009;78:139–144.

Burton C, Heath RA, Weller D, Sharpe M. Evidence of reduced complexity is self-reported data from patients with medically unexplained symptoms. *Nonlinear Dynamics, Psychology, and Life Sciences*. 2010;14(1):15–25.

Carragee EJ, Tanner CM, Khurana S, et al. The rates of false-positive lumbar discography in select patients without low back symptoms. *Spine*. 2000;25:1373–1380.

Carragee EJ, Tanner CM, Yang B, Brito JL, Truong T. False-positive findings on lumbar discography. Reliability of subjective concordance assessment during provocative disc injection. *Spine*. 1999;24:2542–2547.

Dantzer R. Somatization: a psychoneuroimmune perspective. *Psychoneuroimmunology*. 2005;30:947–952.

Deary V, Chalder T, Sharpe M. The cognitive behavioural model of medically unexplained symptoms: a theoretical and empirical review. *Clin Psychol Rev*. 2007;27(7):781–797.

de Kloet ER, Rots NY, Cools AR. Brain–corticosteroid hormone dialogue: slow and persistent. *Cell Mol Neurobiol (Netherlands)*. 1996;16(3):345–356.

Derbyshire SW, Whalley M, Oaklet D. Subjects hallucinating pain in the absence of a stimulus activate anterior cingulated, anterior insula, prefrontal and parietal cortices. *J Pain*. 2003;4(2, Suppl) Abstract 754.

Derbyshire SW, Whalley MG, Stenger VA, Oakley DA. Cerebral activation during hypnotically induced and imagined pain. *Neuroimage*. 2004;23:392–401.

Dimsdale J, Creed F. The proposed diagnosis of somatic symptom disorders in DSM-V to replace somatoform disorders in DSM-IV—a preliminary report. *Psychosom Res*. 2009;66(6):473–476.

Duncan GH, Bushnell MC, Bates R, Dubner R. Task-related responses of monkey medullary dorsal horn neurons. *J Neurophysiol*. 1987;57:289–310.

Engel GL. "Psychogenic" pain and the pain-prone patient. *Am J Med*. 1959;26:899–918.

Engel GL. The clinical application of the biopsychosocial model. *Am J Psychiatry*. 1980;137:535–544.

Ferster CB. A functional analysis of depression. *Am Psychol*. 1973;28(10):857–879.

Flor H, Braun C, Elbert T, Birbaumer N. Extensive reorganization of primary somatosensory cortex in chronic back pain patients. *Neurosci Lett*. 1997;224(1):5–8.

Frances AJ. Foreword. In Frances AJ, First MB, Widiger TA, et al, eds. *Philosophical Perspectives on Psychiatric Diagnostic Classification*. Baltimore: Johns Hopkins University Press; 1994:VII–IX.

Gracely RH, Geisser ME, Giesecke T, Grant MA, Williams DA, Clauw DJ. Pain catastrophizing and neural responses to pain among persons with fibromyalgia. *Brain*. 2004;127:835–843.

Grunel H, Tolle TR. How physical pain may interact with psychological pain: evidence of a mutual neurobiological basis of emotions and pain. In Carr D, Loeser JD, Morris DB, eds. *Narrative Pain and Suffering*. Seattle: IASP Press; 2005:87–112.

Jensen MC, Brant-Zawadzki MN, Obuchowski N, Modic MT, Malkasian D, Ross JS. Magnetic resonance imaging of the lumbar spine in people without back pain. *N Engl J Med*. 1994;331(2):69–73.

Katon W, Sullivan M, Walker E. Medical symptoms without identified pathology: relationship to psychiatric disorders, childhood and adult trauma, and personality traits. *Ann Intern Med*. 2001;134(Suppl Part 2):917–925.

Kramer HH, Stenner C, Seddigh S, Bauermann T, Birklein F, Malhofner C. Illusion of pain: pre-existing knowledge determines brain activation of "imagined allodynia." *J Pain*. 2008;9:543–551.

Laederach-Hofmann K, Ruddel H, Mussgay L. Pathological baroreceptor sensitivity in patients suffering from somatization disorders: Do they correlate with symptoms? *Biol Psychol*. 2008;79(2):243–249.

Lambert GA. The lack of peripheral pathology in migraine headache. *Headache*. 2010;50(5):895–908.

Larauche M, Mulak A, Taché Y. Stress-related alterations of visceral sensation: animal models for irritable bowel syndrome. *J Neurogastroenterol Motil*. 2011;17(3):213–234.

Lewis A. "Psychogenic": a word and it mutations. *Psychol Med*. 1972;2:200–215.

Living E. *On Megrim, Sick Headaches and Some Allied Disorders*. London: J&A Churchill; 1873.

Lutz GK, Butzlaff M, Schultz-Venrath U. Looking back on back pain: trial and error of diagnoses in the 20th century. *Spine*. 2003;28(16):1899–1905.

Macfarlane GJ, McBeth J, Silman AJ. Widespread body pain and mortality: prospective population based study *BMJ*. 2001;323:1–5.

McCracken LM, Faber SD, Janeck A. Pain-related anxiety predicts non-specific physical complaints in persons with chronic pain. *Behav Res Ther*. 1998;36(6):621–630.

McGowan PO, Sasaki A, D'Alessio AC, et al. Epigenetic regulation of the glucocorticoid receptor in human brain associates with childhood abuse. *Nat Neurosci*. 2009;12:342–348.

Melzack R, Casey K. Sensory, motivational, and central control determinants of pain: a new conceptual model. In Kenshalo D, ed. *The Skin Senses*. Springfield, IL: Thomas; 1968.

Merskey H, Bogduk N, eds. *Classification of Chronic Pain*. Seattle: IASP Press; 1994.

Myers B, Greenwood-Van Meerveld B. Role of anxiety in the pathophysiology of irritable bowel syndrome: importance of the amygdala. *Front Neurosci*. 2009;3: article 47, 1–10.

Pavlov IP. *Conditional Reflexes*. New York: Dover; 1927.

Ploghaus A, Tracey I, Gati JS, et al. Dissociating pain from its anticipation in the human brain. *Science*. 1999;284:1979–1981.

Price DD. *Psychological Mechanisms of Pain and Analgesia*. Seattle: IASP Press; 1999.

Price DD. Psychological and neural mechanisms of the affective dimension of pain. *Science*. 2000;288(5472):1769–1772.

Raether M. Psychogene Ischias. (Über psychogene Ischias-Rheumatismus und Wirbelsäulenerkrankungen). Bericht der niederrheinischen Gesellschaft für Natur- und Heilkunde in Bonn. *Dtsch Med Wochenschr*. 1917;50:1576 (quote cited in Lutz et al, 2003).

Raij TT, Numminen J, Närvänen S, Hiltunen J, Hari R. Brain correlates of subjective reality of physically and psychologically induced pain. *Proc Natl Acad Sci U S A*. 2005;102(6):2147–2151.

Reyes Del Paso GA, Garrida S, Pulgar A, Martin-Vazquez, Duschek S. Aberrances in autonomic cardiovascular regulation in fibromyalgia syndrome and their relevance for clinical pain reports. *Psychosom Med*. 2010;72:462–470.

Richarson RD, Engel CC. Evaluation and management of medically unexplained physical symptoms. *Neurologist*. 2004;10:18–30.

Rome H, Rome J. Limbically augmented pain syndrome (LAPS): kindling, corticolimbic sensitization, and the convergence of affective and sensory symptoms in chronic pain disorders. *Pain Med*. 2000;1(2):7–23.

Sawamoto N, Honda M, Okada T, et al. Expectation of pain enhances responses to nonpainful somatosensory stimulation in the anterior cingulate cortex and parietal operculum/posterior insula: an event-related functional magnetic resonance imaging study. *J Neurosci*. 2000;20(19):7438–7445.

Schofferman J, Anderson D, Hinds R, Smith G, White A. Childhood psychological trauma correlates with unsuccessful lumbar spine surgery. *Spine*. 1992;17:S1381–S1384.

Schramme T. On the autonomy of the concept of disease in psychiatry. *Front Psychol*. 2013;4: article 457, 1–9.

Stein DJ, Phillips KA, Bolton D, Fulford KWM, Sadler JZ, Kendler KS. What is a mental/psychiatric disorder? From DSM-IV to DSM-V. *Psychol Med*. 2010;40:1759–1765.

Stein MB, Koverola C, Hanna C, Torchia MG, McClarty B. Hippocampal volume in women victimized by childhood sexual abuse. *Psychol Med*. 1997;27(4):951–959.

Thayer JF, Brosschot JF. Psychosomatics and psychopathology: looking up and down from the brain. *Psychoneuroimmunology*. 2005;30:1050–1058.

Tracey I. Taking the narrative out of pain: objectifying pain through brain imaging. In Carr D, Loeser JD, Morris DB, eds. *Narrative Pain and Suffering*. Seattle: IASP Press; 2005:127–163.

Tracey I. Imaging pain. *Br J Anaesth*. 2008;101:32–39.

van Ravenzwaaij J, olde Hartman TC, van Ravesteijn H, Eveleigh R, van Rijswijk E, Lucassen PLBJ. Explanatory models of medically unexplained symptoms: a qualitative analysis of the literature. *Ment Health Fam Med*. 2010;7:223–231.

Wallace DJ, Linker-Israeli M, Hallegua D, Silverman S, Silver D, Weisman WH. Cytokines play an aetiopathogenetic role in fibromyalgia: a hypothesis and pilot study. *Rheumatology*. 2001;40:743–749.

Watkins LB, Maier SF. The pain of being sick: implication of immune-to-brain communication for understanding pain. *Annu Rev Psychol.* 2000;51:29–57.

Weissbeckera I, Floyda A, Dederta E, Salmona P, Sephtonb S. Childhood trauma and diurnal cortisol disruption in fibromyalgia syndrome. *Psychoneuroendocrinology.* 2006;31:312–324.

Yehuda R, Engel SM, Brand SR, Marcus SM, Berkowitz GS. Transgenerational effects of posttraumatic stress disorder in babies of mothers exposed to the World Trade Center attacks during pregnancy. *J Clin Endocrinol.* 2005;90(7):4115–4118.

Yehuda R, Halligan SI, Bierer LM. Cortisol levels in adult offspring of Holocaust survivors: relation in PTSD symptom severity in the parent and child. *Psychoneuroendocrinology.* 2002;27:171–189.

Zhang T, Meaney MJ. Epigenetics and the environmental regulation of the genome and its function. *Annu Rev Psychol.* 2010;61:439–466.

8 Pain as a Disease

[C]hronic pain [is] the disease of the 21st century, having its own specific cause, symptoms, and signs.
–Michael Cousins (1999, p. 551)

INTRODUCTION

Pain, particularly chronic non-cancer pain, has been viewed in many ways. Most professionals working in this arena and patients themselves with chronic pain tend to see pain as a symptom. However, there has been a shift toward considering pain as a disease entity. In fact, understanding pain as a disease rather than a bothersome symptom can have enormous repercussions. Government funding for research and clinical exploration is finite and tends to focus on disease and its impact (Gillum et al, 2011). Pain as a symptom can be assigned to almost any physical or emotional problem. Indeed, pain is so ubiquitous that it lacks its own identity.

Recognizing pain as a disease would enhance its political posture. Furthermore, conferring disease status to pain would legitimize and enhance its inclusion in medical school education. This would also exonerate the much maligned and stigmatized patient with chronic pain and remove them from the rolls of the weak-willed and weak-minded. In addition, the recognition of pain as a disease carries with it a sense of therapeutic urgency to help minimize the potential catastrophic effects of disease progression. Diabetes, for example, is not treated aggressively because it can be cured but to avoid irreversible consequences, such retinopathy, neuropathy, and organ damage.

In many instances, insurance companies, practitioners, and society do not appreciate any maladaptive consequence to untreated or undertreated pain. Indeed, there is a sense that most patients with pain can manage on their own. A case in point is cancer. There is enormous political, medical, and societal support for cancer research and treatment. Political figures and entertainers enthusiastically and proudly allow their fight with cancer to be publically documented. They are often revered for their courage and indomitable spirit. Yet, the treatment of cancer pain has only become of concern in recent decades. The fact that pain itself can be a disease process and contribute to the development of cancer, immune suppression, and brain damage is often overlooked.

HISTORICAL PERSPECTIVE

John Bonica, considered by many to be the father of the contemporary pain movement, had little to say about pain as a disease process in his 1950 book, though he referred to chronic pain as a disabling disease in 1974. The emphasis on the "whole" person and a biopsychosocial model over the more traditional biomedical-reductionism approach seemed to endow pain with an element of uniqueness yet relative obscurity. In 1974, Richard Sternbach discussed "chronic pain as a disease entity" but mostly in the context of its various physical and psychological components. The International Association for the Study of Pain (IASP) defined pain, in part, as an emotional experience and in 1979 excluded tissue damage as a prerequisite (Merskey and Bogduck, 1994). This further removed pain from being viewed as anything other than a symptom, and a potential psychogenic one at that. Pilowsky (1981) emphasized the concept of "illness behavior" but also noted that "whereas in acute pain the pain is the symptom of a disease, in chronic pain the pain is itself the disease" (p. 31).

In a sense, pain took on the characteristics of a set of behaviors or responses to some type of insult or injury that exceeded expectations and extended beyond the normal healing time, generally defined as 3 to 6 months. Thus, chronic pain was that which was "left over" after the "real" disease resolved. The absence of any means of objectification or verification left pain, especially chronic pain, in a kind of scientific limbo.

The broad range of definitions of pain (see Chapter 1) also created a problem. In addition to the IASP definition of pain as an unpleasant sensory and emotional experience, McCaffery (1968) saw pain as being whatever the patient said it was, existing whenever the patient said it did. Woolf (2004; Woolf and Mannion, 1999) defined pain as a multidimensional sensory experience that is intrinsically unpleasant and is associated with hurting and soreness. Sarno (1998) described pain as being produced in the brain in response to something unconscious, "a manifestation of rage in the unconscious."

By comparison, dictionary definitions described pain as a sensation of consciousness, the opposite of pleasure (*Oxford English Dictionary*, 1989), and "the range of unpleasant bodily sensations produced by an illness or harmful physical contact" (*Oxford Pocket American Dictionary*, 2002). This lack of specificity separated pain further from the general medical and disease-oriented community in which all diseases are defined by some biological marker (biomarker) that is common among its sufferers.

A turning point in our view of pain may have been John Liebeskind's comments in a 1991 editorial entitled "Pain Can Kill." Here he dispelled chronic pain as a benign condition, noting the immunosuppressive and tumor-enhancing effects of pain and its associated stress. In the article "Good Pain: Bad Pain" Isdarola and Caudle (1997) noted that persistent pain caused pathophysiological and chemical changes in the nervous system. Cousins (1999) declared that chronic pain would be the "disease of the 21st century" (p. 551) as he elaborated on the accumulated evidence for pain (persistent nociception) having its own specific causes, symptoms, and signs.

With the beginning of the 21st century neuroimaging studies began to reveal the effects of pain on cortical functioning and central nervous system plasticity (Borsook et al, 2011b; Casey and Bushnell, 2000). Perhaps for the first time, the pervious subjective experience of pain could be objectively observed. Remarkably, pain, especially neuropathic pain, appeared to precipitate a cascade of morphological (structural), physiological (processing), and chemical changes (Backonja, 2003; Bridges et al, 2001; Mendell and Sahenk, 2003). Indeed, black spots suggestive of cell death were identified in the spinal cord.

Loeser (2005) stated, "It is my task today to convince you that pain is in fact a disease." He likened chronic pain to diabetes, multiple sclerosis, and atherosclerosis because of its association with various kinds of impairment and the interruption or modification of vital functions. Many others have described chronic pain as a "fatal disease" (Gallagher and Verma, 2004), a "disease of the nervous system" (Basbaum and Julis, 2006), a "destructive disease process" (Ballantyne, 2006), and as "disease—a result of the neural mechanisms gone awry" (Melzack, 2005). The European Federation of IASP Chapters (EFIC) has also declared chronic pain as a "disease entity in its own right" (Niv and Devor, 2004).

DEFINING DISEASE

There are many philosophical approaches to the concept of disease (Scully, 2004). Essentialists maintain that universals do exist (Scadding, 1996). Therefore, behind every definable object or concept is an ideal form; definitions describe this as an "unchanging essence." Every disease is thought to have an underlying pathological etiology, and the disease should be defined by that essential lesion. The existence of lesion X is considered the cause of disease X; likewise, the presence of disease X implies the presence lesion X. The nominalist, however, tends to label a cluster of symptoms with a disease name without the need to explain the underlying etiology. This is much like the notion of a hypothetical construct, discussed earlier (see Chapter 5). For example, schizophrenia is recognized as a collection of symptoms rather than by any identified lesion.

In the current use of the term *disease*, it is defined as a state in which the person is at increased risk for adverse consequences (Scully, 1996). The World Health Organization (WHO) defines *adverse consequences* as physical or psychological impairment, activity restrictions, and/or role limitations, with the provision that these must be considered within the context of the individual's ethnic and cultural background. The prevention or elimination of adverse consequences becomes the rationale for providing treatment, and not necessarily the eradication of some lesion. Viewed in this framework, genetic mutations do no constitute a disease "until a mutation can be shown to demonstrate a definable risk for developing adverse consequences; individuals carrying the mutation should not considered diseased. Thus, a genetic mutation is not an absolute prerequisite for a disease and cannot be used as the sole defining feature of the disease"

(Temple et al, 2001, p. 808). Therefore, phenotype and genotype are considered as states and not diseases.

There are some agreed-upon criteria to being considered a biomedical disease, including a demonstrable pathophysiology or pathochemistry associated with relevant signs (measurable and objective) and symptoms (clinical presentation). According to Jennings (1986), a pathological diagnosis must be able to be established on the basis of evidence that is independent of the patient's response or actions. Despite this, there are a variety of definitions of disease: "an interruption, cessation, or disorder of body function, system or organ" (*Stedman's Medical Dictionary*, 27th ed., 2000); an "impairment of the normal state of the living animal or plant body or any component that interrupts or modifies the performance of vital functions" (*Webster's 3rd New International Dictionary* [unabridged], 1986); an "unhealthy condition of the body or the mind" (*Oxford Pocket Dictionary*, 2002); "a process-type anomaly...prone to having a dynamic evolving course" (Miettinen and Flegel, 2003); "by the functional meaning of any disturbance for the whole organism" (Horton, 1995); and "if it can be recognized, labeled and understood by physicians...medical intervention helps" (Wylie 1970). Wylie also noted a shift away from considering specific causes for each disease to examining the interplay of host, agent, and environment. Taken together, a disease entity is defined by (a) its own pathology (physiological and/or chemical), (b) being independent and self-perpetuating, (c) a constellation of signs and symptoms, and (d) impairment or modification of vital functions.

EVIDENCE FOR CHRONIC PAIN AS A DISEASE

There is considerable evidence to support viewing pain (chronic pain) as a disease entity, not unlike diabetes, arthritis, and multiple sclerosis. As reviewed earlier, there are four types of pain: acute, chronic, neuropathic, and cancer pain.

Acute pain from tissue injury or inflammation tends to (a) resolve as the injured tissues heals or soon thereafter, (b) is a normal response to damage, (c) serves a protective function, and (d) is often associated with increased autonomic activity. By contrast, chronic pain (a) persists for longer than expected and beyond the time frame for healing, (b) serves no protective function, and (c) is rarely accompanied by increased autonomic nervous system activity.

As discussed in Chapter 3, chronic pain has been conveniently divided into nociceptive and neuropathic types. Nociceptive pain (a) arises from outside the nervous system, (b) is primarily influenced by inflammatory changes, (c) involves neural pathways responding to potentially tissue-damaging stimuli, and (d) results for the activation of nociceptive afferents.

Neuropathic pain arises primarily from a lesion or dysfunction in the nervous system. This damage leads to abnormal peripheral or central somatosensory processing, and the resulting pain is accompanied by neurological symptoms and signs (primarily sensory, but also involving motor control system).

Cancer pain is often viewed as a separate category, as it emerges from the presence of a malignant tumor or process.

Because of the tendency to define chronic pain on the basis of its duration, of 3 to 6 months or beyond the normal healing time, it is often interpreted as a prolonged version of acute pain mixed with some combination of comorbid behavior and psychological factors. According to Brookoff (2000), chronic pain is an entirely different phenomenon. With repeated generated pain signals, neural pathways undergo physiochemical changes resulting in hypersensitivity to the pain (nociceptive) signals, which are resistant to antinociceptive input. He postulated that pain signals become embedded in the spinal cord and in part represent an "anti-nociceptive dysfunction."

Siddall and Cousins (2004) describe the process as beginning with the activation of a specific transmission system involving A-delta and C nociceptive fibers in the periphery. This is followed by a release of neurotransmitters, resulting in inflammatory changes (neurogenic inflammation). Activation of this nociceptive system leads to the release of peptides, such as substance P, neurokinin A, and calcitonin gene–related protein (CGRP), from peripheral terminals of the primary afferent fibers. These events provoke a change in the excitatory sensory and sympathetic neuron fiber, vasodilatation, extravasations of plasma proteins, and the release of chemical mediators. This so-called inflammatory soup consisting of noradrenalin, bradykinin, histamine, cytokines, serotonin, nerve growth factor (NGF), and leukotrienes, to name a few, sensitizes the high-threshold nociceptors, resulting in peripheral sensitization (PS). PS manifests itself clinically as increased sensitivity to mechanical or thermal stimuli. At this point, examination of the patient often reveals the presence of hyperalgesia and allodynia.

There are a number of neurochemical changes that accompany persistent nociception. Repeated activation of α-amino-3-hydroxy-5-methyl-4-isoxazolepropionic acid (AMPA) receptors via increased AMPA, a neurotransmitter generally involved in acute pain, leads to the dislodging of magnesium ions. These ions function like a stopper in the transmembrane sodium and calcium channels of the N-methyl-D-aspartic acid (NMDA) receptor complex. NMDA receptors are usually not functional unless there is a persistent and large-scale release of glutamate, the primary neurotransmitter in the dorsal horn of the spinal cord. This conformational change in the neuronal membrane results in increased susceptibility of the NMDA receptor to stimulation (central sensitization). These peripheral and neurochemical changes mark the initial step in the transition from acute to chronic pain. Even at this juncture, it is apparent that chronic pain is clearly something different and distinct from acute pain.

Prolonged activation of peripheral nociceptors results in a dorsal root reflex response involving antidromic activity (conveying of nerve impulses in a direction opposite of normal). The antidromic impulse triggers the release of inflammatory agents such as substance P and NGF, which in turn increases the excitability of the peripheral nociceptor. In this way, afferents that ordinarily conduct impulses from the periphery to the spinal cord also function as efferents. This process stimulates the growth of peripheral nerve terminals (sprouting) and the accumulation of mast cells further enhancing peripheral sensitization. Thus, there is an increase in afferent signals (ectopic discharges), especially from the dorsal root ganglion (DRG) and the neuromas of both injured and uninjured nerves. In addition, any injury to visceral and neural structures is consequated by alterations in the responsiveness of the autonomic nervous system. Nerve injury is associated with sprouting of sympathetic afferents that form a kind of "basket" around the DRG with resultant peripheral vasomotor and pseudomotor changes manifesting themselves as hyperhidrosis, discoloration, temperature change, alteration in nail and hair growth, and osteoporosis. Such signs are commonly observed among patients with complex regional pain syndromes (CRPS).

This scenario outlines how persistent activation of peripheral nociceptors (pain) can result in chemical, physiological, and morphological changes in the peripheral nervous system. At the level of the spinal cord, there is an increase in glutamate and NMDA activity that stimulates a variety of intracellular events (oncogene induction) and increased production of nitric oxide and secondary messengers, including phospholipases, cyclic guanosine, and protein kinases. A peripheral nerve injury induces heightened AMPA and neurotrophin release, as well as sprouting. The ensuing degradation of the inhibitory neurons containing GABA results in disinhibition and increased responsiveness of central nervous system neurons. The loss of disinhibition creates a type of wind-up effect that culminates in sensitization of the central nervous system to nociceptive input. This is followed by an expansion of the receptor field, afterdischarges, and increased spontaneous neuronal activity.

Clinically, the patient is complaining of spontaneous pain, pain that has spread beyond the original area of injury, hypersensitivity to touch and temperature, and persistent dysesthesias. Similar signs are found in patients diagnosed with whiplash or fibromyalgia and, until recently, were attributed primarily to psychological processes. Changes in the peripheral system that are associated with neuropathic pain include ectopic discharges, spontaneous discharges, alterations in sodium and calcium channel expression, collateral sprouting of primary afferents, sprouting of sympathetic neurons into the DRG, and overall nociceptor sensitization.

This description summarizes some of the critical changes that occur in the peripheral nervous system and the central nervous system at the level of the spinal cord. Pathological changes can also be seen in the brain. Activation of the periaqueductal gray matter (PAG) in the midbrain by persistent nociceptive input disrupts normal autonomic and homeostatic mechanisms. Changes in blood pressure and vasomotor and metabolic activity began to occur. Nerve injury and persistent nociception produce changes in the firing patterns of neurons in the lateral and medial thalamus. Low-threshold and wide dynamic range (WDR) neurons fire more readily. There is an increase in background activity and afterdischarges in response to low-threshold stimuli. Neuroimaging studies have revealed a general increase in cortical and subcortical activity secondary to noxious input. Thalamic response to acute pain is decreased. Brain plasticity, highlighted by cortical reorganization in which cortical representation of bodily structures is altered, is also observed (Apkarian et al, 2004, 2005, 2006; Borsook et al, 2011b).

Apkarian et al (2004) compared patients with chronic low back pain (LBP) with normal controls (NC) in different age groups. A morphometric analysis calculating whole brain gray matter on brain MRI was carried out. The results suggested that whole-brain gray matter volume (GMV) decreased at the rate of about 0.5% in normal persons but at 5–11% in the pain patients over the same period of time. Thus, there is a more rapid onset of cortical atrophy, especially in the areas of the dorsolateral prefrontal cortex (DLPFC) and thalamus. They speculated that this might occur in response to the toxic effects of excessive amounts of pain-associated neurotransmitters. Davis et al (2008) reported that cortical thinning was also found in the anterior cingulated and insula cortex in patients diagnosed with irritable bowel syndrome. In addition, Baliki et al (2006) found heightened medial PFC activity, which is often associated with decreased ability in emotional decision-making, independent of the pain being secondary to fracture or inflammatory joint disease, postsurgical, combined, or idiopathic.

Changes in brain chemistry have also been identified in association with pain. For example, there is decreased N-acetyl aspartate and glucose in DLPF and an altered relationship between chemicals within and across brain regions. Total chemical concentration is 6.5% less in DLPFC, with decreased concentration in glucose (17%) and aspartate (7.8%). Glucose in the thalamus is increased by 11.7% (Apkarian et al, 2004). In one study, positive connectivity was found to be weaker in DLPFC in patients with CLBP than in normal individuals, whereas negative chemical connectivity was stronger in the thalamus and cingulate (Lorenz et al, 2003). Regional chemical changes were correlated with pain and anxiety; the strongest effect was in DLPFC (9 times vs. cingulate; 6 times vs. thalamus). Changes in brain chemistry tended to correlate higher with the affective than the sensory component of pain in CLBP. Even the description of the pain was relevant. Patients noting cramping, gnawing, hot, burning, aching, heavy, tender, and splitting pain had higher levels of DLPFC chemistry than those describing their pain as "shooting, stabbing, sharp."

In general, abnormal brain chemistry and chemical networks are associated with persistent nociceptive input. This abnormal pattern of regional chemistry and chemical connectivity is related quantitatively and qualitatively to pain perception. Moreover, as noted before, unique neurochemical changes have been identified when comparing inflammatory, cancer, sciatic nerve ligation, and sciatic nerve ligature-induced pain (Honore et al 2000). These findings may indicate a higher degree of response specificity rather than a general response to nociception.

In addition to examining these physiological changes that occur in response to nociception, one theory of health and disease emphasizes the complex interactions of multiple control mechanisms that allow the individual to adapt to unpredictable changes. Complexification theory views disease and aging and its associated dysfunctions to be associated with the loss of these dynamic relationships—decomplexification. At times, these complex interactions produce physiological outcomes such as heart rate variability (HRV) that appear random and chaotic. Thus, a somewhat recent interest in chaos theory as it relates to medicine and physiology has emerged, including in relation to health, illness, aging, and disease. The connection to chaos and nonlinear dynamics is obvious given the profound increase in the experience of pain-associated comorbidities and dysfunction as a result of alteration in processing but no change in the provocative stimulus.

Consistent with this growing interest in the complex interactions of multiple control mechanisms, Chapman, Tuckett, and Song (2008) used a systems approach to describe the effects of pain and its associated stress (Figure 8.1). They outlined the interactions of the nervous, endocrine, and immune systems. They postulate the existence of "nested" subsystems or component parts manifesting three essential features: (a) irritability, (b) connectivity, and (c) plasticity. The "supersystem" is made up of the three primary systems interacting via an array of neurotransmitters, peptides, endocannabinoids, cytokines, and hormones. The supersystem governs adaptive response to damage or injury.

Supersystem dysfunction includes failed arousal-to-recovery transition, dysfunctional recovery, or dysfunctional subsystem interface. *Dysregulation* is defined as prolonged dysfunction in the ability of a system to recover its normal relationship (homeostasis) to other systems and its normal level of operation to perturbation (agitation) (Chapman et al, 2008, p. 135). Dysregulation can manifest itself in four ways in patients with chronic pain: (a) biorhythm disturbance, (b) diathesis (increased

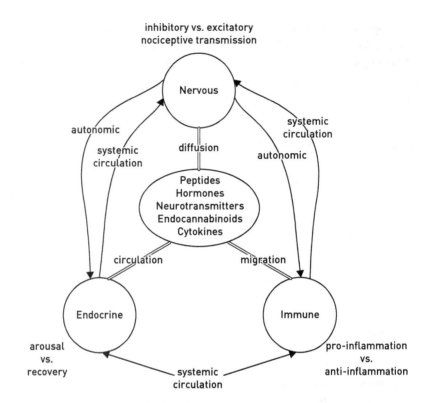

inhibitory vs. excitatory
nociceptive transmission

Nervous

autonomic

systemic
circulation

diffusion

systemic
circulation

autonomic

Peptides
Hormones
Neurotransmitters
Endocannabinoids
Cytokines

circulation

migration

Endocrine

Immune

arousal
vs.
recovery

pro-inflammation
vs.
anti-inflammation

systemic
circulation

FIGURE 8.1

Nervous, endocrine, and immune subsystems communicate dynamically using the language of common chemical substances, as indicated in the center of the figure. The major language elements are peptides, hormones, neurotransmitters, endocannabinoids, and cytokines. These substances are pleiotropic in that they exert different effects depending on context (e.g., phase and location). Circulation, diffusion, and migration are some of the processes of information transmission. Systemic circulation and autonomic nervous system activity are other vehicles of information transmission. Because the nervous, endocrine, and immune systems have constant reciprocal communication, they tend to react to a stressor in a highly orchestrated manner, as a single unit. From Chapman CR, Tuckett RP, Song CW. Pain and stress in a systems perspective; reciprocal neural, endocrine and immune interactions. *J Pain.* 2008;9(2):122–145. Reprinted with permission.

vulnerability to pathological consequences), (c) genetics (interacts with genetically based differences in pain sensitivity and responsiveness to treatments), (d) epigenetics (heritable traits not related to DNA structure, e.g., environmental and ancestral influences). Therefore, ongoing nociception has an impact on the nervous, endocrine, and immune subsystems; their interactions; and their ability to adapt and bring about a "normal" input–output relationship.

PAIN AND STRESS SUPERSYSTEM

Permanent alterations in the nervous system, as described in the caption for Figure 8.1, may lead to persistent dysregulation or decomplexification. A large study of patients with chronic LBP in Norway by Hagen et al (2006) noted increased incidence of pseudo-neurological, gastrointestinal, and allergy-type symptoms as the number of musculoskeletal complaints increased. A significantly higher percentage of LBP patients compared to non-pain normal controls reported complaints in other bodily systems. It appears that patients with LBP suffer from a kind of pain syndrome comprising generalized pain and sleep and mood disturbance, with associated comorbidities involving the neurological, immune, and endocrine systems.

By way of exemplifying the effects of ongoing nociception on the supersystem, Shavit et al (1984) found that uncontrolled pain can inhibit cytotoxic activity of natural killer cells thought to play a surveillance role against tumor development and growth. This suppression or alternation of suppressive immune mechanisms normally serving to defend the body can directly or indirectly contribute to increased tumor growth. Indeed, Lewis et al (1983/84) discovered that pain can actually accelerate the growth of experimentally introduced tumors. Suppression of these natural defenses may also result in a requirement for a higher dose of opioid in an effort to treat the pain. In turn, increased use of opioids can have greater immunosuppressive and tumor-enhancing effects.

It is well known that the use of opioids in the treatment of pain is associated with hormonal alterations. However, pain in and of itself can stimulate hormonal dysfunction and dysregulation in the pituitary–adrenal–gonadal axis. Severe pain as a stressor can overstimulate the pituitary–adrenal axis, causing a release of catecholamines, including adrenaline and noradrenalin. Adrenocorticotrophin hormone (ACTH) released from the pituitary activates the adrenal cortex. The release of glucocorticoids (cortisol and pregnenolone) can be seen in serum levels.

Although a short-term increase in cortisol levels poses little danger, Tennant (2008, 2010) has shown that the effects of sustained elevations in cortisol levels can be quite destructive. Osteoporosis, dental erosion, obesity, hyperglycemia, hyperlipidemia, reduced pain control, more rapid deterioration of the spine, tachycardia, and hypertension are potential consequences. Elevated serum catecholamines can precipitate the development of a myofascial pain syndrome. In the most extreme cases, adrenal exhaustion occurs, highlighted by dangerously low serum pregnenolone and cortisol levels. Pituitary tumors, deficiencies in estrogens and androgens, hormone-induced vegetative state (insomnia, muscle wasting, stares, slow or soft speech, lethargy, diminished functioning, psychomotor retardation), and even unexplained death have been associated with severely depressed serum hormone levels.

One would logically surmise that if pain is a disease causing adverse consequences for the individual, then eliminating or reducing the pain should positively affect or reverse these consequences. This was demonstrated by Smith, Staats, and their colleagues (2002). In a multicenter study, patients with cancer pain treated with intrathecal drug delivery (IDD) therapy were compared to those receiving conventional medical management (CMM). A prospective randomized design was used. The results showed that IDD was more effective than CMM. But more importantly, survival time increased for those patients with the greater level of pain relief. When these results are combined with those from studies showing improved levels of cortical gray matter following a significant reduction in pain as a result of total hip replacement or cognitive behavioral therapy (Baliki et al, 2011; Jokic-Begic, 2010; Rodriguez-Raecke et al, 2009), the evidence linking pain reduction to a decrease in pain-related adverse consequences appears to be mounting.

DYNAMIC VS. GENETIC DISEASE

Diseases are often viewed from a genetic perspective, which involves (a) identifying the abnormality, (b) mapping out the abnormality, (c) determining the genome, and (d) developing a therapy (see Chapter 12). The therapeutic implications include prevention; environmental modifications, such as altering exposure to toxic agents; removing deficient organs; and gene therapy. Mackey and Glass (1977), however, introduced a "dynamical" approach to disease and are credited with introducing the term *dynamical disease*. Dynamical diseases are associated with qualitative changes in the dynamics of an intact physiological system, are studied from the perspective of nonlinear dynamics (Bélair et al, 1995), and can be found within the areas of neurology and psychiatry (Milton and Black, 1995).

A dynamical disease is not a result of some genetic predisposition or external event but emerges from a system operating within is own parameters but which occasionally produces anomalous dynamics (Mackey and Milton, 1987). In essence, the disease is embedded in the physiological system itself. This is exemplified by Lambert's (2010) notion of migraine headache being pathology-free and arising from noise-induced changes; the headache "just happens" as result of random noise in the system. In this approach to disease one analyzes complex rhythms as a means of providing a diagnosis and prognosis, developing methods of control based on the dynamics of the physiological system, improving the identification or perturbing of the dynamics, and finally, adjusting the parameters to their normal range. A fundamental assumption is that the dynamics of chaotic systems are notoriously sensitive to small changes in initial conditions of control parameters of the system. Pooling data may obscure these changes. Increased emphasis is given to examining the individual organism.

A bifurcation (the transition from one dynamic state to another) is said to exist wherein at a given point there is an abrupt change, as seen, for example, in epilepsy, rapid cycling bipolar disease, and migraine headache. Dynamical diseases can arise from pathological alterations in the physiological control system, as might be the case with sudden or ongoing nociceptive activation. Rather than removing "defective" parts or covering up changes in system dynamics, treatment emphasizes restoration of normal, healthy dynamics through the use of pharmacological, electrical, and mechanical interventions. For example, as seen earlier, neuropathic pain has been associated with thalamocortical dysrhythmia (TCD), which may well represent an example of bifurcation (disruption in normal physiological control parameters) in response to changes in the normal dynamics of the physiological system. Traditional pharmacological agents target the transduction and transmission components of the system but not the altered thalamocortical dynamics.

Goldberger (1996; Goldberger and West, 1987) took a slightly different approach, emphasizing the chaotic or complex aspect of the system. He noted that healthy hearts tend to manifest a much greater variability in behavior during a time-series analysis than was previously thought. Hearts at risk seemed overly constrained and ordered. He concluded, "Healthy systems don't want homeostasis, they want chaos" (Goldberger and West, 1987; Lipsitz and Goldberger, 1992).

Similarly, Thayer and Brosschot's (2005) neurovisceral-integration theory illustrated the development of "rigid regularity" as a result of decreased parasympathetic tone and the emergence of sympathoexcitatory (vagal dominance). The loss of the usual reciprocal inhibitory activity ushers in a state of decomplexification. Therapy should focus on resuming the normal dynamics of the systems instead of noting the relative absence of tissue damage to account for the pain of functional or medically unexplained symptoms (MUS). Healthy biological systems are seen as those that are complex, adaptable, and efficient. However, disease and decay are common features of oversimplification (decomplexification) of the dynamics.

CONCLUSION

In general, a biomarker represents an indicator of a biological state and one that can be objectively measured. The presence of certain molecular, anatomical, or physiological characteristics can represent the tendency toward, the existence of, or the rate of progression of a disease. Neuronal degeneration in Alzheimer's disease, blood glucose levels in diabetes, and lymphatic function in cardiovascular disease are common examples. Pundits would argue against pain as a disease given the absence of a biomarker. Cohen et al (2013), for example, reject the notion of pain as a disease, claiming the argument confuses "pain-as-an-experience, pain-as-a-symptom, pain-as-a-pathological-entity, and pain-as-a-cause-of-pathology" (p. 1287). They favor viewing pain as a product of neuroplasticity. Siddall (2013) provides a counterargument supported by data of the type discussed in this chapter. Likewise, Borsook et al. (2011a,b) have identified functional, morphometric, and chemical changes that may serve as biomarkers of pain as a disease state. Changes in synchronization, oscillatory frequency, and coherence (see Chapter 4) may also exemplify "biomarkers" of pain as a dynamical disease. Abnormal physiological rigidity, represented by the neurovisceral-integration model (see Chapter 7) used to explain MUS, provides evidence of decomplexification. The debate over pain as a disease is clouded by a number of definitional issues (Doleys, 2012). However, the need to expand the paradigm through which we view pain (chronic) appears undeniable.

As summarized by Cousins (1999; Siddall and Cousins, 2004), a disease entity (a) has its own pathology (physiological and chemical), (b) is independent and self-perpetuating, (c) consists of a constellation of signs and symptoms, and (d) impairs or modifies vital functions. Chronic pain has been shown to be associated with pathological changes in physiological processing, including those in the peripheral nervous system such as antidromic activity and peripheral sensitization. Central sensitization and altered cortical activity are also seen in the central nervous system (Coderre et al, 1993). The type and amount of alterations in neurotransmitters and inflammatory substances constitute components of chemical-related pathology. Morphological changes are represented by cell death, sprouting, and cortical reorganization. Finally, there is the documented impact of chronic pain on patients, their families, and society. Thus, nociceptive and neuropathic inputs produce altered sensory inputs from the periphery secondary to increased input processing, resulting in pathological changes. The observed signs and symptoms are dependent and unique, physiological and chemical, thus meeting the criteria of a disease entity.

In discussing chronic pain as a disease, it is important not to eliminate the patient from the equation. Viewing chronic pain as merely a failure of homeostasis (homeodynamics) or the homeostatic system de-emphasizes the interaction between the patient and disease process. As illustrated in the pain processing system (see Chapter 5), the amount of overall stress on the system (patient) can influence the ultimate outcome. There are many patients with diabetes and cardiovascular disease who, by virtue of their participation in disease-modifying behaviors (e.g., diet, stress management, weight control, and exercise) alter the trajectory of their disease process. Consistent with quantum theory, the various outcomes following the diagnosis of a disease may be held in a superposition—that which emerges relates to a variety of factors, only one of which is the disease pathology itself.

The issue of persistent (chronic) pain as disease is still being debated. It is a debate worth having, as the process and the outcome will only serve to advance and surely alter our view of pain. Thoughtful deliberation has been a important ingredient in the modern history of investigating pain. Assertions and conjectures may or may not be proven but they are necessary, to avoid theoretical complacency and stagnation.

REFERENCES

Apkarian AV, Bushnell MC, Treede RD, Zubieta JK. Human brain mechanisms of pain perception and regulation in health and disease. *Eur J Pain*. 2005;9:463–484.

Apkarian AV, Scholz J. Shared mechanisms between chronic pain and neurodegenerative disease. *Drug Discovery Today: Disease Mechanisms*. 2006;3(3):319–326.

Apkarian AV, Sosa Y, Sonty S, et al. Chronic back pain is associated with decreased prefrontal and thalamic gray matter density. *J Neurosci*. 2004;24:10410–10415.

Backonja MM. Defining neuropathic pain. *Anesth Analg*. 2003;97:785–790.

Baliki MN, Chialvo DR, Geha PY, et al. Chronic pain and the emotional brain: specific brain activity associated with spontaneous fluctuations of intensity of chronic back pain. *J Neurosci*. 2006;26:12165–12173.

Baliki MN, Schnitzer TJ, Bauer WR, et al. Brain morphological signatures for chronic pain. *PLoS ONE*. 2011:6(10):e26010.

Ballantyne J. Opioids for chronic nonterminal pain. *South Med J*. 2006;11:1244–1255.

Basbaum A, Julis D. Towards better pain control. *Sci Am*. 2006;(June):61–67.

Bélair J, Glass L, an der Heiden U, Milton J. Dynamical disease: identification, temporal aspects and treatment strategies of human illness. *Chaos*. 1995;5(1):1–8.

Bonica J, ed. *Advances in Neurology, International Symposium on Pain*. New York: Raven Press; 1974.

Borsook D, Becerra L, Hargreaves R. Biomarkers for chronic pain and analgesia: part 1. The need, reality challenges, and solutions. *Discovery Medicine*. 2011a;11(58):197–207.

Borsook D, Becerra L, Hargreaves R. Biomarkers for chronic pain and analgesia: part 2. How, where, and what to look for using functional imaging. *Discovery Medicine*. 2011b;11(58):209–219.

Bridges D, Thompson SWN, Rice ASC. Mechanisms of neuropathic pain. *Br J Anesth*. 2001;87:12–26.

Brookoff D. Chronic pain: 1. A new disease? *Hosp Pract*. 2000;35(7);45–52.

Casey KL, Bushnell MC. Pain imaging. *Pain: Clinical Updates*. 2000;8:1–4.

Chapman CR, Tuckett RP, Song CW. Pain and stress in a systems perspective; reciprocal neural, endocrine and immune interactions. *J Pain*. 2008;9(2):122–145.

Coderre TJ, Katz J, Vaccarino AL, Melzack R. Contribution of central neuroplasticity to pathological pain: review of clinical and experimental evidence. *Pain*. 1993;52:259–285.

Cohen M, Quintner J, Buchanan D. Is chronic pain a disease? *Pain Med*. 2013;14:1284–1288.

Cousins M. Pain: the past, present, and future of anesthesiology. *Anesthesiology*. 1999;91:538–551.

Davis KD, Pope C, Chen J, Kwan CL, Crawlet AP, Diamant NE. Cortical thinning in IBS: implications for homeostatic, attention, and pain processing. *Neurology*. 2008;70:153–154.

Doleys DM. How neuroimaging studies have challenged us to rethink: is chronic pain a disease? *J Pain*. 2010;11(4):399–400.

Gallagher RM, Verma S. Mood and anxiety disorders in chronic pain. In Dworkin RH, Breitbart WS, eds. *Psychosocial Aspects of Pain: A Handbook for Health Care Providers, Progress in Pain Research and Management*, Vol. 27. Seattle: IASP Press; 2004:139–178.

Gillum LA, Gouveia C, Dorsey ER, et al. NIH disease funding levels and burden of disease. *PLoS ONE*. 2011;6(2):e16837.

Goldberger AL. Non-lineardynamics for clinicians: chaos theory, fractals and complexity at the bedside. *Lancet*. 1996;347:1312–1314.

Goldberger AL, West BJ. Applications of nonlinear dynamics to clinical cardiology. *Ann N Y Acad Sci*. 1987;504:155–212.

Hagen EM, Svensen E, Erikse HR, Ihlebaek C, Ursin H. Comorbid subjective health complaints in low back pain. *Spine*. 2006;31(12):1491–1495.

Honore P, Rogers SD, Schwei MJ, et al. Murine models of inflammatory, neuropathic and cancer pain each generates a unique set of neurochemical changes in the spinal cord and sensory neurons. *Neuroscience*. 2000;98:585–598.

Horton R. Georges Canguilhem: philosopher of disease. *J Roy Soc Med*. 1995;86:316–319.

Isdarola JM, Caudle RM. Good pain: bad pain. *Science*. 1997;278(5336):239–240.

Jennings D. The confusion between disease and illness in clinical medicine. *CMAJ*. 1986;135:865–865.

Jokic-Begic N. Cognitive-behavioral therapy and neuroscience: toward closer integration. *Psychological Topics*. 2010:19(2):235–254.

Lambert GA. The lack of peripheral pathology in migraine headache. *Headache*. 2010;50:895–908.

Lewis JW, Shavit Y, Terman GW, Gale RP, Liebeskind JC. Stress and morphine affect survival of rats challenged with a mammary ascites tumor (MAT 13762B). *Nat Immun Cell Growth Regul*. 1983/84;3:43–50.

Liebeskind J. Pain can kill. *Pain*. 1991;44:3–4.

Lipsitz LA, Goldberger AL. Loss of "complexity" and aging: potential applications of fractals and chaos theory to senescence. *JAMA*. 1992;267:1806–1809.

Loeser JD. Pain: disease or dis-ease? The John Bonica lecture: presented at the Third World Congress of World Institute of Pain, Barcelona 2004. *Pain Pract*. 2005;5:77–84.

Lorenz J, Minoshima S, Casey K. Keeping pain out of mind: the role of the dorsolateral prefrontal cortex in pain modulation. *Brain*. 2003;126(5):1079–1091.

Mackey MC, Glass L. Oscillation and chaos in physiological control systems. *Science*. 1977;197:287–289.

Mackey MC, Milton JG. Dynamical diseases. *Ann N Y Acad Sci*. 1987;504:16–32.

McCaffery M. *Nursing Practice Theories Related to Cognition, Bodily Pain, and Man-Environment Interactions*. Los Angeles: UCLA Students' Store. 1968.

Melzack R. Evolution of the neuromatrix theory of pain. The Prithvi Raj lecture: presented at the Third World Congress of World Institute of Pain, Barcelona 2004. *Pain Pract*. 2005;5:85–94.

Mendell JR, Sahenk Z. Painful sensory neuropathy. *N Engl J Med*. 2003;348:1243–1255.

Merskey H, Bogduck N. *Classification of Chronic Pain*, 2nd ed. Seattle: IASP Press; 1994:208–213.

Miettinen OS, Flegel KM. Elementary concepts of medicine: V. Disease: one of the main subtypes of illness. *J Eval Clin Pract*. 2003;9(3):321–323.

Milton J, Black D. Dynamic disease in neurology and psychiatry. *Chaos*. 1995;5(1):8–13.

Niv D, Devor M. Chronic pain as a disease in its own right. *Pain Pract*. 2004;4(3):179–181.

Pilowsky I. Chronic pain as a disease entity. *Triangle (Sandoz)*. 1981;20:27–32.

Rodriguez-Raecke R, Nieneier A, Ihle K, et al. Brain gray matter decrease in pain is the consequence and not the cause. *J Neurosci*. 2009;29(44):13746–13750.

Sarno JE. *The Mind-Body Prescription: Healing the Body, Healing the Pain*. New York: Warner Books; 1998.

Scadding JG. Essentialism and nominalism in medicine: logic of diagnosis in disease terminology. *Lancet*. 1996;348:594–596.

Scully JL. What is a disease? Disease, disability and their definitions. *EMBO Rep*. 2004;5(7):650–653.

Shavit Y, Lewis JW, Terman GW, et al. Opioid peptides mediate the suppressive effect of stress on natural killer cell activity. *Science*. 1984;223:188–190.

Siddall PJ. Is chronic pain a dieases? *Pain Med*. 2013;14:1289–1290.

Siddall PJ, Cousins MJ. Persistent pain as a disease entity: implication for clinical management. *Anesth Analg*. 2004;99:510–520.

Smith TJ, Staats PS, Deer T, et al. Randomized clinical trial of an implantable drug delivery system compared with comprehensive medical management for refractory cancer pain: impact on pain, drug-related toxicity, and survival. *J Clin Oncol*. 2002;20:4040–4049.

Sternbach RA. *Pain: Patients, Traits, and Treatments*. New York: Academic Press; 1974.

Temple LKF, McLeod RS, Gallinger S, Wright JG. Defining disease in the genomics era. *Science*. 2001;293(5531):807–808.

Tennant F. Longitudinal study of long-term opioid patients. *Pract Pain Manag*. 2008;8(7):54–58.

Tennant F. Hormone replacements in the treatment of chronic pain. *Pract Pain Manag*. 2010;10(1):36–40.

Thayer JF, Brosschot JF. Psychosomatics and psychopathology: looking up and down from the brain. *Psychoneuroimmunology*. 2005;30:1050–1058.

Woolf CJ. Pain: moving from symptom control toward mechanism-specific pharmacologic management. *Ann Intern Med*. 2004;140:441–451.

Woolf CJ, Mannion RJ. Neuropathic pain: aetiology, symptoms, mechanisms, and management. *Lancet*. 1999;353:1959–1964.

Wylie CM. The definition and measurement of health and disease. *Publ Health Rep*. 1970;85(2):100–104.

9 Pain in Neonates and Infants

Infants that are born pre-term arrive in an untimely manner before their anatomy and physiology are prepared to cope with an extra-uterine environment.
–C.C. Johnston, A.M. Fernandes, and M. Campbell-Yeo (2011, p. S65)

Infant pain is simply not an immature adult one but stems from a quite different underlying structural and functional connectivity within the central nervous system.
–M. Fitzgerald and S. Beggs (2001, p. 254)

INTRODUCTION

Shortly after his premature birth, in 1985, Jeffery Lawson underwent open heart surgery. Incisions were made in both sides of his neck, his right chest, and breastbone around to his backbone. His ribs were pried apart, and an extra artery near his heart was tied off. Another opening was created in his left chest wall for a chest tube. All of this was carried out while he was awake and conscious, as he had only been administered a paralytic agent, Pavulon. Unfortunately, he died 5 weeks later. When asked about the surgery, the anesthesiologist noted that Jeffery was too young to tolerate anesthesia. Plus, it had never been proven to her that premature babies feel pain (JR Lawson, 1986, 1988).

This chapter charts the history of medical attitudes toward and research on infant pain. It addresses both the denial of infant pain and the shift toward acknowledging that neonates and infants do experience pain. The early neurological development of cortical connections relaying pain and the neurophysiological development leading to pain response are also detailed. Finally, the long-term effects of infant experiences of pain are reviewed.

The issue of pain in neonates and infants has had an interesting history. In 1938, Thorek wrote, "Often no anesthesia is required. A sucker consisting of a sponge dipped in some sugar water will often suffice to calm a baby" (p. 2021). Upon discussing neurosurgery in infants and children, Perret and Meyers (1960) commented, "Small infants up to the age of four weeks may be easily managed with a sugar-alcohol nipple narcosis, supplemented by local anesthesia" (p. 545). More recently, Swafford and Allen (1968) contended that "pediatric patients seldom need medication for the relief of pain after general surgery. They tolerate discomfort well. The child will say he does not feel well or that he is uncomfortable or wants his parents, but often he will not relate this unhappiness to pain" (p. 134).

The problem of undertreating pain in children was highlighted by Eland and Anderson (1977) when they reported that, in their study, only 12 of 25 four- to eight-year-olds received postoperative analgesic medications. Eighteen children of this group of 25 were then compared to 18 adults with similar diagnoses. The adults received a total of 372 opioid analgesic doses postoperatively and 299 nonopioid analgesic doses compared to a total of 24 doses for the entire group of 18 children! A survey of neonatal intensive care units (NICUs) in the United States by Frank (1987) revealed that sedatives were as likely to be used for pain as morphine. This would suggest an emphasis on sedating the neonate rather than managing the pain. In France only 20% of pain-producing procedures (heel-sticks, heel-lancing, and venipuncture) are accompanied by any pain management and in Canada less than 50%. Rawlins et al (2007) reported that only 13% of a group of 208 children averaging 5 years of age presenting to an emergency room with burns were provided any analgesic medications. A separate report in 2002 found that less than 50% of children presenting with acute limb fractures received analgesic medications.

It is tempting to consider this apparent lack of attention to pain in infants as a very archaic, if not prehistoric or barbaric, position. Yet, it seems that infants were accorded greater consideration in ancient times than in the 20th century. Even Plato (~400 BCE) believed that the beginning of life (birth) was so violent that for an infant all feelings were essentially painful. In the Middle Ages, when pain was attributed to the wrath of God or the influence of demons, infants were seen as especially vulnerable. In the fifth century, St. Augustine ascribed all the diseases of Christians to demons. These demons tended, Saint Augustine believed, to torment the newly baptized, "yea even the guiltless newborn infant." Hippocrates contended that with experience comes a greater ability to tolerate pain, indicating that even the weak and old tolerate pain better than the young and unaccustomed. In his 1656 book, *The Children's Book*, Felix Wurtz emphasized that infants, especially the premature, by virtue of their immaturity, were particularly sensitive to pain. Many others, including Hess in 1849 and Starr in 1895, called attention to the behavior of infants, such as crying, sleep patterns, and facial expressions, as indicators of their distress.

The 20th century has been coined the "century of infant pain skepticism and denial" (Rodkey and Riddell, 2013). Intended or not, infants were perceived as "a lower animal in human form." In the last hundred years, scientific authorities robbed babies of their cries by calling them "random sound," robbed them of their smiles by calling them "muscle spasms" or "gas," robbed them of their memories by calling them "fantasies," and robbed them of their pain by calling it a "reflex" (Chamberline,1991). In a search for journal articles relating to infant pain, Chamberline was able to identify only 20 publications during the time period 1920–1980, but 4 or 5 in the 1980s alone. This increase appears to reflect a newfound concern and interest in infant pain, perhaps stimulated by the work of Anand and his colleagues (Anand, 2006; Anand and Craig, 1996; Anand and Hickey, 1987; Anand et al, 1987, 1998, 2012; Lowery et al, 2007).

In a review of the pivotal events relating to infant-pain denial during this time period, Rodkey and Riddell (2013) cite the 1873 work of Genzmer. He studied the response of premature infants to pinpricks in sensitive areas and noted the absence of any sign of discomfort despite the presence of droplets of blood. Inexplicably, he apparently ignored the presence of "wetness of their eyes," concluding that pain was not well developed in the neonate. McGraw's related research extended from 1935 to 1969. In one study she stimulated 75 infants with a safety pin, from birth to 4 years of age, for a total of 2,008 observations. The usual response was described as consisting "of diffuse bodily movements accompanied by crying, and possibly a local reflex" (McGraw, 1941). The notion of a "local reflex" reinforced the prevailing medical view that such reactions were mechanical in nature, without any mental or emotional experience. Even if some type of sensitivity to pain existed or was acknowledged it was considered to occur at the subcortical level. Despite the fact that the babies did react, cry, and withdraw their limbs, McGraw asserted only limited sensitivity to pain existed in the first week to 10 days and labeled this a period of "hypesthesia." This assertion soon became an accepted fact.

Pratt et al in 1873 and Crudden in 1937 used thermal stimulation, created by running water of varying temperatures through cylinders attached to various part of the infant's body, to study infant pain. Extreme reactions, especially to cold, were noted. Indeed, any deviation from normal body temperature resulted in a sudden change in respiration and circulation. In his book *Cerebral Function in Infancy and Childhood*, Peiper (1963) summarized his work in the 1920s, noting a distinct physical reaction and crying in response to painful stimulation in premature babies and newborns. Contrary to Genzmer, Peiper claimed that a pinprick would easily arouse any normal infant or immature newborn. A lack of reaction was interpreted as a sign of pathology or illness. Peiper's advocacy for infant pain and the rights of infants were relatively ignored by the medical community, apparently because it clashed with the conventional medical wisdom of the day.

Rodkey and Riddell (2013) point out two factors that may have influenced this indifference to infant pain. First were the writings of Darwin. They noted that "children were lumped together with animals, savages and the insane as primitives whose emotional expression was simply reflex actions reinforced by habit, making them less reliable markers of pain" (Rodkye and Riddell, 2013, p. 343). Second was the behaviorism movement represented by Watson. The behaviorist tendency was to conceptualize infant pain within a simple stimulus–response paradigm. The reductionistic behaviorist perspective was described as searching for reflexes and not consciousness, in a sense decorticating the infant.

The Declaration of Helsinki (1974) re-emphasized the previously muted concerns over infant pain. Research efforts beginning in the mid-1980s led to a much greater appreciation for the impact of noxious stimulation on the neonate and infant and the true complexity of infant pain. Rodkey and Riddell (2013) state that "the sad history of infant pain research reads as an indictment of the modern scientific perspective; the transformation of the infant into a mechanistic scientific object resulted in medical insensitivity and experimental bias" (p. 348). The main medical objections to infant anesthesia were that it was unnecessary and dangerous. Subsequent research has suggested that infants benefit from and tolerate anesthesia well. Those infants previously undergoing surgery without such treatment had probably died of metabolic and endocrine shock following unanesthetized operations.

For example, Anand et al (1987) presented some very compelling data on the benefits of anesthesia for preterm babies and infants. Neonates of about 28.4 weeks' gestation and averaging about 1 kilogram (2.2 pounds) in weight underwent ligation of a patent ductus arteriosus. Each baby was given the standard nitrous oxide and D-tubocurarine (curare) preoperatively. Half of the babies were also given IV fentanyl anesthesia (10 μg/kg). Those receiving fentanyl had a much lower hormonal stress response. The non-fentanyl group was more likely to require ventilator support postoperatively and to have circulatory or metabolic complications. It was concluded that the stress response to surgery was mediated through neural impulses from the site of injury acting on the hypothalamus. This stress response can be avoided by using regional anesthesia at the site of injury, thus preventing the propagation of impulses, or by suppression of hypothalamic and cerebral cortex activity with opioid analgesia. However, Giannakoulopoulos (1994) argued that a hormonal response cannot be equated with the perception (conscious awareness) of pain. Likewise, Lloyd-Thomas and Fitzgerald (1996) stated that if "feeling" and "pain" are properly understood, then the fetus cannot be said to "feel" pain in the ordinary sense of the word.

Although fentanyl appears to suppress a physiological response to nociception, this finding does not ensure total absence of awareness of the pain. At the time of the Anand et al's (1987) study it was believed that (a) newborns are incapable of perceiving and localizing pain because of the relative immaturity of their central nervous system (CNS), and (b) they lacked any memory for a previous painful experience. However, based on (a) the presence of behaviors such as grimacing, vocalization, and withdrawal in response to heel prick and (b) indications of metabolic activity in areas of the brain associated with pain perception, a reconsideration of the attitude toward neonatal pain and the need for anesthesia was urged. Anand et al (1987) also proposed that the degree of analgesia in the paralyzed and ventilated infant could be assessed effectively using biochemical and endocrine markers. They concluded that a newborn's response to pain is "similar to but greater than those in adult subjects."

Researchers in the 19th and 20th centuries discovered the existence and importance of a thin layer of tissue surrounding nerve fibers, the myelin sheath. It was presumed that nerves did not function optimally until the myelination process was completed. Therefore, it was reasoned, because infants have an immature anatomical and physiological nervous system, they are less sensitive to pain. It seems ironic that the same concept of immaturity of the nervous system used by Hippocrates and others in the fourth and fifth centuries to emphasize infants' sensitivity to pain was, some 1,500 years later, used to explain their presumed relative insensitivity to pain.

There appear to be four assumptions, now disproven, that guided early 20th-century thinking about pain in infants and children (Unruh 1992):

(1) Neonates (defined as 1–28 days of age) do not have sufficient neurological or physiological maturity to be capable of pain perception.
(2) Infants (from the Latin word *infants* meaning "speechless," defined as age 1–12 months) and children are less sensitive to and more tolerant of pain than adults.

(3) Pain assessment in infants and children without language is at best unscientific and subjective.
(4) Provisions of pain relief is more injurious than leaving the infant or child in pain.

Scientists and clinicians seem to be in agreement that the fetus, neonate, and infant *do* experience physiological distress and warrant effective treatment (American Academy of Pediatrics, 2006; Barr, 1998; O'Donnell et al, 2002; Schecter et al, 1997; Walco et al, 1994). However, they remain embroiled in the debate as to whether or not what is experienced by the neonate and infant constitutes pain as presently defined by the International Association for the Study of Pain (IASP).

MEANING OF PAIN

The definition and meaning of pain, and its relationship to the fetus and neonate, remains open to question (Anand and Craig, 1996; Cunningham, 1996; Derbyshire, 1996, 2003; Richards, 1985). Even more fundamental to the issue of pain is the manner by which it is determined that the fetus or neonate is in pain. That is, what is it that defines the presence of pain? Options include withdrawal response, arousal, avoidance, verbal report, anticipatory response, physiological reactivity, and an emotional response, to name a few.

Some caution against any definition of pain that requires a verbal report, claiming this excludes animals and nonverbal humans such as infants, and those with various cognitive and communications impairments. This issue might be partially resolved by entertaining B.F Skinner's (1957) definition of verbal behavior as "behavior reinforced through the mediation of other persons. Any movement capable of affecting the behavior of another organism may be verbal" (p. 14). In this context, grimacing, crying, and wincing would be considered verbal behavior if they were associated with a specific behavior response on the part of the observer. The comprehensible utterance of words is certainly a type of verbal behavior, but it is not the only type. Sign language would clearly be considered a type of verbal behavior.

In addition, the infant's verbal response, or its absence, to a presumed noxious stimulus may be influenced by a variety of factors. For example, Brazelton (1961) noted that anesthetics given to the mother during labor can make their way into the infant's system and take up to a week to leave. In discussing the infant's response to circumcision, Goldman (1997) points out Call's report of some infants lapsing into a semi-coma, while Brooks commented that in four of the nine circumcisions she observed, the baby did not cry but rather appeared to be in a state of shock. The evidence suggests that even in the absence of any verbal pain response the blood levels of stress hormones were significantly elevated. Some medical researchers interpret this to be a biological marker and more reliable indicator of pain than even crying itself.

In 1992 Rogers stated that it was "our responsibility to treat pain in neonates and infants as effectively as we do in other patients" (p. 56). This attitude was stimulated by a report from Anand et al (1987) noting improved clinical outcomes in neonates that were given fentanyl anesthesia in preparation for surgery. These data begged the question as to whether fetuses and neonates feel pain (Craig et al, 1993), and if so, if it differed from that of more physiologically mature humans. For some the question appeared absurd and the answer seemed obvious. However, Derbyshire (1998, 2003) argued that our entire concept and definition of pain, particularly when viewed as a conscious phenomenon, can be called into question, depending on our view of infant and neonatal pain. Can a physiologically immature organism such as a fetus be said to "feel pain" in the same way as an adult? If so, how would we know?

DEVELOPMENT OF CORTICAL CONNECTIONS

Upon examining the biological development of the fetus, Fitzgerald (1987, 1994) made the following six observations. First, at 7.5 weeks' gestation there is a reflex response to somatic stimulation. Touching the perioral region produces contralateral bending of the head. Second, at 10.5 weeks, stroking of the hands produces a response. Third, at 13.5 weeks the rest of the body and hind limbs became sensitive. Shortly after the development of sensitivity, hyperexcitability resulting from repeated stimulation can be observed, suggesting a functional pain system and an intact pain response. Fourth, thalamocortical fibers do not penetrate the cortical plane (cortex) until 26 weeks, at which time the response to noxious stimulation can be differentiated from other distress responses. Thus, it can be said that a fetus or premature infant of at least 26 weeks' gestation will respond to invasive procedures in a fashion similar to neonates. Intrauterine needling of the fetus at 20 to 34 weeks' gestation to obtain blood samples from the umbilical vein instead of the umbilical cord produces a hormonal and neural stress response preventable by anesthetics.

Fitzgerald's fifth observation was that cortical regions determined to be important in the processing of the various components of pain (the pain matrix) are not fully responsive until after birth. The use of PET scanning has allowed researchers to track the time periods at which certain cortical structures appear to become activated (Chugani and Phelps, 1986). Glucose utilization is used as a measure of structural activity. Using this technology, in infants 5 weeks of age and younger increased glucose utilization was noted in the sensorimotor cortex, thalamus, midbrain–brainstem, and cerebellar vermis (Klimach and Cooke, 1988). By age 3 months increased activity was found in the parietal, temporal, and occipital cortices and basal ganglia. Activity in the frontal lobe and association regions was not observed until 8 months of age.

Finally, Fitzgerald observed that descending pain inhibitory pathways tend to develop only after the afferent ascending excitatory pathways. The development of the nociceptive system in summarized in Figure 9.1.

The human cerebral cortex has six layers, numbered I–VI, from superficial to deep. The neuronal shapes, sizes, densities, and organization of nerve fibers differ for each layer. Layers I–III (the supragranular region), when mature, allow for communication between one portion of the cortex and other regions. The internal granular layer (layer IV) is most important to our topic of pain. Layer IV is more prominent in the primary sensory cortices and is the primary target of thalamocortical afferents from thalamus type-C neurons. Finally, layers V and VI (the infragranular) connect the cerebral context to subcortical areas and are most appreciated in the motor cortices. Layer V gives rise to the cortical efferent projections to basal ganglia, brainstem, and spinal cord, while layer VI projects primarily to the thalamus.

During fetal development, the immature cerebral cortex (the cortical plate) is positioned between the marginal zone above and the subplate zone, located just below the cortical plate. The fetal subplate zone, a transient structure, and the intermediate zone are the precursors for neonatal white matter (glial cells and myelinated axons). The

Anatomical/ Functional Characteristic	Description	Gestational Age, wk
Peripheral cutaneous sensory receptors	Perioral cutaneous sensory receptors	7.5
	Palmar cutaneous sensory receptors	10-10.5
	Abdominal cutaneous sensory receptors	15
Spinal cord	Spinal reflex arc in response to nonnoxious stimuli	8
	Neurons for nociception in dorsal root ganglion	19
Thalamic afferents	Thalamic afferents reach subplate zone	20-22
	Thalamic afferents reach cortical zone	23-24
Cortical function*	Somatosensory evoked potentials with distinct, constant components	29
	First electrocardiographic pattern denoting both wakefulness and active sleep	30

* Earliest evidence of functional thalamocortical connections required for conscious perception of pain.

FIGURE 9.1
From Lee SJ, Ralston HJP, Drey EA, Partridge JC, Rosen MA. Fetal pain: a multidisciplinary review of the evidence. *JAMA*, 2005; p. 949. Reprinted with permission.

transient fetal subplate zone functions as a waiting compartment for growing cortical afferents. These cells are involved in establishing the initial afferent projections and a transient fetal circuitry.

Subplate neurons are among the first generated neurons in the brain and are critical to establishing the correct wiring and functional maturation of the cerebral cortex. Subplate neurons are the first to form synaptic connection with thalamic neurons. Thalamic afferents begin to reach the somatosensory subplate at about 18 weeks developmental age (20 weeks gestational age). Human studies have generally not demonstrated the existence of functional synapses between thalamic afferents and subplate neurons. Subplate neurons appear to synapse with cortical plate neurons and direct the growth of thalamic afferents to their final synaptic targets in the cortical plate. However, it remains unlikely that these synapses between subplate and cortical plate neurons convey information about pain perception from the thalamus to the developing cortex. Eventually, this temporary relay-type connection gives way to a direct connection between thalamic axons and layer IV of the cortex. The subplate neurons tend to vanish during postnatal development. Highly sensitive to conditions such as hypoxia, damage to these neurons is associated with motor and cognitive defects. Therefore, the best estimates are that it is about 30 weeks' gestation before the connection from the periphery through the brainstem and thalamus onto the cortex is neurologically complete and potentially functional.

Regarding the assessment of pain, Fitzgerald (1987) noted that behavioral observations are relied on up to about age 3 years, the Facial Action Coding System (FACS) or color analogue scale from 3 to 8 years, and more traditional verbal and visual analogue (VAS) and numerical rating (NRS) scales after 8 years of age (see Chapter 6 for more details). The Premature Infant Pain Profile (PIPP; Stevens et al, 1996) has been used with infants as young as 27 weeks of age. It incorporates physiological (heart rate and oxygen saturation) and behavioral (brow bulge, eye squeeze, and nasolabial furrow) responses over a post-stimulation 30-second time period compared to a 15-second baseline. Fabrizi et al (2011) feel that such scales as the PIPP may be assessing "unconscious reflexes," which may or may not reflect the processing of sensory activity in the brain. Therefore, they would extend the assessment of infant pain to include electrical activity in skeletal muscles (electromyography; EMG) and the brain (electroencephalography, EEG). They recorded unique response patterns to non-noxious touch and noxious heel-lance. The data were interpreted as providing evidence that the behavioral observations were indeed associated with cortical activity indicative of the processing of unpleasant sensations.

EARLY NEUROPHYSIOLOGICAL DEVELOPMENT

The pain response can be conveniently divided into three types: the *immediate response*, which lasts a few seconds to a minute; the *persistent response*, lasting days or weeks; and *prolonged response* (anatomical or physiological), which outlasts the clinical period and may continue for years and permanently alter the organism's sensitivity of noxious stimulation.

Immediate Response

Fetuses, preterm infants, and neonates undergo a variety of procedures that might be considered painful. Among them are heel-lancing, venipuncture, and surgery. Their response has usually been measured by their crying, facial expressions, heart rate, respiration, sweating, body movement, hormonal responses, and flexion reflexes (Craig et al, 1993; Granau and Craig, 1987; Johnston et al, 1993). Spinally mediated reflexes are those that occur without any apparent awareness or conscious thought; the term *spinal* implies that it is an automatic response to a stimulus. These reflexive responses are built into the normally functioning organism. Their benefit is obvious in that they protect against tissue damage. These reflexes seem to have lower thresholds and to be more exaggerated, more synchronized, and associated with longer lasting muscle contractions in human infants and animals than in adults. These enhanced spinal reflexes are in contrast to the more subdued facial expression, which tends to strengthen with age. Some have interpreted this to reflect the early onset of the sensory-motor response relative to the affective/emotional response.

Persistent Response

Repeated mechanical stimulation such as tapping the heel with a dull object in a non-painful (innocuous) fashion leads to a stronger (pain) response and at a lesser intensity (decreased threshold) even when compared to the contralateral side. The effect appears to be greatest in the 28–33 weeks post-conception age group and is diminished by 42 weeks. This type of hypersensitivity is seen in response to noxious inflammatory stimuli as well as to mechanical stimulation. The heightened response can also spread outside the immediate area of stimulation (secondary hyperalgesia). Repeated application of the topical anesthetic EMLA (lidocaine and prilocaine) cream patch has been shown to reduce this hypersensitive response.

Prolonged Response

Sensitization to an early injury may persist. For example, circumcised infants demonstrate a stronger response to routine vaccinations at 4 and 6 months of age than that of uncircumcised infants (Romber, 1985; Taddio et al, 1995). Pretreatment with EMLA cream to anesthetize the area attenuates the effect. Infants weighing less than 1000 grams have been found to have lower pain sensitivity, which does not appear to be related to temperament. At 4 months of age these very low-weight infants show a biobehavioral pain response similar to that of infants of normal birth weight, but subtle differences in the autonomic response to heel-lancing remain (Taddio et al, 1995).

Neurobiology and Development of the Pain System

Synaptogenesis (the formation of synapses) is greatest during the first postnatal weeks. In the adult rat, A-beta afferents (generally regarded as responsive to touch and not pain) are restricted to laminae III and IV; however, in the fetus and neonate their terminals extend to laminae I and II (substantia gelatinosa, SG), followed by gradual withdrawal over the first 3 postnatal weeks. Remember that activity in SG is highly correlated with pain. Destruction of C-fibers (pain fibers) via capsaicin leaves more A fibers in the superficial layers in the adult. In the immature rat, excitatory activity can be seen in dorsal horn neurons (SG) elicited by A-beta afferents, whereas in adults rat this is only accomplished by A-delta and C-fiber activation. Expression of c-fos, interpreted as a direct measure of neuronal activity, which is only activated by A-delta and C-fibers in the adult, is activated by A-beta fiber stimulation in the newborn. In general, there is a wider distribution of chemicals associated with pain transmission in the neonatal spinal cord then the adult. The adult-like distribution emerges over the postnatal 3 weeks.

The receptive fields of infant dorsal horn cells are relatively larger. The larger receptive fields lead to lower sensory thresholds and increased excitability of third-order motor neurons (thalamic neurons) in the infant CNS due to convergence of inputs. The large A-fiber-dominated fields increase the chance that CNS cells will be activated by peripheral sensory stimulation and therefore act to increase the sensitivity of infant sensory reflexes. These fields diminish over the first 2 weeks postnatally as a result of a gradual inhibition and reduction of afferent inputs to the dorsal horn, rather than a reduction in receptive field.

The discussion up to this point has focused on the neurobiology and development of the somatosensory system (Klimach and Cooke, 1988), which carries messages from the periphery to the spinal cord and constitutes part of the ascending pain system. Another aspect of the pain system is that of descending inhibition. Activation of this system occurs in higher centers in the adult organism and allows for modulation of spinal nociceptive neurons, thus reducing pain. Descending inhibitory controls (DIC) are immature at birth. This pathway travels from the brainstem via the dorsolateral funiculus (DLF) of the spinal cord. Although axons from the brainstem send neurons down the cord early on in fetal life, they do not send projections into the dorsal horn and thus are not functional until P10 (postnatal day 10) in the rat. Fitzgerald and Koltzenburg (1985) performed a study involving rat pups beginning at P5 of age. They noted the existence of a descending DLF pathway at P6 age comparable to that in the adult, but it was not functional until P10–12. Weak inhibition was noted on day 12. At day 18 the DLF pathway was functional but required high-intensity stimulation. Normal functioning emerged by days 22–24, suggesting the presence of a supraspinal control system capable of influencing nociceptive input.

The relative absence of neurotransmitters like serotonin (5-HT) and noradrenalin (NA) may be partly responsible for this. Interestingly enough, this endogenous analgesic system may be dependent on afferent C-fiber activity, as shown by the lack of DIC in rats whose C-fibers were destroyed by capsaicin. The implication is that infants must have activation of the C-fiber nociceptive, or pain, system in order for the anti-pain system to develop. This delay in the development of the descending inhibitory system may be to allow the more basic reflex patterns to emerge. It may not be coincidental that the DIC system does not appear until the third week along with the emergence of more highly coordinated behavioral patterns.

The type of nervous system plasticity described here appears to be dependent on the glutamate NMDA system. The repetitive activation of nociceptors found in tissue injury results in activation of the NMDA glutamate receptor as a consequence of the following events. First, magnesium ions, which ordinarily help to prevent the membrane from depolarizing, are removed by cumulative depolarization secondary to summation of nociceptor-evoked slow synaptic potentials. In others words, there is an accumulative effect of repeated or prolonged C-fiber activity that dislodges these magnesium ions, much like removing a cork from its bottle, giving way to increased pressure and allowing the liquid to flow. Second, neuropeptides, including calcitonin gene–related protein (CGRP) and substance P (SP), and growth factors such as brain-derived neurotrophic factor (BDNF) released by the C-fibers enhance the release of glutamate and its action on the NMDA receptor. G-protein-coupled receptors may also increase NMDA currents. Fast excitatory synaptic transmission is a result of glutamate acting on AMPA.

The neonate dorsal horn manifests NMDA receptors only—no functional AMPA receptors. This arrangement disappears with age and co-localization of AMPA and NMDA receptors emerges. However, the neonate dorsal horn has a higher concentration of NMDA receptors in the gray matter than that found in the adult. Indeed, all dorsal horn laminae are labeled with NMDA-sensitive glutamate until P10–12, when higher levels appear in the SG. Thus, by P30, binding mimics that of the adult. Furthermore, binding affinity is higher at birth and decreases with postnatal age. NMDA-evoked calcium efflux in the neonatal SG is very high in the first postnatal week, followed by a decline. NK1 G-protein-coupled receptor density, associated with C-fiber activity, is greatest in the first 2 weeks postnatally. Only one-sixth of the binding sites present at P11 are there at P60. In effect, the newborn receptor distribution is the inverse of that of the adult in that the superficial laminae or SG have very few receptors until the second week. In addition, SP levels are also low at birth. This immaturity of the SP/NK1 system may help to minimize the development of central sensitization in the infant nervous system. Thus, while the neonatal somatosensory system may be easily activated by peripheral stimulation, its immaturity may help to protect it from the same hyperreactivity responsible for wind-up and central sensitization seen in the adult.

There also appears to be a strong relationship between pain and physiological correlates of infant temperament (Gunner et al, 1995; Stiffer and Jain, 1996). Stiffer and Fox (1990) examined cardiac responses and vagal tone in a longitudinal study of infants from birth to 5 months of age. At 2 days of age, cardiac activity was measured via ECG 1 hour after feeding. Responses to a pacifier-withdrawal task, in which the pacifier that the infant was allowed to suck for 60 seconds was gently removed, were recorded, along with fussing and crying behavior. Mothers then rated the temperament of their 5-month-old infant. There was a significant correlation between vagal tone, negative reactivity, and the maternal ratings. It was concluded that newborn vagal tone predicted maternal ratings of frustration and fear.

In another study, infants 5 months of age and their mothers participated in laboratory-based activities, including a peek-a-boo game with the mother, peek-a-boo with a stranger, and arm restraint designed to elicit positive and negative reactivity. During the infant arm-restraint, the mother was instructed to hold the infant's arms down for 2 minutes while sitting across from the infant. The infant was released if it demonstrated 20 seconds or less of a distress response. The mother was instructed to begin soothing the infant if the distress response continued for 1 minute. The mothers also rated their infants on a temperament scale. A significant correlation was found between physiological measures, such as vagal tone, and temperament. The infants with higher vagal tone were rated by their mothers as being more fearful and frustrated.

Temperament, however, may be epigenetically influenced by the mother's experience with stressful events (Yehuda et al, 2002, 2005) (see Chapter 7 on psychogenic pain).

LONG-TERM EFFECTS OF EARLY EXPERIENCE

The Hebbian mechanism of cell assemblies and synaptic plasticity suggests that early sensory experience plays a significant role in the development of sensory systems.

Appropriate connections can be strengthened and inappropriate ones eliminated. These activity-dependent changes may involve NMDA receptors, in particular the thalamocortical projections to the somatosensory cortex. This critical period of plasticity is time limited and can be negatively influenced by pharmacological or physical means. Sensory inputs are topographically organized. Initially, these projections are very diffuse and become fine-tuned postnatally. If normal peripheral afferent activity, for example, coddling, stroking, patting, is required to fine-tune normal central connectivity, aberrant activity in the form of tissue damage may alter the normal developmental process.

Tissue damage in the early postnatal period can produce profound and lasting structural and functional changes (Jacquin et al, 1996). Ruda et al (2000) injected P1- and P14-old rat pup left hind-paws with Freund's adjuvant, a substance that causes a painful inflammatory reaction. They applied a staining procedure that allowed them to assess the development of primary nerve afferents. They were able to identify increased growth of primary afferents in lamina I and II of the dorsal horn (SG) of the spinal cord compared to that on the right side. No difference was found in motor neuron distribution. This increase in primary afferent density was also seen at adjacent spinal levels (L4-5; L5-6, L6-S1) (sprouting), though at a progressively lower percentage. A similar increase in the density of primary afferent neurons in lamina I and II was found in adult rats injected at birth (P0) or at day 3 (P3) of age. However, when the injection occurred at P14, no morphological differences were noted on the right or left side or when compared to non-injected animals. When tested as adult rats, the P1 animals had a heighten response to painful and nonpainful stimulation, indicating permanent functional changes.

The explanation or mechanism for this is yet to be worked out. But it appears to involve the release of nerve growth factor (NGF) as a result of peripheral stimulation. The release of NGF seems to stimulate a kind of sprouting wherein neurons grow into areas where they ordinarily would not. Tissue damage in infancy leads to substantial up-regulation of neurotrophins (such as NGF) in the skin at almost four times the rate seen in adults. Neurotrophic factors can (a) influence the physiological properties of primary sensory neurons, (b) affect sensory nerve survival, and (c) regulate physiological phenotypes, that is, deafferentation, and the mechanical sensitivity of A-beta and C-fiber nociceptors. Thus, increased levels of NGF proteins may produce permanent changes in nociceptors and low-threshold mechanoreceptors, rendering the organism more sensitive to peripheral stimulation. Neurotrophin levels also affect innervation density of the skin. High levels of NGF and BDNF can result in hyperinnervation that persists and is associated with hypersensitivity in the injured area.

These functional and structural changes can produce long-lasting consequences, including increased sensitivity to stimulation and more widespread pain.

Anand et al (1999) studied six groups of neonatal rat pups undergoing daily stimulation from P0 (day of birth) to P7. It was speculated that the plasticity of the developing rat brain during this period approximates that of the premature human infant from 24 to 36 weeks. The paws of the rat pups were stimulated 1, 2, or 4 times with non-noxious tactile stimulation using a cotton-tipped swab or noxious stimulation consisting of inserting a 25-gauge needle rapidly through the paw. The animals were reared under normal conditions with their mothers from P7 to P23, at which time they were weaned. Pain thresholds were assessed on P16, P22, and P65 using the hotplate test. Other behavioral tests, including alcohol preference testing, defensive withdrawal testing, social discrimination testing, and air-puff startle response, were conducted during adulthood. Decreased pain thresholds, increased preference for alcohol, increased anxiety and defensive withdrawal, and social hypervigilance were found in those exposed to repetitive neonatal pain. It was concluded that "repetitive pain may be associated with lower pain thresholds during development and lead to stress vulnerability and anxiety-mediated adult behavior" (Anand et al, 1999, p. 633).

Johnston and Stevens (1996) found increased physiological responses coupled with decreased behavioral responses to repetitive heel-sticks in preterm neonates in an NICU. This pattern seemed to mimic Seligman's (1975) concept of "learned helplessness," which is characterized by a developed lack of motivation to response to an aversive event, and a retarded ability to learn that responding works in avoiding discomfort, resulting in emotional disturbance, generally depression and anxiety. Pain experienced during circumcision in neonates appeared to correlate with increased behavioral responsiveness to vaccination pain at 4 to 6 months of age (Johnston and Stevens, 1996).

In their review article, Johnston and her colleagues (2011) note the effects of untreated procedural pain in neonates. A blunting of the behavioral response to repetitive tissue-damaging procedures was found to be correlated with the number of procedures performed in the NICU. This diminished response was also associated with less recovery time between procedures in preterm neonates. In general, the studies reviewed showed decreased behavioral response to pain in infants that did not receive morphine for procedural pain compared to those that did. Furthermore, at 18 months of age, the NICU survivors appeared relatively insensitive to pain. Interestingly, thermal but not mechanical hypersensitivity have been demonstrated in 11- to 16-year-olds who had NICU experience or surgery as pre- or full-term neonates. Full-term neonates who received no procedure-associated anesthesia or morphine showed increased crying, sensitivity, and anticipatory distress to immunization during infancy. In addition, the magnitude of the response appeared to correlate with the number of painful procedures despite the use of an analgesic.

Repeated tissue damage will activate primary sensory neurons in the skin. There are six ways in which tissue damage can influence peripheral sensory structure and function: (1) skin wound, (2) sensitization of receptors, (3) altered phenotype of receptors, (4) hyperinnervation of damaged tissue, (5) local release of neurotrophins, and (6) altered gene expression in the dorsal root ganglion. C-fiber polymodal nociceptors, which respond to mechanical, thermal, and chemical noxious stimuli, manifest mature firing patterns and thresholds at birth. However, high-threshold A-delta mechanoreceptors and low-threshold rapidly adapting A-beta mechanoreceptors, which respond to touch and brush, are both relatively immature. In the adult, the inflammatory response is neurogenic, arising from the release of substance P from peripheral C-fibers. However, the levels of this neuropeptide in the C-terminal remain low and are not released in sufficient quantities to produce neurogenic activity until P10 in animal models.

In general, hypersensitivity is a product of peripheral sensitization, central sensitization, or both. "Activation of these central cells by repetitive A-delta and C-fiber inputs initiates sensitization such that they respond to normal inputs in an exaggerated and extended manner and allow inputs that were previously ineffective to activate the neurons" (Fitzgerald and Beggs, 2001, p. 249). The results are hyperexcitability, enlarged receptive fields, increased spontaneous activity, enhanced discharges to mechanical, thermal, and electrical stimulation, and possible decreased thresholds These changes are also associated with increased neuronal activity transmitted to supraspinal sites and thus increased pain intensity and duration. Therefore, exposing neonates or infants to certain types of noxious stimulation, such as injection, surgery, or drawing of blood, especially without adequate analgesia, may produce abnormal development of nociceptive neurons in the spinal cord, rendering them more susceptible and hyperresponsive to pain as adults.

Given the developmental sequence of the nociceptive system, neonates of younger gestational age are more likely to experience non-noxious stimulation as painful and have more widespread sensitivity because of the broader receptive fields. The relative absence of a descending pain inhibitory system leaves the preterm neonate vulnerable to increased nociception and primary hypersensitivity.

There also appears to be a blunting of the hypothalamus–pituitary–adrenal (HPA) response in infants who have undergone multiple painful procedures while in the NICU. Children and adolescents with a history of NICU procedures showed enhanced activity in the anterior cingulate cortex and insula in response to experimentally induced pain. The accumulated evidence suggests that painful procedures affect preterm neonates differently than full-term neonates. This effect seems to be associated with younger age at birth, more days on oxygen, and larger number of skin-breaking procedures.

Evidence that environmental manipulations in newborn rat pups can influence behavioral reactivity of adult rats is also mounting. For example, the impact of maternal separation was studied by Coutinhol et al (2002). Rat pups were separated from their mothers for 3 hours a day from days P2 to P14. At 2 months of age they demonstrated increased visceromotor responses to colorectal distension and increased stress-induced fecal pellet output. These observations led the authors to conclude that early life events predispose the individual to visceral hyperalgesia and increased colonic motility in response to psychological stress. Using a different methodology, Randich et al (2006; DeBerry et al, 2007) showed how early insult to the bladder in the neonatal but not the adolescent-age rat can predispose the animal to the development of bladder hypersensitivity in adulthood. Taken together, these findings indicate that early traumas can have a long-term effect on visceral hypersensitivity of the type seen in functional bowel disorders such as irritable bowel syndrome and in painful bladder disorders.

These researchers also noted that neonatally stressed adult rats demonstrate decreased exploratory behavior in novel environments, a lower threshold for learned helplessness, and increased loss of hippocampal neurons associated with early-onset cognitive defects, compared to a control groups of adult rats. Endocrine changes included increased HPA axis responses to emotional stressors and impaired negative feedback control mechanisms in the hypothalamus. These long-term changes have been attributed to plasticity in the neonatal hypothalamus, forebrain, prefrontal cortex, and hippocampus, and were related to the expression of glucocorticoid and other receptor systems involved in regulation of the HPA axis, the autonomic nervous system, and adult stress behavior.

CONCLUSION

The experience of pain is a complex integration of cognitive, affective, and sensory components occurring at the cortical level. Pain is considered to be a conscious and dynamic experience modulated by a variety of mental, emotional, psychological, and sensory mechanisms. The precise interpretation of altered physiological, hormonal, and behavioral activity in response to activation of the nociceptive system continues to be debated. To the extent that pain is understood to be a biopsychosocial and multidimensional (sensory, affective, cognitive) experience it challenges whether or not what the fetus and neonate feels is pain, at least as it is current defined by the IASP.

One might argue the notion of "a rose by any other name," and that by any definition the fetus and neonate clearly demonstrate distress and should be treated accordingly. Accepting the notion of fetal and neonatal pain, however, has stimulated a concern about returning to the thoroughly discredited "specificity" theory which, intentionally or not, encourages a linear model that presumes the severity of pain to be related to the strength of the noxious stimulus. The absence of this linear correlation has been well documented. Accepting either position, that infant and neonatal pain does or does not mimic that of the adult, leaves one with a sense of satisfaction that is unsettling in terms of how neonates' and infants' pain is understood and treated.

The first comprehensive textbook on this topic was not published until 1987: *Pain in Children and Adolescents*, by P.J. McGrath and A.M. Unruh. Our understanding of the development, structure, and function of the human neonatal nociceptive and pain system is, itself, in its infancy. It depends in large part on the accuracy of extrapolating data from animal research to humans. It is in this arena that discussions of the role of conscious awareness become relevant (Block, 2007; Chalmers, 1995). The likelihood that more a highly developed and psychologically sophisticated organism reveals different ontological patterns is hard to ignore.

As it stands, the topic of neonatal and infant pain has been addressed in a dichotomous fashion: do they feel pain or do not. Leventhal (1984) and Derbyshire (1999) presented a developmental model of pain on the basis of a continuum (see Figure 13.1 in Chapter 13). This model proposes the presence of a gradually organized and elaborated stimulus information-processing network in the CNS involving three hierarchical mechanisms: (a) innate expressive-motor, (b) schematic processing, and (c) conscious abstract. The first two of these are considered preconscious perceptual-motor processing. A dimmer-switch analogy is used to help illustrate the transition from one phase or process to another. Consciousness is regarded as moving gradually from fully "off" to fully "on." The innate set of expressive-motor mechanisms appears with the first signs of movement in response to sensory stimulation, occurring at about 7 to 14 weeks of gestation. Schematic processing involves the automatic encoding in memory of the experience in order to produce a categorical structure representing the general informational and sensory aspects of pain experiences. A set of conscious abstract rules about emotional episodes and associated voluntary responses is proposed to arise over time as a consequence of self-observation and conscious efforts to cope with aversive situations. Therefore, the conscious pain experience is dependent upon the acquisition of certain developmental markers, tentatively described as being available by 12 months of age.

This developmental approach may provide a temporary diversion, but there are many questions that need to be answered. If the neonate and infant do not feel pain, what do we call what they do feel? Is there a need to consider the experience of pain in the context of the cognitive and affective sophistication of the organism, or degree of system complexity? Some argue that even fish experience pain and demonstrate consciousness by virtue of the fact that they can learn to avoid harmful stimuli (see Rose, 2002, for a review). Should all types of responses to nociception—verbal, hormonal, physiological, behavioral—be assumed to be equally representative of the organism's experience in response to nociception? What role can or should neuroimaging play in addressing the issue of fetal pain? To the extent that pain is a conscious experience (see Chapter 13) can any organism that emits a pain response be said to have had a conscious experience? These and many other philosophical and practical questions invite investigation and consideration. In doing so, the dynamic and complex nature of pain and the need to expand the paradigm through which pain is viewed will likely become even more apparent.

REFERENCES

American Academy of Pediatrics, Committee on Fetus and Newborn, Section on Surgery, and Section on Anesthesiology and Pain Medicine; Canadian Paedictric Society, Fetus and Newborn Committee. Policy statement: prevention and management of pain in the neonate: an update. *Pediatrics.* 2006;18(5):2231–2241.

Anand KJ. Fetal pain? *Pain: Clinical Updates.* 2006;14(2):1–4.

Anand KJ, Bergquist L, Hall RW, Carbajal R. Acute pain management in newborn infants. *Pain: Clinical Updates.* 2012;19(6):1–6.

Anand KJ, Carr DB. The neuroanatomy, neurophysiology, and neurochemistry of pain, stress and analgesics in newborns and children. *Pediatr Clin North Am.* 1998;36(4):795–822.

Anand KJ, Coskun V, Thrivikraman KV, Nemeroff CB, Plotsky PM. Long-term behavioral effects of repetitive pain in neonatal rat pups. *Physiol Behav.* 1999;66(4):627–637.

Anand KJ, Craig KD. New perspectives on the definition of pain. *Pain.* 1996;67:3–6.

Anand KJ, Hickey PR. Pain and its effects in the human neonate and fetus. *N Engl J Med.* 1987;317(21):1321–1329.

Anand KJ, Sipple WG, Green AA. Randomized trial of fentanyl anesthesia in preterm babies undergoing surgery: effects on the stress response. *Lancet.* 1987;1(8524):62–66.

Barr RG. Reflections on measuring pain in infants: dissociation in responsive systems and "honest signalling." *Arch Dis Child Fetal Neonatal Ed.* 1998;79(2):F152–F156.

Block N. Consciousness, accessibility, and the mesh between psychology and neuroscience. *Behav Brain Sci.* 2007;30:481–548.

Brazelton TB. Psychophysiologic reactions in the neonate. II. Effects of maternal medication on the neonate and his behavior. *J Pediatr.* 1961;58:513–518.

Chalmers DJ. Facing up to the problem of consciousness. *Journal of Consciousness Studies.* 1995;2(3):200–219.

Chamberline DB. Babies don't feel pain: a century of denial in medicine. Presented at the Second International Symposium on Circumcision, San Francisco, California, May 2, 1991. http://www.nocirc.org/symposia/second/chamberlain.html. Accessed April, 28, 2013.

Chugani HT, Phelps ME. Maturational changes of cerebral function in the infant determined by FDG positron emission tomography. *Science.* 1986;231:840–843.

Coutinhol SV, Plotsky PM, Sablad M, et al. Neonatal maternal separation alters stress-induced responses to viscerosomatic nociceptive stimuli in rat. *Am J Physiol Gastrointest Liver Physiol.* 2002;282:G307–G316.

Craig KD, Whitfield MF, Grunau RV, Linton J, Hadjistavropoulos HD. Pain in the preterm neonate: behavioral and physiological indices. *Pain.* 1993;52(3):287–299.

Crudden C. Reactions of newborn infants to thermal stimuli under constant tactual conditions. *J Exp Psychol.* 1937;20:350–370.

Cunningham N. Comments on Derbyshire, *Pain*, 67 (1996) 210–211. *Pain.* 1998;74:102–104.

DeBerry J, Ness TJ, Robbins MT, Randich A. Inflammation-induced enhancement of the visceromotor reflex to urinary bladder distention: modulation by endogenous opioids and the effects of early-in-life experience with bladder inflammation. *J Pain.* 2007;8(12):914–923.

Derbyshire SWG. Comments on editorial by Anand and Craig. *Pain.* 1966;67:210–211.

Derbyshire SWG. Reply to N. Cunningham. *Pain.* 1998;74:104–106.

Derbyshire SWG. Locating the beginnings of pain. *Bioethics.* 1999;13(1):1–31.

Derbyshire SWG. Fetal "pain"—a look at the evidence. *APS Bull.* 2003;13(4):6–12.

Eland JM, Anderson JE. The experience of pain in children. In Jacox AK, ed. *Pain: A Source for Nurses and Other Health Care Professionals.* Boston: Little, Brown; 1977:453–473.

Fabrizi L, Worley A, Patten D, et al. Electrophysiological measurements and analysis of nociception in human infants. *J Vis Exp.* 2011; Dec 20:58.

Fitzgerald M. Pain and analgesia in neonates. *Trends Neurosci.* 1987;10:344–346.

Fitzgerald M. Neurobiology of fetal and neonatal pain. In Wall P, Melzack R, eds. *Textbook of Pain.* Edinburgh: Churchill Livingstone; 1994:153–163.

Fitzgerald M, Beggs S. The neurobiology of pain: developmental aspects. *Neuroscientist.* 2001;7(3):246–257.

Fitzgerald M, Koltzenburg M. The functional development of descending inhibitory pathways in the dorsolateral funiculus of the newborn rat spinal cord. *Dev Brain Res.* 1985;24:261–270.

Frank LS. A national survey of the assement and treatment of pain and aggitation in the neonatal intensive care unit. *J Obstet Gynecol Neonat Nurs.* 1987;16:387–393.

Giannakoulopoulos X, Sepulveda W, Kourtis P, Glover V, Fisk NM. Fetal plasma cortisol and beta-endorphin response to intrauterine needling. *Lancet.* 1994;344(8915):77–81.

Goldman R. *Circumcision: The Hidden Trauma.* Boston: Vanguard; 1997.

Granau RV, Craig KD. Pain expression in neonates; facial action and cry. *Pain.* 1987;28:395–410.

Gunnar MR, Porter FL, Wolf CM, Rigatuso J, Larson MC. Neonatal stress reactivity: predictors to later emotional temperament. *Child Dev.* 1995;66:1–13.

Jacquin MF, Renehan WE, Klein BG, Mooney RD, Rhoades RW. Functional consequences of neonatal infraorbital nerve section in rat trigeminal ganglion. *J Neurosci.* 1996;6(12):3706–3720.

Johnston CC, Fernandes AM, Campbell-Yeo M. Pain in neonates is different. *Pain.* 2011;152:S65–S73.

Johnston CC, Stevens BJ. Experience in a neonatal intensive care unit affects pain response. *Pediatrics.* 1996;98:925–930.

Johnston CC, Stevens B, Craig KD, Grunau RVE. Developmental changes in pain expression in premature, full-term, two- and four-month-old infants. *Pain.* 1993;52:201–208.

Klimach VJ, Cooke RWI. Maturation of the neonatal somatosensory evoked response in preterm infants. *Dev Med Child Neurol.* 1988;30(2):208–214.

Lawson JR. Letter. *Birth.* 1986;13:124–125.

Lawson, JR. Correspondence. Pain in the neonate and fetus. *N Engl J Med.* 1988;318:1398–1399.

Lee SJ, Ralston HJP, Drey EA, Partridge JC, Rosen MA. Fetal pain: a systematic multidisciplinary review of the evidence. *JAMA.* 2005;294(8):947–954.

Leventhal H. A perceptual motor theory of emotion. In Scherer KR, Ekman P, eds. *Approaches to Emotion.* Hillsdale, NJ: Lawrence Erlbaum; 1984:271–291.

Lloyd-Thomas AR, Fitzgerald M. Do fetuses feel pain? Reflex responses do not necessarily signify pain. *BMJ.* 1996;313(7060):797–798.

Lowery CL, Hardman MP, Manning N, Hall RW, Anand JK. Neurodevelopmental changes of fetal pain. *Semin Perinatol.* 2007;31:275–282.

McGrath PJ, Unruh AM. *Pain in Children and Adolescents.* Amsterdam: Elsevier; 1987.

McGraw M. *Growth: A Study of Johnny and Jimmy.* New York: Appleton-Century-Crofts; 1935.

McGraw M. Neural maturation as exemplified in the changing reactions of the infant to pin prick. *Child Dev.* 1941;12:31–42.

McGraw M. *The Neuromuscular Maturation of the Human Infant.* New York: Hafner; 1969.

O'Donnell J, Ferguson LP, Beattie TF. Use of analgesia in a paediatric accident and emergency department following limb trauma. *Eur J Emerg Med.* 2002;9:5–8.

Peiper A. *Cerebral Function in Infancy and Childhood.* New York: Consultants Bureau; 1963.

Perret G, Meyers R. Neurosurgery in infants and children. *Pediatr Clin North Am.* 1960;7(3):545–582.

Pratt KC, Nelson AK, Sun KH. The behavior of the newborn infant. *Ohio State University Studies Contributing to Psychology.* 1930; No. 10.

Randich A, Uzzell T, DeBerry JJ, Ness TJ. Neonatal urinary bladder inflammation produces adult bladder hypersensitivity. *J Pain.* 2006;7(7):469–479.

Rawlins JM, Khan AA, Shenton AF, Sharpe DT. Epidemiology and outcomes analysis of 208 children with burns attending an emergency department. *Pediatr Emerg Care.* 2007;23:289–293.

Richards T. Can the fetus feel pain? *BMJ.* 1985;291:1220–1221.

Rodkey EN, Riddell RP. The infancy of infant pain research: the experimental origins of infant pain denial. *J Pain.* 2013;14(4):338–350.

Rogers MC. Do the right thing—pain relief in infants and children. *N Engl J Med.* 1992;326:55–56.

Romber R. *Circumcision: The Painful Dilemma.* South Hadley, MA: Bergin and Garvey; 1985.

Rose JD. The neurobehavioral nature of fishes and the question of awareness and pain. *Rev Fisheries Sci.* 2002;10(1):1–38.

Ruda MA, Ling Qing-Dong, Hohmann AG, Peng YB, Tachibana T. Altered nociceptive neuronal circuits after neonatal peripheral inflammation. *Science.* 2000; 289:626–630.

Schecter NL, Blankson V, Pachter LM, Sullivan CM, Costa L. The ouchless place: no pain, children's gain. *Pediatrics.* 1997;99(6):890–894.

Seligman MEP. *Helplessness.* San Francisco: WH Freeman; 1975.

Skinner BF. *Verbal Behavior.* New York: Appleton-Century-Crofts; 1957.

Stevens B, Johnston C, Petryshen P, Taddio A. Premature Infant Pain Profile: development and initial validation. *Clin J Pain.* 1996;12(1):13–22.

Stiffer CA, Fox NA. Infant reactivity: physiological correlates of newborn and 5-month temperament. *Dev Psychol.* 1990;26(4):582–588.

Stiffer CA, Jain A. Psychophysiological correlates of infant temperament: stability of behavior and autonomic patterning from 5 to 18 months. *Dev Psychol.* 1996;29(4):379–391.

Swafford LI, Allen D. Pain relief in the pediatric patient. *Med Clin North Am.* 1968;52(1):131–135.

Taddio A, Goldbach M, Ipp M, Stevens B, Koren G. Effect of neonatal circumcision on pain responses during vaccination in boys. *Lancet.* 1995;345(8945):291–292.

Thorek M. *Modern Surgical Technique,* Vol. III. Montreal: Lippincott; 1938.

Unruh AM. Voice from the past: ancient views of pain in childhood. *Clin J Pain.* 1992;8:247–254.

Walco GA, Cassidy RC, Schechter NL. Pain, hurt, and harm; the ethics of pain control in infants and children. *N Engl J Med.* 1994;331:541–544.

Yehuda R, Engel SM, Brand SR, Marcus SM, Berkowitz GS. Transgenerational effects of posttraumatic stress disorder in babies of mothers exposed to the World Trade Center attacks during pregnancy. *J Clin Endocrinol.* 2005;90(7):4115–4118.

Yehuda R, Halligan SI, Bierer LM. Cortisol levels in adults offspring of Holocaust survivors: relation in PTSD symptom severity in the parent and child. *Psychoneuroendocrinology.* 2002;27:171–189.

10 Pain and Religion

Science without religion is lame, religion without science is blind.
–Albert Einstein (1941)

INTRODUCTION

It would be difficult to discuss pain, and especially its associated suffering, without invoking the topics of religion and spirituality. The word *pain* comes from the Greek *poine* and the Latin *poena* (Loeser, 2005). Both of these terms derive their meaning from "punishment." *Algos*, which is linked to neuralgesia and analgesia, relates to a physiological process such as impulse transmission, absent any reference to its meaning or purpose, that is, punishment. *Suffering* comes from the Greek term *pherein* and the Latin term *terre*, which translates to carry, bear, or endure. The Greeks and Romans tended to separate pain and suffering. Pain was considered more material and to be of the body and brain, while suffering was of the spirit and mind. This dichotomy extended even to the heart, as the ancients made a distinction between the physical heart and spiritual heart. Similarly, the French term *la douleur* refers to somatic (nociceptive or neuropathic) pain, and *les douleurs* refers to spiritual pain and human suffering.

Though seemingly separated by irreconcilable differences, science and religion bear a number of commonalties. Each, in its own way, seeks to explain the mysteries of life, to answer major philosophical questions, and bring clarity to that which appears confusing. Both strive to account for our very beginnings and provide a sense of the future. Humans appear drawn to both to determine the meaning of life. In them we expect to find consolation and hope—something to sink our teeth into. For some, science and religion (spirituality) are inexorably at odds with one another. For others, the one (science) is taken as a magnificent manifestation of the other.

PAIN, RELIGION, AND SPIRITUALITY

The Christian Bible speaks often of suffering, rarely of pain. However, in Genesis, Adam and Eve disobeyed God's commandment not to eat the forbidden fruit. After being rebuked, God proclaimed that women would forever deliver children in pain. Therefore, pain became associated with punishment. The Bible suggests that pain, and by extension, suffering, may be a direct consequence of God's displeasure. In *Applications Commentary*, Jon Courson (2003) describes the complaining of the Israelites in response to the hardships encountered during their exodus from Egypt after being freed from bondage as "sinful" and leading to suffering. By contrast, Job's steadfastness in the face of what appeared to be unjustified and capricious pain and suffering was richly rewarded by the return of his losses many times over, giving those who endure, hope. This meaning revolves around the notion of redemptive suffering. Even today, psychologists recognize the potential failure of otherwise proven pain reduction treatments with patients in pain who believe their pain to be a just punishment for some transgression.

The Christian Bible also gives numerous examples of disease and suffering. Jesus was noted to have cured many afflictions. The emphasis appeared to be on the disease entity, whether a naturally occurring phenomenon or indicative of demonic possession. Absolution of sin or curing of the disease resulted in relief. C.S. Lewis (1940) argued that pain is God's "megaphone calling a person back to his spiritual foundations." It is easy to understand how one so indoctrinated would, upon committing a sin, think themselves a fugitive from justice until some type of pain or suffering would befall them. During the Dark Ages, pain and suffering were interpreted as visible evidence that the person had committed some type of transgression. Some Christians believed pain and suffering to be the consequences of original sin and necessary to prove one worthy of salvation. Examples of self-flagellation and martyrdom are common in the history of Christianity.

The Christian emphasis on the punitive aspects of pain and suffering was not unlike that of the Greeks and Hebrews. Pain was often ascribed to the invasion of the body by evil demons or spirits, a tradition not totally abandoned even in the 21st century. Regarding the suffering of Christ, in *Jesus Among Other Gods*, Ravi Zacharias (2000) stated: "Looking at the cross, evil becomes a mirror of fearsome reality. But by carefully looking into the cross, we discover that it is not opaque but translucent, and we are able to glimpse true evil through it. The suffering of Jesus is a study in the anatomy of pain. At its core, evil is a challenge of moral proportion against a holy God. It is not merely a struggle with our discomfort" (p. 131). Zacharias appears to see the suffering and pain experienced by Christ as indicative and a consequence of evil in the world. It is not a matter of evil directly entering the body but rather it is the driving force, seen or unseen, that can inflict pain. The pain and suffering that we encounter may be a means by which evil can strike at God and cause one to question God's existence and involvement in the lives of humans. There is an implied mandate to seek out and confront evil in its various forms, even at the risk of one's own physical discomfort.

According to Hinduism, mental or physical suffering and pain are not viewed as punishment but as natural consequences of the moral laws of the universe. Pain and suffering are seen as the unfolding of karma in response to mentally, verbally, or physically inappropriate actions in one's current or past life. In a sense, suffering is the debt brought on by past negative behavior. One must accept suffering as a just consequence and as an opportunity for spiritual progress. "Hindu tradition holds that as we are in human form on earth, we are bound by the laws of our world and will experience physical pain. Pain is truly felt in our current physical bodies; it is not illusory in the sense of not really felt. But while the body may be in pain, the Self or soul is not affected or harmed" (Whitman, 2007, p. 609). By contrast, the Christian view sees the soul as threatened and at risk, based in part on how one responds to their painful circumstances. For Hindus the soul or true self is free from suffering. When the soul manifests itself in the person, he or she achieves liberation (moksha). Abstinence from causing pain or harm to other beings (ahimsa) is a central tenet of Hinduism.

In Hinduism all things are manifestation of God/The Ultimate, and God/The Ultimate encompasses everything, including pain and suffering. Thus pain and suffering are not seen as wholly good or bad. Rather, they may provide an opportunity to progress along one's spiritual path. The objective is to detach one's self from the things of this world, including pain and suffering, by recognizing that the self is not of this world. No circumstance, including pain, can cause one to suffer once perfect detachment is achieved. When a person is equally comfortable with suffering and joy he or she is said to be fit for immortality.

Relief of pain and the lessening of suffering is to be pursued, but with the goal of becoming neutral to it and whatever outcomes emerge as a result of treatment. Likewise, practitioners are not to become frustrated at their failures. Rather, all must recognize the outcome to be part of the person's karma, and therefore not known or controlled by the individual. There appears to be a high premium on becoming neutral and nonreactive, at least emotionally, in the presence of pain. Mindfulness meditation and yoga are used to achieve detachment. Some pray to God/The Ultimate for support in their efforts to become detached from their one earthly circumstance, including pain, and focus their life on God/The Ultimate.

The Hindu philosophy can be interpreted as being rather fatalistic because of the nature of karma. However, the individual is encouraged to live his or her life in a positive manner, that is, in accordance with dharma. It is the effort, trying one's best, and not the outcome, that is emphasized. There are many parallels here to the acceptance-based treatments researched and development by McCracken and his colleagues (2005). Acceptance is not giving in to the pain but rather a disengaging from an unrelenting struggle with the pain. Understanding one's condition, developing realistic appraisals and goals, and being willing to perform everyday positive activities despite the pain are emphasized.

Regarding the Judaic view, pain is seen as an event that can serve a variety of purposes, including to cleanse negativity, break negative shells (*kilpot*), or help one to experience Light. What is difficult for the body can be joy for the soul. Whitman (2010) lists several functions that pain and suffering can serve, including bringing one closer to God, self-improvement, a test of faith, or an opportunity to learn about life, and it may occasionally by redemptive. When asked about some of the past and present hardships faced by many of the Jewish faith, Levi Chazen (2008) noted that these events serve to teach the lesson that the land of Israel is acquired only through suffering, as the Talmud says. This is true whether one interprets the "land of Israel" literally or metaphorically. Only by first tearing down the house can the gold be found. The Torah is said to teach that anything of real value sometimes has a price to it, sometimes requiring self-sacrifice and even pain.

Rabbi Noah Weinberg outlines 48 ways to wisdom. Number 25 is entitled "No Pain No Gain." He describes pain as an unavoidable reality of life, and that one of the keys to success is to accept and grow from it. Comfort is presented as the opposite of pain. However, comfort is not the ultimate pleasure or goal, and those who seek it are likely to be disappointed. He notes that achieving many of the good things in life requires a substantial effort, which can seem painful. For Rabbi Weinberg, pain and pleasure are inexorably linked together. Fear of pain is regarded as worse than the pain itself. Tziv Freeman notes that pain and suffering occur when the body and soul are dissonant with one another. The Baal Shem Tov, a Jewish mystical rabbi, considered to be the founder of Hasidic Judaism, taught that one should embrace pain with joy. The meaning of painful events is seen as being beyond human comprehension and may or may not ultimately be revealed.

The Jewish Kabbalah is a set of teachings that attempt to explain the relationship between God the Creator and the finite universe. It endeavors to define the nature of the universe and of human beings (the nature and purpose of existence). Some Jews accept the Kabbalah as representing the true meaning of Judaism, while others reject its doctrines as antithetical to Judaism. The Kabbalah states that the only reason for pain is to make us think about its cause, meaning, and purpose (Berg, 2007). Specifically, Creator-bestowed pain is designed to propel us beyond our focus on our earthly existence to a higher level of existence and awareness of hidden causes wherein the purpose of the pain is revealed. The Kabbalah seems to support the notion that God suffers when God's people suffer. God (Shekhinah) is available to assist in dealing with the ever-present realities of the world, including pain. The prevailing sentiment appears to be that the real treasures of life are beyond our mortal existence and are acquired through suffering and pain or are not acquired at all.

Within Judaism, the topic of circumcision has brought science and religion to somewhat of an impasse. As written in the Torah, God created a covenant with Abraham in which God promised Abraham would be the father of many offspring from whom nations and kings would emerge and reside in the land of Canaan, where He would be their God. It is also written that "Such shall be the covenant between Me and you and your offspring to follow which you shall keep: every male among you shall be circumcised" (Genesis 17:10). Notwithstanding the debate over the definition of pain in infants (see Chapter 9), there is significant scientific data to support the potentially traumatic effects of circumcision. Indeed, Anand and Hickey (1987) reported that an infant's response to a painful event is greater even than an adult's, and Ryan and Finer (1994) have described circumcision as being among the most painful procedures in neonatal medicine.

Goldman (1999) has reviewed the effects of circumcision on infants and the concerns relating to the welfare of the infant and Jewish tradition. He also addresses a forgotten and often unwitting participant in this ritual, the mother. For some mothers, this is a sacred and time-honored commemoration of Abraham's covenant with God. Others hope they will have a daughter and be spared the agony of having their son circumcised. Yet others spend their pregnancy in tearful and quiet desperation ruminating over the apparently unavoidable. While the accounts of the response of the infants undergoing circumcision vary, Goldman reported one mother to say, "The screams of my baby remain embedded in my bones and haunt my mind....His cry sounded like he was being butchered. I lost my milk" (see Chapter 11 on empathy and pain).

The debates surrounding circumcision in the Jewish community contain many religious, moral, and ethical issues. For our purposes, it is sufficient to note the unmistakable impact and importance of the scientific data regarding infant pain, and the potential short- and long-term physiological effects of such procedures. In some instances, long-standing religious traditions are called into question and even modified when the impact on the organism is fully understood. In the same fashion that religious beliefs have at times overshadowed the scientific enterprise, as in the case of Galileo, scientifically sound data may be used to refute or reinforce certain religious traditions. This is no more in evidence than with the ongoing debate regarding the origin of the universe. The influence of scientifically generated data on our view and treatment of the infant provides another example, and is discussed in greater detail in Chapter 9.

This discussion may also reflect the distinction made in the Jewish faith between how one responds to one's own pain and that of another's pain. When the individual is the one suffering, he or she is encouraged to find the strength to use the suffering as an opportunity for growth and purification. It is to be understood that God loves each individual and thus must be giving or allowing the pain to exist for the individual's own good. However, in the same manner as Moses is perceived to have done when encountering another in pain, one is urged to "feel the other's pain" and provide strength and comfort. It is important to be present with the person and provide comfort in any way possible.

Regarding animals' pain during experimentation, Rabbi J. David Bleich (1986) presented his related concerns and findings to the Senate Judiciary Committee when the Pain Relief Promotion Act was being proposed. He noted that Judaism (a) places the highest importance on palliation of pain, particularly in the case of terminal patients, and (b) that Jewish law regards "pain suffered by terminal patients as life-threatening, in the sense that such pain has the potential for compromising the brief longevity anticipated for the terminal patient." He went on to note that in consideration of the "life-threatening nature of pain," Judaism not only permits but mandates that pain-relieving methods, especially those for patients in "extremis," be undertaken even if they violate religious restrictions, including those related to the Sabbath. In summary, he noted that "Jewish law and tradition would enthusiastically endorse the provisions of H.R. 2260 designed to encourage more extensive and more effective palliation of pain." This position appears to give priority to the relief of suffering and pain, even if such endeavors appeared at odds with long-standing religious traditions. Perhaps the well-being of the individual in pain assumes greater importance than adherence to a religious custom. It may, in fact, be an expression of one's religious convictions.

RELIGIOUS VIEWS ON ANIMAL SLAUGHTER

Jewish and Muslim religious traditions view animals as creatures of God and deserving of appropriate treatment and care. A guiding principle is that of preventing the suffering of living creatures. The codes put forth by both religions represented a significant advancement with respect to the proper treatment of animals in ancient times. Animal cruelty was viewed with great disdain. Unnecessary cruelty to animals was strictly forbidden, and in many cases, animals were accorded the same sensitivity as human beings. Judaism does not give a specific opinion as to whether animals experience physical or psychological pain in the same manner as humans. However, it recognizes a relationship between the way a person treats animals and the way they treat other humans. That is, anyone willing to be cruel to a defenseless animal is more likely to be cruel to another human. For Muslims, if animals have been subjected to cruelties in their breeding, transport, slaughter, or general welfare, meat from them is considered impure and unlawful to eat. They note that Allah has "prescribed benevolence toward everything." So great is the concern for the animal's well-being that the slaughterer is prohibited from sharpening the knife in front of the animal to be slaughtered for fear of "killing the animal twice." Furthermore, it is forbidden to kill one animal in the presence of other animal awaiting the same fate.

For both Jews and Muslims, dietary restrictions and requirements extend to the manner in which animals to be consumed are to be slaughtered. The Jewish dietary code is described in the original five books of the Holy Scriptures. The Muslim code is found in the Quran. The Torah prohibits consumption of blood (Leviticus 7:26–27; Leviticus 17:10–14), as it was thought to contain the life or soul of the animal. The Jewish Talmud and Muslim Quran both contain specific rules regarding the slaughtering of animals. The Jewish codes require that acceptable animals be slaughtered by a specially trained Jewish male, the "shochet." He is to use a very sharp knife, the "chalef," and with a single stroke cut through the trachea and esophagus, severing the jugular vein and carotid artery. This is thought to lessen the animal's suffering while allowing the blood to escape. Muslins prefer that animals be slaughtered by a person of the Muslim faith. Any Muslim may slaughter an animal while invoking the name of Allah. In cases where Muslims cannot kill their own animals, they may eat meat killed by a "person of the book" (a Christian or a Jew). Instructions are provided to minimize the pain and ensure humane slaughtering. A sharp knife is to be used and the animal cannot be made to wait or "tied up and bound."

While stunning of animals before slaughter is commonplace in most Western countries, pre-slaughter stunning was not practiced by Jews or Muslims, as it was thought to conflict with their respective religious mandates. In addition, it was thought by many that animals did not experience pain. As one can imagine, evaluation of religious slaughtering methods by those concerned over the impact on the animal was a very delicate matter. Objectivity, sensitivity to religious tradition, and emotional restraint were required by all involved.

Zimmerman (1986) has defined pain in animals as an aversive sensory experience caused by actual or potential injury that elicits protective motor and vegetative reactions, results in learned avoidance, and may modify species-specific behavior, including social behavior. Daly et al (1986) and Hemsworth and Mellor (2009) were able to identify electrical brain wave patterns associated with the apparent experience of pain in animals. When the throats of calves were cut in the manner prescribe by Jewish and Muslim customs, brain activity associated with pain persisted for up to 2 minutes. They also demonstrated that the patterns corresponding to pain disappeared when the animal was concussed using electrical stunning methods 5 second after the incision. They showed that slaughtering of animals, no matter how efficient, without stunning was indeed painful.

In response to these and other data, The Muslim World League, consisting of some 55 prominent community leaders, scientists, and Muslim theologians, met with the World Health Organization in 1986 to develop guidelines regarding stunning in the slaughter of animals. An updated report in 1997, the Islamic Ruling on Animal Slaughter, notes that pre-slaughter stunning by electric shock would be lawful if it was proven to lessen the animal's suffering, used the weakest electrical current, rendered the animal unconscious, and did not result in the animal's death or make the meat harmful to the consumer. Indeed, Muslim slaughter without stunning is now forbidden in New Zealand (Hemsworth and Mellor, 2009).

PAINFUL RITUALS

In addition to the Judaic and Islamic practice of circumcision, there are many religious observances and rituals that would be considered painful. On the Day of Ashura, Shi'a Muslims engage in self-flagellation with chains and spikes during the Zanjeer Zani ritual. Some Muslim flagellants are known to injure themselves in mourning of Hussein and the massacre at Karbala. Hindus make a barefoot 40-mile pilgrimage over hot ground, with little or no water or food, to Sabari Malai. The accompanying injuries, suffering, and pain are seen as expressions of their devotion. During the Sundance ceremony of the Plains Indians, young men are attached to a pole, representing the Tree of Life, a direct connection to the the Creator, by a skewer piercing their chest, honoring ancestors and communities (Bolelli). Some reports indicate that at the end of the dance they literally attempt to tear themselves free, leaving pieces of their flesh behind. After undergoing chest piercing, a participant in the Sundance ceremony was quoted as saying, "I felt pain, but I also felt that closeness with the Creator. I felt like crying for all the people who needed my prayers … it brought tears to my eyes."

Religious masochism such as self-inflicted pain and suffering in the form of mortification (to punish one's body or control one's passions by self-denial) and self-flagellation (whipping or flogging oneself) is not uncommon. Its primary purpose is to gain some type of transcendent state thought to bring one closer to their deity. Christianity, for example, has a long tradition of mortification, including self-denial, fasting, self-flagellation, and even self-castration. Catholic monks and nuns take vows of celibacy and poverty, forgoing the usual human comforts and pleasures of this world in an effort to mimic the life of Christ and in the hope of the ultimate reward in the life hereafter. During the festival of Thaipusam, Hindu yogis engage in a ritual known as Kavadi. The ritual practices can involve carrying heavy weights up a hill, piercing various body parts with skewers, or suspending themselves by meat hooks penetrating the flesh of the back and legs. "The greater the pain," one text says, "the greater the god-earned merit."

On the Day of Ashura, some worshipers whip their own backs with bunched knives, known as *zanjirs*. The appearance of body marks or wounds resembling those suffered by Christ during the crucifixion are referred to as *stigmata*. Such marks may be accompanied by the experience of pain. The hands, feet, and chest areas of Christ's body that were pierced by nails or a spear are considered the five Holy Wounds. Tears of blood, sweating of blood, wounds on the back mimicking the effects of scourging, cuts on the forehead like those caused by the crown of thorns, and pain without any visible wound have also been noted. Sometimes the wounds did not clot, remained "fresh" and uninfected. One might consider this to be a form of self-flagellation in the sense that stigmatics eagerly sought to suffer pain and harm in a manner similar to Christ.

Stigmata are primarily, though not exclusively, associated with the Roman Catholic faith. Perhaps the first reported stigmatic was Saint Paul: "I bear on my body the marks of Jesus" (Galatians 6:7). A religious explanation for this phenomenon is offered by theologian Ivan Illich (1987), in a paper entitled "Hospitality and Pain": "Compassion with Christ…is faith so strong and so deeply incarnate that it leads to the individual embodiment of the contemplated pain." Saint Francis of Assisi and Padre Pio of Pietrelcina may be two of the more notable stigmatics. During a 40-day fast in 1224, two years before his death, while praying, Saint Francis experienced the presence of an angel being crucified. Humbled by this vision, he was beset with joy, pain, and suffering. Thereafter, he manifested wounds in his hands, feet, and side. Padre Pio's stigmata emerged early in his life, persisted for over 50 years, and were the object of study by several reputable physicians in the 1920s. The wounds were described as unexplained, subject to healing and then reappearing. No diagnosis was ever rendered, and X-rays of the hands in 1954 revealed no bony abnormalities (Ruffin, 1991).

From a scientific perspective, there is a tendency to dismiss such reports as some form of hysteria or to offer up a plausible scientific explanation. Alternative explanations to the supernatural origin of stigmata have included the presence of a dissociative disorder, self-starvation, self-mutilation (conscious or unconscious), comorbid medical conditions (i.e., skin ulcers, purpura—purple hemorrhage of blood into the skin), and a psychosomatic reaction (psychogenic purpura). Another possibility is that of a psychophysiological reaction. For example, biofeedback research (Miller, 1978) has documented the ability of the rodent to learn to increase the flow of blood to one ear or the other. Given the remarkably greater sophistication of the human brain, one might speculate that these observations are a consequence of mental focus so intense as to produce chemical and cellular changes in the skin. The possibility of stigmata representing the most extreme form of mirror-pain (touch) synesthesia (Fitzgibbon et al, 2010, 2012; see Chapter 11) should be considered. Our scientific minds would tell us that the statistical probability of stigmata is so low as to question its existence. Our religious or spiritual mind uses the same data to make the case for divine intervention or a miracle.

Many attempts have been made to replicate these types of religious experiences in the laboratory or through the use of psychoactive substances. The use of sensory-deprivation environments, controlled use of hallucinogenic, and physiological monitoring of experienced yogis and mystics represent a few such models. However, does replicating the physiological parameters of the experience constitute the totality of the experience? William James (1902/2009) labeled this "medical reductionism." He argued that it would be "logically fallacious" to assume that there is nothing beyond the physical state or that which can be fully described in the context of a neurological event. James felt that one must consider the possibility that such altered states of consciousness make the individual more receptive to the metaphysical and uniquely personal religious experience.

ACADEMIC STUDIES

Religion can be defined as a belief in or recognition of the existence of God, gods, spirit, deity, or higher power influencing or having control over the universe and one's life or destiny. Research in the area of pain and religion has gone in many different directions. In most cases religion is viewed as a complex multidimensional concept involving cognitive, emotional, behavioral, and motivational components. These aspects of religion may act individually or in concert. Their impact can be directly on the patient's pain perception, mood states, and overall sense of well-being, or indirectly through the interpretation, attribution, and meaning the patient ascribes to their pain or pain causing disease. For example, some patients may feel they are being justifiably punished for a past transgression and therefore must bear their pain until God decides otherwise. Others may view coping with pain as an opportunity to witness to God's unfailing support. Religiosity or spirituality (R/S) can also be seen as a mechanism for coping with pain such as through the use of prayer.

In *Sacred Pain: Hurting the Body for the Sake of the Soul*, Ariel Glucklich (2001) outlines five different models from which to approach pain within a religious context. The *juridical model* views ritual pain as a form of self-punishment and penance for past transgressions and sin, and as means of removing punishment imparted by God, karma, or one's own guilt. The *military model* is based on the Christian and Muslim traditional view of the embodied soul as the enemy. Hurting the flesh, and pain, are weapons used against this enemy and by which the soul is liberated. Christian ascetics highly valued pain. Indeed, it is said that the Catholic Saint Simeon the Stylite tortured himself to death because of his love of pain. The more common *athletic model* sees pain as a tool for training the body. The transformative experience often described by mystics illustrates the *magical model*. Finally, the *psychotropic/ecstatic model* emphasizes the importance and meaningfulness of euphoric states and altered level of consciousness to the individual.

Dezutter et al (2010) explored the impact of patients' image of God on their response to their pain and illness. For example, is God seen in a positive light as a kind, caring, loving, benevolent God, or negatively as an angry, dissatisfied, and punishing God? Patient responses to questionnaires and the frequency of religious behaviors, such as attending religious services, were interpreted as representing one's image of and relationship with God. As might be expected, a patient's sense of well-being is associated with the meaning given to their disease and their image of God. Reappraising pain as an opportunity for growth and learning, and the presence (real or imagined) of social support, resulted in a greater sense of one's ability to cope with the pain and a reduction in the perceived suffering. Those who tended to blame God, express anger toward God, and discover God not to be the benevolent deity they had thought, experienced a greater degree of pain and suffering. What remains to be explored is the relative importance of patients' image of God image in relation to their attachment or relationship with God. In other words, is God some remote, distant deity who chooses or not to inflict disease or pain for some unknown reason, or is God part of our experience, available to provide guidance, support, and a safe harbor? In a sense, is one's attachment more intellectual and cognitive or emotional?

A study by Weich et al (2008) exposed participants to pictures of two women with similar appearance. Both pictures showed a young woman wearing a veil or head-covering looking downward as though in a state of contemplation. One picture was an image of the Virgin Mary ("religious condition") the other was Leonardo da Vinci's "Woman with Ermine" ("non-religious condition"). Some of the participants were Catholic, others were identified as non-religious. Each participant viewed the image for 30 seconds before and then during exposure to a series of electric shocks. Participants rated their pain level as well as their emotional experience. While the Catholics reported a sense of reverence when viewing the Virgin Mary, the non-religious participants reported indifference and some even disdain. When the image of the Virgin Mary was present, Catholics reported a decrease in subjective pain compared to when having viewed "Woman with Ermine," 75/100 vs. 65/100. Though seemingly small, this level of pain reduction was statistically significant and rivaled that of some traditional pain therapies. No differences in pain ratings were noted among the non-religious participants when viewing one picture or the other. Furthermore, the use of fMRI revealed altered activity in the right ventrolateral prefrontal cortex (VLPFC) in those reporting a reduction in their pain. This area of the brain is known to be activated when cognitively oriented therapies have been effective in reducing pain, which suggests that viewing a religiously significant image activated a well-recognized neural mechanism involved in pain modulation.

Spiritual beliefs can influence the cognitive and emotional components of pain and therefore the activity of the involved neurophysiological processes. The relationship between spirituality, coping, and pain is often cast within the usual biopsychosocial model, appealing to the gate control theory of pain as an explanatory mechanism. That is, the instigation of a set of beliefs resulting in a reformulation of the meaning of the pain, along with the use of prayer and spiritual support as coping strategies, modulates activity at the cortical level and thus dampens the experience, especially the affective component, of pain.

The relationship between spirituality, coping, and pain has been examined by several researchers (Bush et al, 1999; Wachholtz et al, 2007). Religious or spiritual (R/S) coping can be divided into passive or active, positive and adaptive (God as benevolent and loving), or negative and maladaptive (deferring to or blaming God, feeling abandoned or punished by God). Expressions of positive spirituality, through the use of prayer, hope, participation in religious services, religious-based attributions, or seeking spiritual support, are considered to be *active* coping responses. These active coping responses have generally been associated with longer survival time, enhanced sense of relaxation, decreased muscle tension, better mental health, fewer postoperative complications, less depression, and delayed onset of physical disability. Negative R/S coping, by contrast, tends to be related to poorer mental and physical health, as well as higher mortality rates. In some cases, praying and hoping were associated with increased pain, functional impairment, and disability. However, it may be that these patients were already in ill health and found themselves turning to religion as a source of solace. There is some suggestion that positive spirituality and the sense of well-being may influence serotonin receptor activity in the brain (Borg et al, 2003).

Prayer has been found to be either the first or second most commonly used pain-related coping strategy (Ashby and Scott, 1994; Roenstiel and Keefe, 1983). Determining whether prayer is used as an active coping strategy (to reduce the pain experience) a or passive one (to cope with the pain and suffering) may help to explain some of these different findings. Furthermore, it is unclear if it is pain intensity or pain tolerance that is being influenced by prayer. Longitudinal studies have found a correlation between day-to-day spiritual coping activity and pain. The possible contribution of distraction has yet to be determined. In general, it is thought that R/S behaviors may affect pain in any of a number of ways: distraction, attributions, self-efficacy, social support, instrumental support, and relaxation.

Rippentrop et al (2005) attempted to characterize religiousness and spirituality in a group of 122 patients with chronic pain. Over 65% had had pain for at least 1 year, a third for 3 years or more. Some 70% lived in rural areas or small towns, 87% had 12 years or more of formal education, and 72% described themselves as Christian. Their responses to the Brief Multidimensional Measure of Religiousness/Spirituality (BMMRS) were compared to those of 1,445 individuals in the general population used in the development of normative data for the BMMRS. Among other areas, the BMMRS questionnaire probes the person's values and beliefs, attitudes toward forgiveness, and private religious practices, including prayer, meditation, and reading religious material.

The authors reported a number of unexpected findings. For example, patients with a longer history of pain tended to be less forgiving of themselves and others, experienced less support from their religious congregation, and became increasingly more bitter and angry. Those reporting lower levels of overall mental health status tended to feel punished and abandoned by God and avoided any reliance on God. The less forgiving patients perceived themselves to be and the more negative their religious coping strategies, the greater their pain intensity and interference levels, the greater their feelings of being punished and abandoned by God, and the greater the lack of any daily spiritual experiences. In general, patients with chronic pain reported less desire to reduce their pain and suffering. It was as though they became "so consumed by their own suffering that they may have nothing left for others who are hurting. Such persons feel alone and abandoned by others as well as God" (Rippentrop et al, 2005, p. 319). Persons receiving money from entitlement programs because of their pain and disability were also found to be less forgiving and have more negative religious coping attitudes, appeared more angry with themselves, others, and God, and seemed to harbor more resentment, frustration, and disappointment.

CONCLUSION

There appears to be no evidence that the Jewish, Christian, Muslim, or Hindu religions find suffering and pain, in and of themselves, to have any intrinsic value. Rather, there is likely to be a deeper meaning and an opportunity for spiritual growth through the circumstances a person is exposed to and the responses made to them. Pain and suffering are often regarded as manifestations of the evil and sin in the world. Pain is recognized as part of a learning process, a warning that something is wrong. For some, to ask "Why?" assumes an ability to comprehend and understand the mind of God.

The physiological and neurochemical mechanisms of nociception are fairly well understood. From an objective or scientific perspective, pain can be viewed as a product of the activation of nociceptors, resulting in a variety of neurochemical and physiological processes involving central nervous system structures. The release of adrenalin and endorphins creates a characteristic state of hyperarousal and hyperexcitability. It is, however, the context in which this occurs that greatly influences the meaning, interpretation, intensity, and impact of pain on the individual. This is no more evident than in the setting of religion and religious rituals. To this day, despite the availability of a modern pain unit, some 49% of patients interviewed in Maputo, Mozambique follow the ancient religious lure to the "nyanga" (healer), where the use of traditional treatments including scarification and expulsion of spirits are common (Ferreira et al, 2013).

Rituals involving pain are found in many cultures and across many different religions. Ritualized self-inflicted pain and suffering may occur for many reasons, including exploring religious experience and a transcendental state, penance or punishment, identification with the divine, ritual observance, or honoring one's ancestors. In the proper context, the mind appears capable of turning pain into bursts of ecstasy, an emotional release, an altered state of consciousness, or a temporary high mimicking a feeling of transcendence; pain of this type seems highly desirable to those who experience it. Perhaps John Milton was right when, in *Paradise Lost*, he described the mind as its own place, and in itself can make a heaven of hell.

The relationship of religious experiences and mental (brain) activity has created such interest that it has spawned a new area of investigation, neurotheology (Joesph, 2002; Persinger et al, 2010). The term *neurotheology* was coined by Ashbrook in 1984, in the hope that ongoing exploration of religion-related brain functions would lead to renewed, scientific appraisal of theistic beliefs. Neurotheology represents another example of William James' notion of medical materialism (reductionism). That is, it is an attempt to reduce a religious experience to its neurological and physiological, if not cellular, aspects. The implied assumption is that such experiences can be so described—that anyone manifesting a like experience will demonstrate the same physical substrate, and anyone manifesting these aspects will experience them in the same manner. If that is the case, then there is little room for individually assigned interpretation or meaning.

Yet no one would assert that everyone with increased blood pressure and heart rate would consider themselves as having a panic attack or that every panic attack has the identical physiological profile. Indeed, certain therapies are designed to help people reinterpret physical symptoms in a more adaptive fashion. Accepting such a notion of an infallible, reproducible physiological substrate would eliminate the need for any consideration of meaning, the mind, or consciousness. A neurological profile would tell us all we need to know about the individual and the problem in question. However, if the exploration of pain has done nothing else it has highlighted the sometimes vast discrepancy between the medical and neurological data and the patient's experience of pain. The continued exploration for so-called biomarkers need not be abandoned, but caution should be exercised in the interpretation of the findings and the discrediting of other more phenomenological data.

REFERENCES

Anand K, Hickey P. Pain and its effects in the human neonate and fetus. *N Engl J Med.* 1987;317:1326.

Artson BS, Glazer M. *The Bedside Torah: Wisdom, Visions, and Dreams.* New York: McGraw Hill; 2001.

Ashbrook, J. Neurotheology. The working brain and the work of theology. *Zygon.* 1984;19:331–350.

Ashby JS, Scott LR. Prayer as a coping strategy for chronic pain patients. *Rehabil Psychol.* 1994;39(3):205–209.

Berg Y. *Kabbalah on Pain: How to Use it to Lose it (Technology for the Soul).* Los Angeles: Kabbalah Publishing; 2007.

Bleich JD. Judaism and animal experimentation. In Regan T, ed. *Animal Sacrifices—Religious Perspectives on the Use of Animal in Science*. Philadelphia: Temple University Press; 1986.

Borg J, Andree B, Soderstrom H, Farde L. The serotonin system and spiritual experiences. *Am J Psychiatry*. 2003;160:1965–1969.

Bush EG, Rye MS, Brant CR, Emery E, Pargament KI, Riessinger CA. Religious coping with chronic pain. *Appl Psychophysiol Biofeedback*. 1999;24:249–260.

Chazen L. Judaism: *Metzora*: no pain, no gain. *Israel Nation News*. April 10, 2008. www.israelnationalnews.com/Articles/Article.aspx/7897. Retrieved October 9, 2013.

Courson J. *Applications Commentary: The New Testament*. Nashville, TN: Thomas Nelson; 2003.

Daly CC, Gregory NG, Wotton SB, Whittington PE. Concussive methods of pre-slaughter stunning in sheep—assessment of brain-function using cortical evoked responses. *Res Vet Sci*. 1986;41:349–352.

Dezutter J, Luyckx K, Schapp-Jonker H, Bussing A, Corveleyn J, Hutsebaut D. God image and happiness in chronic pain patients: the mediating role of disease interpretation. *Pain Med*. 2010;11:765–773.

Einstein A. Science, Philosophy and Religion: a Symposium. 1941. www.sacred-texts.com/aor/einstein/einsci.htm. Retrieved February 20, 2013.

Ferreira K, Schwalbach MT, Schwalbach J, Speciali J. Chronic pain in Maputo, Mozambique: new insights. *Pain Med*. 2013;14:551–553.

Fitzgibbon BM, Enticott PG, Rich AN, Giummarra MJ, Georgiou-Karistianis N, Bradshaw JL. Mirror-sensory synaesthesia: exploring "shared" sensory experiences as synaesthesia. *Neurosci Biobehav Rev*. 2012;36(1):645–657.

Fitzgibbon BM, Giummarra MJ, Georgiou-Karistianis N, Enticott PG, Bradshaw JL. Shared pain: from empathy to synesthesia. *Neurosci Biobehav Rev*. 2010;43:500–512.

Freeman T. Embracing pain with joy—Kabbalah, Chassidism and Jewish mysticism. http://www.chabad.org/library/article_cdo/aid/1407611/jewish/Embracing. Accessed October 14, 2013.

Glucklich A. *Sacred Pain: Hurting the Body for the Sake of the Soul*. New York: Oxford Press, 2001.

Goldman R. The psychological impact of circumcision. *BJU International*. 1999;83(Suppl 1):93–102.

Hemsworth PH, Mellor DJ. A scientific comment on the welfare of sheep slaughtered without stunning. Animal Welfare Science Centre (AWSC), Melbourne, Victoria, Australia, July 14, 2009. http://www.daff.gov.au/animal-plant-health/welfare/aaws/a_scientific_comment_on_the_welfare_of_sheep_slaughtered_without_stunning. Accessed October 23, 2013.

Illich I. Hospitality and pain. Presented at the McCormick Theological Seminary, Chicago, November, 1987. http://ournature.org/~novembre/illich/1987_hospitality_and_pain. PDF. Accessed October 14, 2013.

Islamic Ruling on Animal Slaughter. World Health Organization, Regional Office for the Eastern Mediterranean, Alexandria, Egypt, 1997.

James W. *The Varieties of Religious Experience: A Study in Human Nature*. Seven Treasures Publications; 1902/2009.

Joseph R (ed.). *Neurotheology: Brain, Science, Spirituality, Religious Experiences*. San Jose, CA: University Press; 2002.

Lewis CS. *The Problem of Pain*. New York: Harper Collins; 1940.

Loeser JD. Pain, suffering, and the brain: a narrative of meaning. In DB Carr, JD Loeser, DB Morris, eds. *Narrative, Pain, and Suffering*. Seattle: IASP Press; 2005:17–29.

McCracken LM, Vowles KE, Eccleston C. Acceptance-based treatment for persons with complex, long-standing chronic pain: a preliminary analysis of treatment outcome in comparison to a waiting phase. *Behav Res Ther.* 2005;43:1335–1346.

Miller NE. Biofeedback and visceral learning. *Annu Rev Psychol.* 1978;29:373–404.

Muslim World League. Recommendation about pre-slaughter stunning. 1986; No. 3:1. WHO-AM/FOST/1-E, p. 8.

Persinger MA, Saroka K, Koren SA, St-Pierre LS. The electromagnetic induction of mystical and altered states within the laboratory. *J Conscious Expl Res.* 2010;1(7):808–830.

Rippentrop AE, Altmaier EM, Chen JJ, Found EM, Keffala VJ. The relationship between religion/spirituality and physical health, mental health, and pain in a chronic pain population. *Pain.* 2005;116:311–321.

Rosenstiel AK, Keefe FJ. The use of coping strategies in chronic low back pain patients: relationship to patient characteristics and current adjustment. *Pain.* 1983;17(1):33–44.

Ruffin B. *Padre Pio: The True Story.* Huntington, IN: OSV Press; 1991:160–163.

Ryan C, Finer N. Changing attitudes and practices regarding local analgesia for newborn circumcision. *Pediatrics.* 1994;94:232.

Wachholtz A, Pearce M, Koenig H. Exploring the relationship between spirituality coping, and pain. *J Behav Med.* 2007;30:311–318.

Weich K, Farias M, Kahane G, Shackel N, Tiede W, Tracey I. An fMRI study measuring analgesia enhanced by religion as a belief system. *Pain.* 2008;139:467–476.

Weinberg N. The 48 ways to wisdom. http://www.aish.com/sp/48w/. Accessed October 14, 2013.

Whitman SM. OUCH: How three religions view pain and suffering. March 2, 2010. www.pendlehill.org/lectures/feb2010/343-how-three-religions-viewnpain-and-suffering. Accessed October 16, 2013.

Whitman SM. Pain and suffering as viewed by the Hindu religion. *J Pain.* 2007;8(8):607–613.

Zacharias R. *Jesus Among Other Gods.* Nashville, TN: W. Publishing Group; 2000.

Zimmerman M. Physiological mechanisms of pain and its treatment. *Klin Anaesthesiol Intensivther.* 1986;32:1–19.

11 Empathy and Pain

I pity the man who does not feel the pain of the lash on another's man back.
–Abraham Lincoln

INTRODUCTION

Empathy is characterized by a sense of knowing or sharing the experience of another; another's feeling becomes "contagious" and resonates within us. There are many types of empathy. Empathy can exist for a situation (a personal loss) or an emotion (suffering). According to Gallese (2000), empathy comes from the German word *Einfühlung* and was introduced by Theodor Lipps in 1903 as a way of referring to the interaction between a work of art and its observer—that is, the manner in which the observer imaginatively projected himself into the contemplated object. The concept of Einfühlung was later extended into the domain of intersubjectivity, which he characterized in terms of inner imitation of the perceived movements of others. When watching an acrobat perform, Lipps noted that he felt as though he was performing the acrobatics. In all likelihood, much of what we think of as empathy is processed at the nonconsciousness level (Yamada and Decety, 2009).

The importance of the awareness of the acting body and a mechanism for accomplishing this has become a major field of study for social-cognitive neuroscience (Decety and Batson, 2007; Decety and Meyer, 2008). However, this concept is also relevant in the area of pain, as it addresses social interaction as a potential pain-producing event occurring without any physical injury or activation of the peripheral nociceptive system (pain without nociception).

TERMS AND DEFINITIONS

The synchronization of biological functions among humans may represent a type physiological empathy. McClintock (1971) reported a study involving female room-mates at Wellesley College. Although the timing of their menstrual cycles was disparate upon moving in together, they appeared to become more coordinated over time. In fact, some 30% became synchronized within 3 months. Moreover, there was a greater likelihood of this occurring among those considering themselves to be friends. While the debate over the extent of this phenomenon continues, it seems to be related to the release of and exposure to pheromones to which the brain reacts in an unconscious fashion.

According to Decety and Jackson (2004, 2006), the ability to understand the emo-tions and feelings of another, whether witnessed firsthand as in watching a distressed child, or secondhand via pictures, book, or the imagination, refers to the experience of empathy. Empathy is described as having two components. The *affective* compo-nent requires the ability to share in the emotional experience of another; the *cogni-tive* component involves understanding another person's perspective. This ability to "mind-read" appears to be hard-wired in the brain and develops through social inter-actions. Understanding and comprehending another's feelings does not imply that any action will be taken.

In addition to perspective-taking, self-awareness, and emotional reappraisal, empa-thy also has a representational component and a processing component. The *represen-tation component* consists of memories localized in distributed neural networks of the brain that encode information and, when temporarily activated, enable access to this stored information. The *process component* involves computational procedures that are localized and independent of the nature or modality of the stimulus being processed. *Mentalizing*, or what is called *theory of mind (ToM)*, denotes the ability to explain and predict our own behavior and that of others by appealing to desires, intentions, emo-tions, and beliefs.

Emotional resonance refers to the congruence between the emotions expressed by another and the observer. It may be a precursor to empathy. For example, new-borns cry more in reaction to cries of distress from other newborns than they do when hearing their own crying or that of a 5-month-old. Emotional resonance is also reflected in the type of affective synchrony regularly observed in mother–infant pairs at 2–3 months of age. By 2 years of age, children experience emotional concerns on behalf of a victim, appear to comprehend other's emotional difficulties, and act in a prosocial manner, providing comfort and help (Hutman and Dapretto, 2009). This emotional resonance incorporates both emotional contagion and intersubjective sym-pathy. *Emotional contagion* denotes the tendency to automatically mimic and synchro-nize facial expressions, vocalizations, postures, and movements with those of another and, consequently, to converge emotionally with the other person. *Intersubjective sympathy* implies having an innate predisposition to being sensitive and responsive to the subjective states of another. Infants (36 hours old), for example, can discriminate happy, sad, and surprise facial expressions.

These observations of the behavior of infants would lead one to speculate that there is a built-in, shared representational mechanism. In this model, perception of the emotions of another would activate the neural mechanisms responsible for the generation of emotions in the observer. This system would then prompt the observer to resonate with the state of the person being observed. The observer would then activate the motor representation and associated autonomic and somatic responses that stem from the observed target.

In general, empathy responses tend to involve the emotional and not the sensory aspects of another's pain. There is evidence, however, of mirror-pain synesthesia (discussed later in the chapter) in which the individual experiences some or all of the painful physical sensations when observing another in pain (Fitzgibbon et al, 2010, 2012). Single-unit recordings have suggested activation of pain-related neurons in the anterior cingulate cortex (ACC; Hutchinson et al, 1999) in response to actual thermal stimulation or when observing another being so stimulated. ToM research has shown that the prefrontal cortex, especially the right side, is involved in the capacity to reason about the emotional and feeling states of others, including the ability to adopt another's perspective (Decety and Chaminade, 2003). Individuals appearing to lack the ability to simulate emotions they cannot experience must rely on cognitive input to the ToM mechanisms. Sociopathic patients, autistic children, Asperger's patients, and individuals with certain types of neurological injuries manifest the failure of a mentalizing mechanism (ToM module) (Leslie, 1991). Prefrontal, paracingulate, and amygdala dysfunction appear to be common in these patients.

EMPATHY RESEARCH

Animal Studies

Langford and colleagues (2006) explored the concept of empathy in mice through conducting a series of studies. They theorized that if empathy existed in mice, then observing pain in one mouse should affect the behavior of its conspecific to a painful stimulus. After obtaining a baseline frequency of writhing, a classic pain behavior of isolated mice, an inflammatory substance was injected into the paw. Then, two same-sex mice, from the same or different cages, were placed in a transparent Plexiglas cylinder, one at each end, so they could easily observe one another. One or both of the mice were injected. When compared to the isolated mouse, there was no difference in the amount of pain behavior, regardless of whether one or both of the mice from different cages received the injection. However, if the two injected mice had resided together in the same cage for 14 to 21 days, they exhibited substantially more writhing behavior than a single isolated mouse or two mice from separate cages. Furthermore, this increased pain behavior was observed in cage-mates whether they were genetically related or not. Indeed, when the dyad was made up of strangers, the writhing behavior of the injected mouse was lower than that seen in the isolated mouse, but only in males. This was interpreted as distraction and perhaps stress-induced analgesia created by the presence of a stranger.

In an effort to determine how the mice were communicating with one another, Langford et al systematically blocked sight, smell, and hearing. When a visual barrier was positioned between the mice, their pain behavior tended to mimic that of an isolated mouse. They concluded that the socially mediated hyperalgetic response in the presence of a conspecific appeared to be tied to visual cues. However, they could not completely control for the possibility of pheromonal communication.

A second study used the injection of an inflammatory agent (formalin) into the foot. Mice pairs placed in individual cylinders, but in clear view of one another, were injected. There was a remarkable concordance (synchrony) of pain behavior (licking the injected foot). Most interesting was the observed reduction in pain behavior in the mouse receiving a higher concentration of the formalin when it observed a cage-mate getting a lower and thus less painful concentration.

In the final experiment in this series, mouse dyads were tested as in the second study, and one or both mice were injected. Their paw withdrawal response to a laser heat stimulus was then tested. The degree of thermal hyperalgesia was determined by time-to-paw withdrawal, relative to the socially isolated mouse. Predictably, the mice in dyads formed of cage-mates showed a heightened sensitivity to the heat stimulus, whether both or only one of the dyad was injected, compared to a social isolated mouse or a dyad made up of strangers. Finally, the researchers demonstrated that the increase in pain sensitivity occurred even when the two mice were exposed to different painful stimuli, for example, injection of an inflammatory substance or thermal pain.

Langford et al interpreted their data as indicating that the pain system is sensitized by observing pain in a familiar conspecific. Furthermore, this socially mediated hyperalgesia cannot be accounted for on the basis of stress, imitation, or conditioning. Appealing to activation of mirror neurons as an explanation was deemed inadequate because the socially mediated hyperalgesia occurred when each mouse was exposed to a different stimulus. In addition, theorizing the presence of sympathy, altruism, or some conscious (cognitive) representation did not appear necessary. Instead, they turned to the perception-action model (PAM) of Preston and de Waal (2002). The PAM theory states that attended perceptions of the object's state automatically activates the subject's representations (i.e., mental) of the state, situation, and object, and that activation of these representations automatically primes or generates the associated autonomic and somatic responses, unless inhibited. The observer's response is also affected by the familiarity and similarity of experience between him or her and the conspecific.

Studies by Rice and Gainer (1962) have shown that rats will press a bar to lower a distressed conspecific harnessed and suspended in the air, back to safety all the while remaining close to and oriented toward it. In a separate instance, Church (1959) examined the behavior of one rat as it observed another receiving an electric shock. Rather than pressing a bar to discontinue the shock, it runs to the furthest corner from the distressed rat and crouches, motionless. This response occurs without prior exposure to the shock, is intensified following exposure to the shock, and is stronger when the previous shock has occurred at the same time as the conspecific. This behavior is contrary to the phenomenon of shock-induced aggression (Azrin et al, 1963, 1964; Whitman and Doleys, 1973), in which animals in a confined space reflexively attack one another when simultaneously shocked through a gridded floor.

Masserman et al (1964) used monkeys trained to pull chains to deliver different amounts of food. The situation was then altered such that when one monkey pulled the chain presenting the larger reward, a second monkey, in clear view of the first, received a brief electric shock. After witnessing this, two-thirds of the monkeys chose the non-shock chain, even though it was attached to the lesser food reward. Indeed, one monkey stopped pulling either chain for 5 days and another for 12 days. These animals appeared to be starving themselves to avoid shocking their conspecific. Starvation was more associated with visual than auditory cues and was more likely if the monkeys had experienced the shock themselves. Starvation was enhanced by familiarity of the shocked monkey.

Siebenaler and Caldwell (1956) reported on two separate episodes of empathetic, altruistic, and cooperative behaviors among dolphins. In one instance a school of dolphins was stunned by a blast of dynamite. In the second case a dolphin was rendered unconscious when it struck its head while being lowered into a holding tank. In both situations two dolphins immediately appeared. They positioned themselves one under each of the stunned animal's pectoral fins, supporting the unconscious animal until it could swim on its own. Of note is the apparent realization that the efforts of a single animal would be worthless as it would be unable to keep the blow-hole of the injured animal from submerging. There are many stories of seemingly spontaneous assistance offered by dolphins to endangered swimmers. Other species of fish and mammals would abandon the scene or attack the swimmer.

Chimpanzees in the Yerkes colony have demonstrated empathy for another suffering from hunger. The chimp with abundant food (the rich one) would often share its food with a less fortunate chimp when it exhibited begging behavior. If the two were friends, the food was shared more freely than if they were not. In some cases, the rich animal was approached by a stranger. Although still finding the begging behavior irresistible, the rich animal would share some food but gave less of it and actually threw it with apparent indignation at the begging stranger (Nissen and Crawford, 1936).

Human Studies

Loggia and his colleagues (2008) studied the effects of empathy on pain perception in a group of non-pain males and females. The subjects were exposed to painful or nonpainful thermal stimuli while observing an actor, assumed to be another participant, relating a personal tragedy designed to elicit high or low levels of empathy and compassion. Subjects rating their empathic response to the story as high reported that the painful thermal stimulus to which they were briefly exposed was more intense and unpleasant than reported by those noting a low empathic response. Moreover, the higher the degree of empathy felt by the subject, the greater their pain rating.

Singer et al (2004, 2006) analyzed the empathic neural responses in a group of non-pain males and females engaged in an economic game. An experimental confederate participated in the game with the actual subject and was instructed beforehand to play the game either fairly or unfairly. A brief electric shock designed to elicit a pain response was administered to the experimental confederate after the game. Brain activity of the actual subjects was monitored by fMRI neuroimaging. As expected, increased activity was noted in the anterior and frontal insula as well as the ACC, parts of the brain's well-known pain network, when subjects were exposed to a painful stimulus. Both genders showed an empathic response in the insula cortex and brainstem when observing an unfamiliar but likeable (one who played a game fair) person in pain. Increased activity in ACC was more pronounced in females but borderline in males. Those scoring higher on an empathy scale had higher empathy activity in the ACC and the insula cortex. Subjects were less empathic toward unfair players. The relative lack of empathy was manifested by lower amounts of empathetic brain activity when observing them in pain. This suppressed or modulated empathetic response was more true of male than female subjects.

The ventral striatum, nucleus accumbens, and orbitofrontal cortex are regions of the brain known to be part of the reward processing network. Increased activity in these areas has been associated with the high reported by drug addicts. Men, more than women, demonstrated increased activity in these reward processing areas when observing an unfair player in pain. Furthermore, the magnitude of this response correlated with their composite revenge score. Thus, cooperation, as shown by fair play, tends to nurture an empathic response in the brain, while selfish or unfair behavior effectively diminishes the empathetic response. In a sense, increased activity in the reward processing circuit of the brain suggests that humans, especially males (Han et al, 2008), derive a feeling of satisfaction simply from seeing justice performed (e.g., the punishment of an unfair player). This appears to extend to the feeling of envy wherein the envious person derives a feeling of satisfaction when the object of their envy encounters some misfortune (Takahashi et al, 2009).

Empathy for pain, like pain itself, is a two-component process—affective and cognitive. Research by Lamm et al (2007a,b, 2011) and that of Jackson et al (2006) have identified the neural correlates of these two components. The affective component is represented by the emotional response to the distress and pain of another. It has been associated with activity in the anterior insula and anterior medial cingulate cortex. By comparison, the cognitive (top-down modulatory system) aspect involves the prefrontal dorsolateral and median prefrontal cortices, known to participate in emotional regulation, as well areas associated with mentalizing, including the temporoparietal junction, the temporal poles, and the precuneus/posterior cingulate cortex (PCC). The relative contributions of these two components have been shown to be influenced by attention. With the redirection of attention, the autonomic affective response to another's pain is dissociated from the more cognitive empathic response.

There appears to be a developmental aspect to empathy. Steinberg (2005) and Mella et al (2012) demonstrated a stronger automatic affective component in response to observing another in pain in adolescents than that in adults. This is assumed to be the consequence of a relative immature mechanism for the down-regulation of emotional responses and an underdeveloped mentalizing cortical network. The exact age at which the latter matures is unclear, but Mella et al (2012) found a significant difference when comparing a group averaging 13 years of age to one 34 years of age. In this instance, after completing questionnaires relating to emotional responsiveness and empathy, subjects viewed a series of colored pictures depicting one hand or two hands in either painful or neutral situations. In addition to the pictures there were descriptions of common accidents, such as catching a hand in a door or cutting it with a pair of scissors. Subjects rated both the pain they thought the person in the picture would feel and their own degree of self-unpleasantness. EEG recording were used to obtain event-related potentials (ERPs). Adolescents showed an earlier automatic emotional response than that of young adults. In general, adolescents have been found to show enhanced activity in the amygdala relative to that in adults and younger children, which suggests that emotional information is highly relevant to them. This appears particularly true for females.

Taken as a whole, research on empathy shows that adolescents tend to demonstrate a heightened emotional response combined with an underdeveloped prefrontal control system. There is also less frontolimbic connectivity than that found in adults. The cognitive abilities necessary to moderate the emotional response emerge over time. Whereas the adolescent is especially vulnerable emotionally, an adaptive balance between the cognitive and emotional (affective) components of empathy is achieved by young adulthood. This is accompanied by a reduction in personal distress, increased perspective-taking, more mature reasoning, and appropriate behavioral responses.

Research involving recordings of single-neuron activity in the brains of macaque monkeys has demonstrated the existence of an execution-matching system (Iacoboni et al, 2005; Iacoboni and Dapretto, 2006). Although this system appears to reside in the premotor cortex (Rizzolatti et al, 1996), the parietal lobule, supplementary mortar area, and the cerebellum are also involved. As implied by its name, activity in the premotor cortex is associated with and tends to precede the eventual performance of an action. However, a subset of these neurons becomes activated when one monkey observes another performing an action. These have been referred to as *mirror neurons* (MN). Canonical neurons (Grezes et al, 2003) are stimulated by looking at a graspable object, while MNs discharge only when the observed monkey is actually performing an action such as grasping, holding, tearing, or manipulating an object. Thus, MNs respond to specific, goal-oriented motor acts.

Research conducted on MNs often involves a subject (monkey) observing an agent (another monkey) and an object (orange). In order for the MNs to be activated there must be an interaction between the other monkey (agent) and the object. These MNs are not activated merely by the sight of the agent (monkey) and its object (orange). Likewise, the degree to which the MNs are engaged is less when the agent is mimicking the action without the target object (grasping an imagined object) or is using a tool of some type. Toddlers, unlike monkeys, seem to actually grasp the intent of an action. This is illustrated by 18-month-old children successfully pulling a dumbbell apart even after observing a demonstrator being unsuccessful at the task. However, this only occurred when there was a direct interaction between the agent (demonstrator) and object (dumbbell) (Meltzoff, 1995). Such was not the case if the demonstrator used a tool or mechanical device.

Jeannerod et al (1995) and di Pellegrino et al (1992) have proposed that MNs constitute an internal representation of the observed goal-directed behavior, enabling the observer to understand and imitate the behavior of others. PET scan studies have shown activation in the bilateral dorsolateral prefrontal cortex and in presupplementary motor area in subjects observing an action with the intent to imitate it. fMRI data indicated activation of the left frontal cortex and right superior parietal lobe when subjects observed a finger movement and when re-creating that movement under different conditions. Iacoboni et al (1999, 2005) interpreted these data to indicate a common code, or direct matching hypothesis, of perception and action. Taken together, the left frontal area of the brain encodes for the goal of movement and understanding the meaning of one's actions. The right parietal lobe encodes for the precision of the movement that would be involved in memorization or imitation of an observed act. Thus we have *shared representations* for perception and action, although the brain areas activated while observing the act and those used in imaging the act are somewhat different.

These areas of the brain also appear to be involved in cognitive empathy processing. In this state, the observed circumstances are held in the mind as alternative interpretations, and actions are considered by activation of somatosensory, limbic, and response areas of the brain. Long- and short-term goals and outcomes (cost-benefit ratio of a given response) are processed in the ventromedial prefrontal cortex. Therefore, empathy seems to involve two parallel processes. The first is a rapid, reflexive subcortical process from sensory to thalamic to amygdala and finally to response cortices representing the apparent reflexive, contagious, or resonant emotional empathic response. The second process is somewhat slower and involves the thalamus-to-cortex-to-amygdala connection and represents the more cognitive or understanding form of empathy.

The purpose for this mirror-matching mechanism remains unclear. However, the capability of individuals to adapt to a particular social environment relies on the ability to select a certain type of behavior on the basis of an understanding of the behavior of others. Gallese and colleagues (Gallese, 2000; Gallese and Goldman, 1998; Gallese et al, 1996) proposed that action understanding relies heavily on a neural mechanism that matches, in the same neuronal substrate, the observed behavior with the one executed. When a given action is planned, its expected motor consequences are forecast. Thus the individual that is going to execute a given action can predict its consequences. Through a process of motor equivalence this information can be used to predict the consequences of the actions performed by others. This implicit, automatic, and non-conscious process of motor simulation enables the observer to use his or her own resources to penetrate the world of another without the need to theorize about it. A process of action simulation automatically establishes a direct, implicit link between agent and observer. Action is the a priori principle enabling social bonds to be initially established. In sum, Gallese and colleagues suggest that through a process of motor equivalence a meaningful link between agent and observer can be established.

Mirror-Pain Synesthesia

Synesthesia is defined by the occurrance of unusual perceptual experiences in response to ordinary stimulation. There may be a many as 63 variants of synesthesia. The estimated prevelance ranges from 1.6 to 30% depending on the type. Mirror-sensory synesthesia is a specific type, of which mirror-pain synesthesia is a subtype. Mirror-pain synesthesia (MPS) is demonstrated when an observer witnesses a noxious stimulus being applied to another (inducer) and actually experiences the pain (the concurrent). This may be considered a kind to physical empathy (see Fitzgibbon et al., 2010, 2012, for a detailed description and review). Ramachandran (2000) and others have identified cells in the human anterior cingulate that are activated not only when the individual pokes a person with a needle (pain neurons) but also when merely watching another being poked. These mirror neurons were affectionately refered to as *empathy neurons*, or the Dalai Llama neurons.

Activation of the somatosensory cortex has been noted when watching a needle enter the hand of another. In one instance, the subject reported feeling as though being touched when observing another being touched. This was also associated with increased somatosensory cortex activity.

Amputees have reported increased phantom limb pain when viewing or just imagining another amputee in pain. One study by Osborn and Derbyshire (2001) found that responders to images depicting injury to another showed increased activity in the anterior midcigulate, anterior insula, prefrontal cortex, and S1 and S2. The nonresponderes failed to demonstrate any changes in insular cortex, S1, or S2.

MPS may represent an extreme form of the otherwise normal process. Fitzgibbon et al (2012) have proposed that this phenomenon is a consequence of the disinhibition of systems involved in empathy for pain. It may occur developmentally or can be acquired as a result of brain injury, sensory deafferentation, or amputation or in the case of intense, traumatic, or chronic pain. Although individuals manifesting MPS score higher on tests of empathy and tend to be more emotionally reactive, this is not likely to be the basic mechanism. The reduced inhibitory control of normal connections, particularly those involving S1, S2, and the insula cortex, results in a hyperactivity of the somatosensory mirror system. The hypervigilance to pain cues associated with various pain conditions could further intensify this hyperactivity.

Fitzgibbon et al have also hypothesized potential genetic and epigenetic factors. Thus, an activity that ordinarily occurs at the nonconscious level comes to exceed the threshold for the conscious perception of pain.

LACK OF EMPATHY AND HURT FEELINGS

There appears to be a neural substrate for empathy for or feeling another's pain. But what of the relationship of "hurt feelings" to the activation of pain-related cortical structures? Eisenberger et al (2003) have studied whether social comments or actions, perceived as negative, stimulate a painful emotional experience within the framework of social rejection. Subjects were either socially included (SI), explicitly socially excluded (ESE), or implicitly socially exclude (ISE) in a social activity. Those who were ESE were prevented from participating by the others engaging in the social activity, that is, an individual was intentionally not invited or was asked to leave a social gathering. The ISE subjects were unable to participate because of external circumstances unrelated to the others involved in the social activity.

Using fMRI technology, the authors recorded increased activity in the ACC, primarily the dorsal aspect, and in the right ventral prefrontal cortex (RVPFC). The ACC encodes for the affective or distressing component of pain. When ablated in animal mothers, it disrupts the maternal behavior of keeping their pups near or in re-establishing contact in response to a separation cry. Activation of the RVPFC helps to regulate or dampen the pain-distress and negative emotional responses. When activity in the ESE subjects was compared with that in the IS and ISE groups, much greater activity in the dorsal ACC was found, suggesting emotional distress similar to that of physical pain. Those reporting the higher degree of "having their feelings hurt" also had less activation in the RVPFC. Some activity was noted in the insula cortex, but it was not related to the degree of distress. The ISE subjects showed some less ACC activation than that in the ESE subjects, however, the RVPFC was silent. These data suggest that both groups felt hurt, but that the degree of pain-distress in the ESE group was strong enough to provoke an inhibitory response from the RVPFC, not unlike that recorded in response to painful physical stimulation. Indeed, the right PFC has been shown to be involved in the suppression of emotional memories. The authors concluded that "social pain is analogous in its neurocognitive function to physical pain, alerting us when we have sustained injury to our social connections, allowing restorative measures to be taken" (Eisenberger et al, 2003, p. 292).

Eisenberger and colleagues (Way et al, 2009) also examined if social rejection–induced pain had a genetic component. She focused on the mu-opioid receptor gene (*OPRM1*), which has frequently been associated with physical pain. Subjects socially excluded from a game and scoring high on measures of sensitivity were studied with fMRI and genetic testing. The results revealed that persons possessing a rare form of the *OPRM1* gene previously shown to be associated with increased sensitivity to physically induced pain reported higher levels of rejection sensitivity. Furthermore, increased activity was found in the "social pain–related" regions of the brain, including the dorsal anterior cingulate cortex and anterior insula, in those who were socially excluded.

This appears to be the first study linking the mu-opioid receptor gene to social sensitivity in response to rejection. Way et al (2009) have noted, "These findings suggest that the feeling of being given the cold shoulder by a romantic interest or not being picked for a schoolyard game of basketball may arise from the same circuits that are quieted by morphine." Indeed, Raz and Berger (2010) found that socially isolated rats consumed significantly more morphine when given ad lib access than did paired animals. In addition, a mere 60 minutes of social contract per day abolished this difference. In regard to the obvious overlap in the neurobiology of physical and social pain, Eisenberger and Lieberman (2004) have suggested that the ability to feel the pain of social rejection may be an adaptive way of ensuring they are maintained. Over time, the evolutionary advantage of social connection may have prompted the social-attachment system to share some of the mechanisms of the pain system.

THREAT DETECTION SYSTEM (TDS)

Price (2000) has emphasized the importance of perceiving threat to the experience of pain; activation of a threat detection system (TDS) is very primitive and primal. At the same time that it forces attention to the threatening stimulus or situation, it evokes an avoidance or escape response, which has obvious survival consequences. Decety and Jackson (2004) and others have demonstrated that much of this processing is unconscious. In their two-stage process theory of empathy for pain, Fan and Han (2008) suggest that the early stage involves unconscious detection of the inherent threat value. The later stage incorporates prosocial and motivational value judgments.

From a developmental perspective, it would be tempting to postulate the presence of some type of TDS during infancy, if not the prenatal period (see Chapter 9). Although not able to withdraw, except by a basic reflex response, from a threatening stimulus, infants clearly communicate their discomfort, unrest, and pain. This may form the rudimentary or unconscious aspect of the TDS. Over time, and with the development of an expanded repertoire of physical capabilities, children learn by instruction, conditioning, and modeling how and when to escape or avoid anticipated or experienced physically or interpersonally based pain. The TDS may well be an important modulation of the experience of pain.

The TDS may contribute to our understanding of why one person might disregard a personally life-threatening situation to save another person, and a second individual would stand by or flee. It might be reasonable to speculate on the "unconscious" activation of a TDS by physical or social stimuli. The TDS may well ignite parallel processing of emotional (empathy), behavioral, and value judgment systems—not unlike in Melzack's neuromatrix theory (Melzack, 1999). The demands of the situation (extracting an injured person from a burning automobile) would be compared to the risks (being injured or dying during the rescue effort). The outcome could be influenced by the characteristics of the injured person (one's own child, compared to a fleeing convicted felon). A behavioral response would then emerge. The initial response might be checked by a reconsideration of the consequences, resulting in a type of approach–avoidance conflict. Resolution of the conflict might require ignoring certain facts or information, or reformulating their relative value, therefore re-engaging the cyclical-parallel processing-system. The more the behavioral outcome is determined by a fixed principle (all life is worth saving no matter what the cost), the more deliberate and rapid the response. Therefore, the TDS may well function as a mediator between the degree of empathy for a given situation and the individual's behavioral response. Needless to say, this complicated and complex processing is often conducted in a matter of seconds or less, at times appearing reflexive in nature.

THEORY OF MIND AND MIRROR NEURONS

Gallese and Goldman (1998) have defined *mind-reading* "as the activity of representing specific mental states of others, for example, their perceptions, goals, beliefs, expectations and the like" (p. 495). There are two principle theories of mind-reading, or theory of mind (ToM): the theory theory (TT) and the simulation theory (ST). Within TT there are two perspectives, domain-specific ability and developmental process. Domain-specific ability suggests the existence of an innate, encapsulated, and specific cortical module, whose function is segregated from the other intellectual capacities of the individual. Alternatively, the developmental process views ToM as the final stage of a process in which different scientific theories about one's environment are tested and eventually discarded and new ones adopted (Baron-Chon, 1991; Fodor, 1992; Harris et al, 1989).

The TT proposes that people ordinarily accomplish the act of mind-reading through the development and acquisition of a type of common-sense theory of the mind sometimes referred to a "functional philosophy of the mind." It is thought that individuals possess a set of causal and explanatory laws that connect certain external stimuli with certain inner states. These inner states relate to other inner states, which in turn are connected to certain behaviors. For example, if asked to "read the mind" of a shopper purchasing an object, TT theorists would suggest that while looking the shopper came upon a desirable object (perception or inner state). This particular perception was linked to a desire for the object (a second inner state). This desire activated another inner state associated with decision making and ultimately to the act of purchasing the object. It can therefore be assumed that once the shopper saw an object he or she was sufficiently attracted to it to justify the expenditure. Further, if one's desire or need for an object is strong enough, one will purchase it, and vice versa. Therefore, if we see someone purchasing an object, this implies that the person holds a strong desire or need for it. It is the application of such commonly accepted or "tacitly known casual laws" that TT says allows us to assign certain mental states, attributions, and motivations to another.

In effect, ST claims that we pretend to have the desires, beliefs, preferences, and feelings of another; we put ourselves in their shoes. The attempt is to simulate another's thought process, or what we imagine our thoughts or feelings would be in that situation. This is not unlike playing chess, where White tries to imagine (simulate) Black's strategy. White does not actually make Black's move, but employs this mind-reading process to calculate a counter strategy. These pretended states trigger an internal decision-making mechanism that produces a pretend outcome. This mentalizing process is taken off-line, allowing for the prediction of the mental state of another without engaging in the predicted response. Imagine the chaos that would be created if a person acted out or acted on all of the beliefs, desires, preferences, and feelings they imagined another to have. Further evidence for off-line processing is the relative inability of patients with prefrontal lesions to prevent the compulsive imitating of gestures and complex behaviors performed in front of them.

A major difference, then, between TT and ST is that TT tends to make mind-reading a scientific and dispassionate exercise highlighted by the application of accepted rules or laws to understand another's mind. By contrast, ST views mind-reading as an attempt to mimic, replicate, and impersonate the mental life of another.

It is easy to see how this attempt to simulate or match the mental state of another would relate to the discovery of MN. Perhaps, in the same way that observing a person performing a specific act can activate MNs in the premotor cortex of the observer, imagining or attempting to simulate the mental state of another may activate a type of affective/cognitive mirror neuron (A/C-MN) associated with desires, preferences, beliefs, and feelings. Indeed, it may, in fact, "hurt" to watch someone walking with a painful limp, or observe a patient with rheumatoid arthritis attempting to button their clothes. Parents often find it hard to stand back and let a child struggle though some difficult task, even knowing that it would be in the child's best interest to learn for themselves, even if it involves some hardship.

In all likelihood, if such A/C-MNs exist, they will be found in the prefrontal, cingulate, and/or insular cortices—areas of the brain known to involve cognitive and emotional or affective processes (Gallagher and Firth, 2003). Persons appearing somewhat dispassionate to the plight of others may lack some integral connection or aspect of this system, or have effectively learned to suppress its activation. In the same way that premotor MNs are not activated unless the person attends to the action of another, ignoring certain key features (external stimuli) of another person's behavior may prevent activation of A/C-MNs. By contrast, those motivated toward mind-reading, such as mental health practitioners, may acquire a keen sense of what another is thinking or feeling at the time of a specific act.

CONCLUSION

Patients whose spouses are more attentive and sympathetic appear to have a greater response to painful stimulation. Persons feeling social rejection, isolation, and/or exclusion have activation in many of the same regions of the pain network as those responding to physical trauma. Grieving over the loss of a loved one, observing pain in a liked conspecific, and negative social comparisons are each associated with increased brain activity, especially in the ACC and insula cortex. This empathetic brain response can be seen in precognitive infants and cannot be explained entirely on the basis of stress, imitation, conditioning, cognitive (conscious) representations, sympathy, or altruism. Thus, humans appear to be endowed with an innate capacity for empathy that can only be deactivated by deliberate and conscious inhibition.

Shared representations entail a complex interconnection among various networks of neurons involved in the processing or representation of motor and emotional components and thus do not exist in one area of the brain. Premotor areas are involved in planning, sequencing, and executing behaviors. Temporal lobes are the repository for long-term memories of objects, places, and people. Consolidation of such memories is facilitated by the amygdala and processed in the hippocampus. The perception and regulation of emotions is carried out in the limbic system, particularly the cingulate and orbitofrontal cortices. The prefrontal cortex guides emotional-regulation skills necessary for controlling the degree of emotional distress and the ability to remain focused. Dorsolateral and ventromedial prefrontal regions participate in the maintenance and manipulation of information in working memory.

The accumulated data to this point identify the somatosensory cortex, ACC, insula, thalamus, and periaqueductal gray area as definite parts of the pain network. Many of these same areas can be activated by observing pain and distress in familiar, particularly likeable, conspecifics, experiences of social exclusion, bereavement, being treated unfairly, and negative social comparison, and thus can be said to constitute an empathy network. Lieberman and Eisenberger (2009) stated that "the brain may treat abstract social experiences and concrete physical experiences as more similar than is generally assumed. The link between social and physical pains and pleasures adds to the growing chorus of neurocognitive findings that point to the critical importance of the social world for the surviving and thriving of humans" (p. 891). The interaction of the pain matrix with MNs and the TDS provides yet another example of the complex nature of the experience of pain.

The systematic review of the experimentally based literature by Krahé et al (2013) on the social modulation of pain leaves little doubt as to the validity of this concept. Interpersonal situations such as empathy and social rejection are generally not considered part of the pain classification system, unless subsumed under the heading of psychogenic pain. However, the data would seem to indicate that the pain associated with empathy, particularly in the form of mirror-pain synesthesia, and the pain experienced in response to social rejection involve activation of cortical structures similar to those activated by pain associated with stimulation of the peripheral nociceptive system. To the extent that socially mediated pain is associated with the activation of aspects of the pain matrix representing the sensory and emotional components of pain, they appear to meet the IASP definition of pain. They also provide additional examples of a type of pain that emerges as a result of the activation and interactions of widespread cortical networks and does not require any apparent stimulation of the peripheral nociceptive system. Furthermore, there may be a group of individuals much like those with congenital insensitivity to pain (see Chapter 12) who possess such a highly developed empathy and sensitivity to rejection that they ultimately display the behavioral, physiological, and psychological manifestations associated with chronic pain. The need to expand the understanding of pain and to incorporate such socially mediated pain into the pain lexicon would seem obvious.

Nothing in this discussion of empathy and ToM should be construed as indicating that we understand or know what "the mind" is. Some consider it an emergent phenomenon, others what the brain does, some a pseudo-phenomenon, others the inner or cognitive self. It is in this arena that reductionism and materialism often lose traction. The existence of the mind is rarely doubted. In fact, we sometimes wonder if a particular person may have lost theirs. The apparent absence of a rigorous means of defining and measuring the mind should not deter our continued exploration of it.

REFERENCES

Azrin NH, Hutchinson RR, Hake DF. Pain-induced fighting in the squirrel monkey. *J Exp Anal Behav.* 1963;6:620–626.

Azrin NH, Ulrich RE, Hutchinson R, Norman DG. Effect of shock duration on shock-induced fighting. *J Exp Anal Behav.* 1964;7:9–11.

Baron-Cohen S. Precursors to a theory of mind: understanding attention in others. In Whiten A, ed. *Natural Theories of Mind: Evolution, Development and Simulation of Everyday Mindreading.* Oxford: Basil Blackwell; 1991:233–251.

Church RM. Emotional reactions of rats to the pain of others. *J Comp Physiol Psychol.* 1959;52:132–134.

Decety J, Batson CD. Social neuroscience approaches to interpersonal sensitivity. *Soc Neurosci.* 2007;2:151–157.

Decety J, Chaminade T. When the self represents the other: a new cognitive neuroscience view on psychological identification. *Conscious Cogn.* 2003;12:577–596.

Decety J, Jackson PL. The functional architecture of human empathy. *Behav Cogn Neurosci Rev.* 2004;3:71–100.

Decety J, Jackson PL. A social-neuroscience perspective on empathy. *Curr Direct Psychol Sci.* 2006;15(2):54–58.

Decety J, Meyer M. From emotion resonance to empathic understanding: a social developmental neuroscience account. *Dev Psychopathol.* 2008;20:1053–1080.

di Pellegrino G, Fadiga L, Fogassi L, Gallese V, Rizzolatti G. Understanding motor events: a neurophysiological study. *Exp Brain Res.* 1992;91:176–180.

Eisenberger NI, Lieberman MD. Why rejection hurts: a common neural alarm system for physical and social pain. *Trends Cogn Sci.* 2004;8:294–300.

Eisenberger NI, Lieberman MD, Williams KD. Does rejection hurt? An fMRI study of social exclusion. *Science.* 2003;302(5643):290–292.

Fan Y, Han S. Temporal dynamic of neural mechanisms involved in empathy for pain: an event-related brain potential study. *Neuropsychologia.* 2008;46:160–173.

Fitzgibbon BM, Enticott PG, Rich AN, Giummarra MJ, Georgiou-Karistianis N, Bradshaw JL. Mirror-sensory synaesthesia: exploring "shared" sensory experiences as synaesthesia. *Neurosci Biobehav Rev.* 2012;36(1):645–657.

Fitzgibbon BM, Giummarra MJ, Georgiou-Karistianis N, Enticott PG, Bradshaw JL. Shared pain: from empathy to synesthesia. *Neurosci Biobehav Rev.* 2010;43:500–512.

Fodor JA. A theory of the child's theory of the mind. *Cognition.* 1992;44:283–296.

Gallagher HL, Firth CD. Functional imaging of "theory of mind." *Trends Cogn Sci.* 2003;7:77–83.

Gallese V. The acting subject: towards the neural basis of social cognition. In Metzinger T, ed. *Neural Correlates of Consciousness. Empirical and Conceptual Questions.* Cambridge, MA: MIT Press; 2000:325–333.

Gallese V, Fadiga L, Fogassi L, Rizzolatti G. Action recognition in the premotor cortex. *Brain.* 1996;119:593–609.

Gallese V, Goldman A. Mirror neurons and the simulation theory of mind-reading. *Trends Cogn Sci.* 1998;2:493–501.

Grezes J, Armony JL, Rowe J, Passingham RE. Activations related to "mirror" and "cononical" neurones in the human brain: an fMRI study. *Neuroimage.* 2003;18(4):28–937.

Han S, Fan Y, Mao L. Gender difference in empathy for pain: an electrophysiological investigation. *Brain Res.* 2008;1196:85–93.

Harris P, Johnson CN, Hutton D, Andrews G, Cooke T. Young children's theory of mind and emotion. *Cogn Emot.* 1989;3:379–400.

Hutchinson WD, Davis KD, Lozano AM, Taker RR, Dostrovsky JO. Pain-related neurons in the human cingulated cortex. *Nat Neurosci.* 1999;2:403–405.

Hutman T, Dapretto M. The emergence of empathy during infancy. *Cogn Brain Behav.* 2009;13:367–390.

Iacoboni M, Dapretto M. The mirror neuron system and the consequences of its dysfunction. *Nat Rev Neurosci.* 2006;7:942–951.

Iacoboni M, Molnar-Szakacs I, Gallese V, Buccino G, Mazziotta JC, Rizzolatti G. Grasping the intentions of others with one's own mirror neuron system. *PLoS Biol.* 2005;3(3):e79.

Iacoboni M, Woods RP, Brass M, Bekkering H, Mazziotta JC, Rizzolatti G. Cortical mechanisms of human imitation. *Science.* 1999;286:2526–2528.

Jackson PL, Brunet E, Meltzoff AN, Decety J. Empathy examined through the neural mechanisms involved in imagining how I feel versus how you feel pain. *Neuropsychologia.* 2006;44:752–761.

Jeannerod M, Arbib MA, Rizzolatti G, Sakata H. Grasping objects: the cortical mechanisms of visuomotor transformation. *Trends Neurosci.* 1995;18:314–320.

Krahé C, Springer A, Weinman JA, Fotopoulou A. Social modulation of pain: others as predictive signals of salience—a systematic review. *Front Hum Neurosci.* 2013;7 (article 386):1–20.

Lamm C, Batson CD, Decety J. The neural substrate of human empathy: effects of perspective-taking and cognitive appraisal. *J Cogn Neurosci.* 2007a;19:42–58.

Lamm C, Decety J, Singer T. Meta-analytic evidence for common and distinct neural networks associated with directly experienced pain and empathy for pain. *Neuroimage.* 2011;54:2492–2502.

Lamm C, Nusbaum HC, Meltzoff AN, Decety J. What are you feeling? Using functional magnetic resonance imaging to assess the modulation of sensory and affective responses during empathy for pain. *PLoS ONE.* 2007b;2:e1292.

Langford DJ, Crager SR, Shehzad Z, et al. Social modulation of pain as evidence for empathy in mice. *Science.* 2006;312:1967–1970.

Leslie AM. Theory of mind impairment in autism. In Whiten A, ed. *Natural Theories of Mind: Evolution, Development and Simulation of Everyday Mindreading.* Oxford: Basil Blackwell; 1991:63–77.

Lieberman MD, Eisenberger NI. Pains and pleasures of social life. *Science.* 2009;323:890–891.

Lipps T. *Ästhetik: Psychologie des Schönen und der Kunst: Grundlegung der Ästhetik, Erster Teil.* Hamburg: L Voss, 1903.

Loggia ML, Mogil JS, Bushnell MC. Empathy hurts: compassion for another increases both sensory and affective components of pain perception. *Pain.* 2008;136:168–176.

Masserman JH, Wechkin S, Terris W. "Altruistic" behavior in rhesus monkeys. *Am J Psychiatry.* 1964;121:584–585.

McClintock MK. Menstrual synchrony and suppression. *Nature.* 1971;229:244–245.

Mella N, Studer J, Gilet A, Labouvie-Vief G. Empathy for pain from adolescence through adulthood: an event-related brain potential study. *Front Psychol.* 2012;3 (article 5):1–9.

Meltzoff AN. Understanding the intentions of others: re-enactment of intended acts by 18-month-old children. *Dev Psychol.* 1995;31:838–850.

Melzack R. From the gate to the neuromatrix. *Pain.* 1999;6:S121–S126.

Nissen HW, Crawford MP. A preliminary study of food sharing behavior in young chimpanzees. *J Comp Psychol.* 1936;22:393–419.

Osborn J, Derbyshire SWG. Pain sensation evoked by observing injury in others. *Pain.* 2001;148:268–274.

Preston SD, de Waal FBM. Empathy: its ultimate and proximate bases. *Behav Brain Sci.* 2002;25:1–72.

Price DD. Psychological and neural mechanisms of the affective dimension of pain. *Science.* 2000;288(5472):1769–1772.

Ramachandran VS. Mirror neurons and imitation learning as the driving force behind "the great leap forward" in human evolution. *The Edge.* May 29, 2000.

Raz S, Berger BD. Social isolation increases morphine intake: behavioral and psychopharmacological aspects. *Behav Pharmacol.* 2010;21:39–46.

Rice GEJ, Gainer P. "Altruism" in the albino rat. *J Comp Physiol Psychol.* 1962;55:123–125.

Rizzolatti G, Fadiga L, Fogassi L, Gallese V. Premotor cortex and the recognition of motor actions. *Cogn Brain Res.* 1996;3:131–141.

Siebenaler JB, Caldwell, DK. Cooperation among adult dolphins. *J Mammol.* 1956;37:126–128.

Singer T, Seymour B, O'Doherty P, Stephen KE, Dolan RJ, Firth CD. Empathic neural responses are modulated by the perceived fairness of others. *Nature.* 2006;439:466–469.

Singer T, Seymour B, O'Doherty P, et al. Empathy for pain involves the affective but not sensory component of pain. *Science.* 2004;303:1157–1161.

Steinberg L. Cognitive and affective development in adolescence. *Trends Cogn Sci.* 2005;9:69–74.

Takahashi H, Kato M, Matsuura M, Modds D, Suhara T, Okubo Y. When your gain is my pain and your pain is my gain: neural correlates of envy and Schadenfreude. *Science.* 2009;323:937–939.

Way BM, Taylor SE, Eisenberger NI. Variation in the μ-opioid receptor gene (*OPRM1*) is associated with dispositional and neural sensitivity to social rejection. *Proc Natl Acad Sci U S A.* 2009;106(35):15079–15084.

Whitman RM, Doleys DM. Escape as an alternative to shock-induced fighting in rats. *Psychol Rep.* 1973;32:511–515.

Yamada M, Decety J. Unconscious affect processing and empathy: an investigation of subliminal priming on the detection of painful facial expressions. *Pain.* 2009;143:71–75.

12 Genetics and Pain

If it were not for the great variability among individuals, medicine might as well be a science and not an art.
–Sir William Osler, 1892 (quoted in A.D. Roses, 2000, p. 857)

Each neuron in the ascending nociceptive pathway can change its phenotype in the face of sustained peripheral injury....Noxious stimulation always results not only in a new gene expression in the spinal cord and brain but also in a pattern of gene expression that changes substantially over time.
–S.P. Hunt and P.W. Mantyh (2001, p. 83)

INTODUCTION

Research and clinical observations have repeatedly demonstrated the lack of a correlation between the degree of tissue damage and pain. Only 15% of those undergoing damage to a peripheral nerve develop neuropathic pain. Many patients with radiographic evidence of osteoarthritis and degenerative lumbar disc disease are asymptomatic for pain. Although psychosocial factors have been found to be important, they only account for about 25% of the variance among individuals. In addition, there is considerable variability in the amount of analgetic medicine required by different patients. Genetics may play a role in explaining these discrepancies. But how much emphasis should be put toward identifying a pain gene? Assuming a pain gene can be identified, under what conditions should genetic engineering be acceptable?

Mapping of the human genome has greatly expanded the vistas of pain research and treatment (Altshuler et al, 2008) and prompted a reconsideration of how we define a disease (Temple et al, 2001). One obvious goal of genetic research is the prevention or elimination of pain, especially chronic pain. In an effort to eliminate pain, it is easy to overlook its protective functions. Brand and Yancey (1993) have chronicled the unimaginable infection, loss of limb(s), suffering, and death in a group of patients in India who had lost their ability to feel pain as a result of damage caused by leprosy. Studies of those unfortunate few with congenital insensitivity to pain (CIP) have revealed a drastically reduced lifespan because of their inability to detect painful injuries.

Sequencing of the human genome was completed in 2003. The number of protein-coding genes in the human genome approximates 23,000. Pollard (2009) reported a 99% concordance between the chimpanzee and human genome. Of the three billion letters that make up the human genome, less than 1% (a mere 15 million) are different from those of the chimpanzee. Researchers uncovered 118 base pairs that appeared to be a part of a rapidly evolving sequence, referred to as the *human accelerated region 1* (HAR1). Neurons that play a specialized role in development of the cerebral cortex contain HAR1. Other HARs included FOXP2, which contains a rapid changing sequence associated with speech, and ASPM, which is linked to brain size. No one would argue the enormity of the difference in intellectual capacity between that of the human and the chimpanzee. Therefore, although HARs make up a relatively minute portion of the human genome, their impact is profound. (See the Appendix and "Introduction to Genetics" for a basic summary of definitions and methodology in genetic research.)

ROLE OF GENETICS

Much of the work discussed in this section was carried out or summarized by Fillingim et al (2008), Diatchenko et al (2005, 2006, 2007), and Kim et al (2004, 2009; Kim and Dionne, 2005). There are three main approaches to the study of genetics and pain: (a) experimental pain models, (b) specific clinical pain states such as postoperative pain following hernia repair, and (c) well-defined disease states. The ability to generalize from one approach to the other remains dubious.

Genetic-molecular changes occurring in response to a brief thermal or electrical stimulus, for example, will likely differ from those changes that follow the removal of an appendix. Changes associated with an external stimulus or prompted by a surgical procedure, in turn, will differ from those associated with chronic pain conditions. Changes in genetic expression can occur in a matter of a few hours or over several days. Furthermore, although genetics may play a significant role in terms of the disease state, such as rheumatoid arthritis, its contribution to the level of pain and disability is less certain. Levels of pain and pain-related disability are typically influenced by psychological and environmental variables. Defining the disease to be studied can itself be difficult. For instance, the results of studies examining the role of genetics in temporomandibular joint (TMJ) pain vary widely due to the use of differing diagnostic criteria. In the case of low back pain (LBP), there are many potential causes and mechanisms. Finding a common pathophysiology could prove to be an arduous task.

Pain genetics involves the exploration of two main areas: (a) genes related to the mechanisms involved in pain (pain mechanism genes) and (b) polymorphic genes related to the differences in response to various experimental stimuli and pathological conditions (pain sensitivity genes). Target molecules for genetic variations related to pain sensitivity include (a) those involved in transduction, (b) pain modulatory molecules expressed peripherally and centrally, including opioid receptor genes, and (c) molecules involved in neurotransmitter metabolism. These populations of molecules may be associated with alterations in pain sensitivity resulting from common genetic variations, usually a single-nucleotide-polymorphism (SNP). There may be as many as seven million SNPs existing across some 5% of the human population.

Mutations resulting in decreased pain sensitivity occur in less than 1% of the population (Kim et al, 2009). Pain-related genetic-based research has focused on pain-sensitive and pain-insensitive phenotypes. Some of the more commonly phenotypes explored include COMT (SNP met158val), which has been associated with lower pain sensitivity and higher brain mu-opioid activity; OPRM1 (SNP A118G), associated with pain sensitivity; and GCH1 (GT cyclohydrolase), which was found to relate to lower levels of experimentally induced pain in normal individuals and lower levels of persistent pain following lumbar surgery.

Other studies have examined the association between genetic markers and nociceptive processing. For example, TRPV1 (transient receptor potential V subtype 1), also referred to as vanilloid receptor ionophore 1 (VR1), exists in primary afferent neurons and is a polymorphism (allelic variation) that has been linked to alterations in the process of transduction of noxious stimuli in the periphery. OPRD1 (delta opioid receptor) appears to be involved in pain processing, perhaps at the cortical level. *Hereditary sensory and autonomic neuropathy* (HSAN) refers to a group of genetic-based disorders characterized by abnormalities in nociceptive processing and autonomic function (discussed later in the chapter). Three SNPs in NTRK1 have been found in HSAN type IV. This mutation at the molecular level results in a group of peripheral neuropathies in which there is a congenital insensitivity to pain resulting from the loss of nociception.

Another area of study has been the development and survival of small-diameter nociceptors necessary for normal pain transmission and responsiveness. Knockout technology has been used to delete genes that encode for neurotrophins. *Neurotrophins* are part of a group of growth factors involved in the development, function, and survival of neurons. Neurotrophic factors are secreted by certain tissues and prevent neurons from initiating apoptosis (programmed cell death). There are four structurally related neurotrophins (neurotrophic factors): nerve growth factor (NGF), brain-derived neurotrophic factor (BDNF), neurotrophin-3 (NT-3), and neurotrophin-4 (NT-4) (Indo, 2004).

NGF is a protein secreted by a neuron's target cell and is critical to the survival of sympathetic and sensory neurons; it was first isolated from snake venom in 1956. NGF is significantly elevated in the first year of life. NGF supports both the growth and survival of sympathetic ganglion neurons and nociceptive sensory neurons in the DRG. NGF also regulates the differentiation of peripheral nerves throughout the organism's life and is an inflammatory mediator and capable of activating primary sensory nociceptors. NGF knockout mice lack both sensory and sympathetic ganglia. Thus, it appears to be necessary for the survival of peripheral sensory and sympathetic neurons (NGF-responsive neurons). Elevated NGF has been implicated in interstitial cystitis, chronic prostatitis, osteoarthritis, psoriasis, and diabetic neuropathy (Kumar and Mahal, 2012).

BDNF is found primarily in the brain, especially in the hippocampus, cortex, cerebellum, and forebrain. BDNF stimulates the growth and differentiation of new neurons and synapses through the sprouting of axons and dendrites. BDNF appears to be vital to learning, memory, and higher levels of cognitive processing. BDNF is one of the most active substances to stimulate neurogenesis. Mice genetically altered to lack the ability to make BDNF suffer developmental defects in the brain and sensory nervous system and usually die soon after birth. Neurotrophins bind to the p75 and tyrosine kinase (Trk) receptors, including TrkA, TrkB, and TrkC. NGF binds to TrkA, BDNF and NT-4 bind to TrkB.

NT-3 neurotrophic factor is found in central and some peripheral nervous system neurons. It activates both TrkB and TrkC receptors. Mice born without the ability to make NT-3 suffer the loss of proprioceptive and some types of mechanoreceptive sensory neurons.

The *TrkA* gene has been associated with colon and thyroid cancers, and a mutation of the TrkA (Ntrk1) gene has been associated with congenital insensitivity to pain with anhidrosis (CIPA). TrkA and TrkC gene expression has been shown to be related to a positive prognosis of neuroblastoma and medullablastoma, respectively. TrkA neurons co-express the neuropeptide transmitters CGRP and substance P (SP).

TrkA-deficient mice show a lack of small-diameter sensory afferents and manifest a significant loss of responsiveness to an otherwise painful pin-prick and heat. This may also be responsible for the loss of the normal neurogenic inflammatory response and a relative insensitivity to self-inflicted pain. NGF-null mice were found to lack the TrkA-expressing cells in the DRG. However, there was no change in the TrkB or TrkC cells, indicating the lack of compensatory response. CGRP (calcitonin gene-related peptide) typically found in small-diameter sensory afferents was virtually absent. The few null mice that survived long enough to be tested failed to show any response to noxious mechanical stimulation and had a delayed response to noxious heat.

TrkA knockout mice are prone to severe sensory and sympathetic neuropathies and die within 4 weeks. The presence of skin ulcers and self-mutilation by 3 to 4 weeks testifies to the lack of any acute neurogenic inflammatory response, which is dependent on the release of peptides in the periphery from small-diameter afferents. These animals also show cell loss in the trigeminal and sympathetic ganglia. CRGP and SP are significantly reduced or eliminated in the dorsal root ganglion (DRG).

The similarity of phenotypic presentation between the TrkA knockout mice and patients with CIPA is uncanny: abnormal pain and temperature sensation, injury and ulcers on the digits, self-mutilation, abnormal DRG, and small peripheral nerve fibers are but a few of the similarities. The NGF-TrkA systems regulate both nociceptive and sympathetic neurons during embryonic development and in the adult animal. Their potential as contributing factors to several clinical pain states is obvious (Kumar and Mahla, 2012).

EXPERIMENTAL PAIN: ANIMALS

It is estimated that heritability in pain accounts for some 28–76% of pain sensitivity in animal models (Mogil, 1999, 2008). The most commonly used animal in pain genetics research is the mouse. Surprisingly, the human genome was found to contain largely the same genes as those in the mouse. Many of the same types of genes appear relevant to pain. This does not however, ensure that the genes play the same role in both species or that the same genetic polymorphisms will be responsible for the same pathology. In most instances there is no adequate model for many painful conditions suffered by humans. Nevertheless, animal models of nociceptive, inflammatory, and neuropathic pain do exist and provide a reasonable starting point for study of the role of genetics in pain mechanisms and treatment in humans. The translational aspects may be accomplished by identifying potential candidate genes to be targeted in human association studies. While no reasonable person would argue that an animal model can replicate the human condition, it would be rather parochial to deny the potential value of such research.

Genetic engineering of the laboratory animal, especially the mouse, can produce a strain that is exquisitely sensitive or resistant to noxious stimuli or opioid drugs. Mutant strains of mice, whether discovered as a result of spontaneous mutation or created using transgenic (Mogil et al, 2000) or knockout technology, provide a building block for understanding the role of genetics and the physiological mechanisms involved in pain transmission, modulation, and maintenance. Some mutant strains, including Jimpy, Wallerian, and CXBK, manifest an altered response to noxious stimuli or opioid drugs. A mutation, however, may also affect more than one trait (pleiotropic). Each trait, such as the pain response, involves a complex interaction among a variety of genes (epistasis). Selective breeding and inbreeding have both been used. Selective inbreeding is used to produce an isogenic (genetically identical) strain, but such animals tend not to be very robust because of the sibling mating process. Furthermore, it can take 20 generations to get the desired effect. Selective breeding has successfully produced mouse strains that manifest extremes in pain response (high analgesia [HA] vs. low analgesia [LA]) and genetic sensitivity to opioids (high analgesic response [HAR] vs. low analgesic response [LAR]).

Mogil and his collaborators (1999) tested 11 inbreed strains of mice across an array of stimuli and painful pathological conditions including neuropathic pain models. They identified five types of nociception and hypersensitivity thought to be genetically distinct: (1) baseline thermal nociception, (2) spontaneous response to noxious chemical stimuli, (3) thermal hypersensitivity, (4) mechanical hypersensitivity, and (5) afferent input-independent hypersensitivity. There was a range of 1.2- to 54-fold variability in response depending on the particular strain. Furthermore, pain sensitivity appeared more genetically related than pain responsivity with heritability estimates ranging from 0.3 to 0.8.

Diphtheria toxin has been used to kill (knockout) the postmitotic sensory nerves in the mouse that express the sodium channel $Na_v1.8$. Although the mice responded normally to low-threshold mechanical and acute noxious heat, they did not respond to noxious mechanical pressure or cold. Their response to inflammatory insults was also blunted. This suggests that the cells responsible for detecting noxious acute heat are, in fact, different from those involved in inflammatory thermal hyperalgesia. Nerve injury, however, produced the normal enhanced pain sensitivity to thermal and mechanical stimuli. Therefore, while $Na_v1.8$-expressing neurons appear necessary for mechanical, cold, and inflammatory pain, their absence had no effect on neuropathic pain or heat sensation (Abrahamsen et al, 2008).

By creating different animal models of pain such as inflammatory and neuropathic models, specific receptor and neurotransmitter changes and activity can be identified. Different pain phenotypes including thermal or mechanical sensitivity, allodynia, and hyperalgesia can also be determined and studied. For example, it has been found that certain mutant types lacking the gene for the temperature-activated TRPV1 respond differently to stimuli exceeding 50°C than to stimuli less than 50°C. This finding implicates the TRPV1 receptor as one, though clearly not the only, thermal nociceptive mediating receptor.

Genetic involvement in the effects of opioids has also been investigated (Stamer and Stüber, 2007b). Of the three primary classes of opioid receptors mu, kappa, and delta, the mu- receptor has garnered the greatest attention by virtue of its clinical relevance. Genetic studies have confirmed that each of the receptor classes participates in pain control. Knockout studies targeting the *mu opioid receptor gene (OPRM)* have documented the loss of morphine-based analgesia without any significant alteration in pain sensitivity to noxious stimuli. However, these animals retained their ability to respond to kappa and delta opioids. The same was true for the effects of mu and delta opioids when kappa receptors were knocked-out. These findings suggest the presence of multiple parallel pain processing systems presumably to ensure survival via the enhanced probability of detecting a life threatening injury.

In *The Genetics of Pain*, Mogil (2004) points out at least four noteworthy findings that have emerged from pain genetic animal research. First, the genetic mediators may vary according to the particular stimulus. Mogil et al (1999) studied 12 inbred mouse strains and found that it was the stimulus rather than the condition that was important. That is, an analysis of 24 different tests of nociception including nerve injury, abdominal constriction, and hot plate yielded five symptom clusters: (1) mechanical allodynia, (2) afferent dependent, (3) thermal hyperalgesia, (4) thermal, and (5) chemical. Thus, not all nociceptive tests are unique unto themselves. Several tests shared a particular physiological mechanism as depicted by the same or different pain responses among the different mouse strains.

A second significant finding was that mouse strains sensitive to pain were also resistant to morphine analgesia and vice versa. Furthermore, the genetic correlation between nociception and analgesia depended on the type of pain involved. For example, the correlation between the hot-plate test and morphine analgesia in certain strains was high whereas in other strains it was low. Thus, different genes are relevant to morphine analgesia depending on the type of pain being used. The reason for a genetic variation in the mu-opioid receptor (OPRM) being selective to one type of pain over another is unclear. Perhaps there are other non-mu-opioid-based analgesics. Indeed, cholinergic, adrenergic, and cannabinoid agonists, along with antiepileptic drugs, have proven analgesic properties.

The third finding was that sex-related differences in pain sensitivity and analgesic responsiveness have long been appreciated. Across species, females tend to be more pain sensitive than males. But males tend to be more sensitive to certain opioid agonists than females, except in humans; women are more responsive to mu- and kappa-opioid agonists than men. However, research with different animal strains has revealed inconsistent findings. Male Sprague Dawley rate are more sensitive to noxious thermal stimulation than females, but the findings are reversed in the Long Evans strain.

Chesler et al (2002) appear to have confirmed an important interaction of sex, strain, and environmental factors. They analyzed some 8,043 observations of thermal nociceptive sensitivity in 40 different mouse strains collected over an 8-year period. The impact of study factors such as sex, age, weight, testing facility, cage density, season, time of day for testing, temperature, humidity, experimenter, and within-cage order of testing was evaluated. In general, they noted that the genotype of the animal strain accounted for 27% of the observed pain response variability, environment 42%, genotype × environment 18%, and residual or error 13%. Females were more sensitive than males; the first mouse tested from a cage containing several mice showed a higher latency (greater pain tolerance) than subsequently tested ones; and animals tested later in the day, in the springtime, and under higher levels of humidity tended to be more sensitive to thermal nociception. Cage density primarily affected males, as they appeared to become stressed over maintenance of a dominance hierarchy. Females, by contrast, seemed to find the presence of others calming. Regarding the order in which the animals were tested, the first mouse tested was not only more pain tolerant but had a 50% greater response to an analgesic drug like morphine compared to the fourth mouse tested. Whether by release of some pheromonal substance or unique vocalization, interanimal communication appears to be a reality (see Chapter 11). The most significant environmental factor was the experience of the tester. This may reflect the degree of stress imposed by an inexperienced handler.

Finally, Mogil (2004) noted that the manner in which different strains of mice process nociceptive information appears to vary (Chesler et al, 2002). One remarkable finding is that Sprague Dawley rats obtained from one source had neurons projecting from a particular area of the brain to the spinal cord via an entirely different route compared to rats obtained from a different source.

Furthermore, data have shown that heroin's analgesic effect is accomplished by activating different receptor populations in different mouse strains. In one strain the delta-opioid receptor is activated, in another it is the kappa-opioid receptor. The mechanism of morphine analgesia may also have some strain-dependent characteristics. If these data are extended to humans, an admittedly large leap, it would mean that individuals might be differentially responsive to different classes, as well as dosages, of analgesic drugs.

EXPERIMENTAL PAIN: HUMANS

A case for the role of genetics in the pain experienced by humans can be made solely on the basis of the vast interindividual differences noted in acute, clinical, and experimentally induced pain (EIP) (Nielson et al, 2009; Patsopoulos et al, 2007). EIP research in humans has taken advantage of the use of cold, heat, electrical, pressure, ischemic, and chemical stimuli; exercise; and saline injections. In most instances, normal individuals without any painful condition or disease have been recruited to participate; other studies have used patients with acute postoperative or chronic pain.

A number of studies have examined pain sensitivity among healthy subjects. Coghill et al (2003) presented a brief 49°C stimulus to the leg and noted pain ratings ranging from 1/10 to 8/10. Furthermore, brain imaging studies revealed an associated variability in cortical activation, indicating a relationship between the subjective report and cortical activity. Kim et al (2004) recorded pain rating ranging from 0 to 100 in a group of 500 healthy individuals exposed to heat stimulus to the forearm. Fillingim (2004) noted that the heat-pain threshold varied from 34.1°C to 48.0°C. Diatchenko et al (2005) examined 16 different measures across 202 subjects and reported pain sensitivity scores ranging from −20 to 30 (integral Z-score). These data highlight the enormous range of pain sensitivity, even in highly controlled conditions, among healthy individuals.

It has been estimated that heritability accounts for some 11–23% of the variability in experimental thermal pain sensitivity in humans. Twins studies have noted heritability to account for 22–55% in pain sensitivity to various stimuli among women (Norbury et al, 2007). Nielsen et al (2008) studied cold and heat pain in identical (monozygotic, MZ) and fraternal (dizygotic, DZ) twins. Substantial variability to heat and cold pain was noted in both groups. They estimated that 60% of the variance to cold pain but only 26% of heat pain variance was genetically mediated. Surprisingly, genetic factors common to both modalities explained only 7% of the cold and 3% of heat pain variance. Furthermore, environmental factors common to both modalities explained only 5% of cold pain variance and 8% of heat pain variance. Upon examining pressure pain threshold in adult twins, MacGregor et al (1997) reported that the shared environmental factors were more influential than genetic factors.

Genetic Contributions to Experimental Pain Responses

One approach to study of the role of genetics in humans is to focus on the processing of painful stimuli rather than on genes linked to an underlying disease associated with pain. That is, are there specific pain-sensitivity genes that function to increase the individual's experience of pain to a particular stimulus over that of another? One study examined this issue using 98 pairs of female twins (51 MZ and 47 DZ) (Norbury et al, 2007). The authors reported significant heritability estimates ranging from 22 to 55% for several experimental pain measures, including responses to heat pain and chemically induced pain. A separate report by Nielsen et al (2008) noted significant heritability for sensitivity to both cold pain (60%) and heat pain (26%). Thus, human twin studies, on balance, suggest significant heritability for experimental pain responses. This apparent heightened pain sensitivity, which is at least partially determined by genetic factors, has been postulated as a risk factor for future development of chronic pain (Diatchenko et al, 2005, 2006; Edwards, 2005).

Multiple factors influence pain sensitivity, perception, and tolerance. Kim et al (2004) undertook a study of the effects of genetics in association with gender, ethnicity, and psychological temperament on pain sensitivity in an experimental setting. Five-hundred volunteers, including 306 females, consisting of European Americans, African Americans, Asian Americans, and Hispanics, participated. The subjects completed a temperament inventory designed to rate them on four dimensions: novelty-seeking, harm-avoidance, reward-dependence, and persistence. Cold-pain intensity and tolerance were measured by the amount of time they kept their hand submerged in freezing water (cold pressor test) and their pain intensity rating upon withdrawing their hand from the cold water, or at 30 seconds. The subjects also experienced 5 seconds of exposure to eight different thermal stimuli ranging from 35° to 49°C. Genotyping scanned for two SNPs of *TRPV1* and *OPRD1* and a common functional polymorphism of the *COMT* gene, *COMT Val[158]Met*. Heat-pain sensitivity was determined primarily by gender, an *OPRD1* polymorphism, and temperament. Gender, ethnicity and temperament interacted with *TRPV1* and *OPRD1* SNPs to account for individual variations in thermal pain sensitivity.

Six studies used *COMT*-related genotypes and found it to be associated with pain sensitivity. In one instance, low levels of catechol-*O*-methyltransferase (COMT) were found to be associated with high pain catastrophizing. Fillingim et al (2008; George et al, 2008) examined patients with shoulder pain and found that those with both high levels of catastrophizing and a pain-sensitive *COMT* genotype reported the greatest pain. *COMT* was unrelated to cold-pain tolerance, but contributed to sensitivity to cold but not heat pain in females.

OPRM variations were studied in five different projects. SNPs of *OPRM* were linked to mechanical pain and possibly heat pain but in a gender-specific manner. The G-allele was associated with a reduced response to analgesics. Eleven SNPs from *OPRD1* were unrelated to cold- and heat-pain variability.

MC1R has been linked to ischemic pain tolerance and ratings. *MC1R* was also associated with analgesia derived from the use of pentazocine (a mixed agonist-antagonist opioid) in women as well as mu-opioid drugs in both men and women.

An interesting study by Mogil et al (2011) examined the effects of a synthetic vasopressin analog, desmopressin, administered intranasally, on pressure and heat-pain threshold and tolerance following the application of capsaicin cream. The authors were interested in the involvement of an SNP of the *AVPR1A* gene which had been found only in males, and only if they were stressed at the time of testing. The results revealed that desmopressin inhibited capsaicin-induced pain, but only for the non-stressed subjects. The non-stressed subjects were identified as those having had previous experience with capsaicin-induced pain and found it to be tolerable, whereas the stressed subjects feared the worst. Mogil et al speculated that activation of the "stressed-induced" endogenous analgesic system offsets the effects of the *AVPR1* gene on desmopressin-related analgesia. This was one of the first studies to report a gene × drug × environment (stress) interaction. The authors also suggested that the low rate of replication in some genetic studies may, in fact, be related to the stress level of the subjects at the time of testing.

Candidate Gene Studies: Experimentally Induced Pain

There has been a fair amount of effort put into researching specific candidate genes and their relationship to different responses to EIP. As noted in the previous section, *COMT* is one of the more frequently studied candidate gene. One SNP of this gene (met158val) involves the substitution of valine for methionine, which results in lower enzymatic activity due to thermal instability of the enzyme. Zubieta et al (2003) reported that valine homozygotes showed lower pain sensitivity and significantly greater brain μ-opioid receptor activation in response to experimental muscle pain induced via injection of hypertonic saline into the masseter muscle. However, this SNP was not associated with ratings of cold pain in a subsequent study (Kim et al, 2006). *COMT* haplotypes were associated with overall pain sensitivity. The haplotype that was characterized by low pain sensitivity also seemed to confer protection against subsequent development of temporomandibular disorder (TMD).

Another candidate gene associated with experimental pain responses is the μ-opioid receptor (*OPRM1*) gene, which has been suggested as a promising candidate gene for pain sensitivity (Uhl et al, 1999). A common SNP of *OPRM1* is A118G. The G-allele has been associated with significantly higher pressure pain thresholds than those with the major allele (Fillingim et al, 2005), especially for males. Subsequently, it was shown that pain-related evoked-potential responses were lower among individuals with at least one G-allele compared to those carrying two A-alleles (Lötsch et al, 2006). Thus, two studies using vastly different experimental pain models suggest that this G-allele is associated with reduced pain sensitivity. The frequency of the G-allele was found to be significantly lower among patients with chronic pain than in a postsurgical patient population (Janicki et al, 2006), which suggests a possible association with the development of chronic pain.

Based on preclinical data from rodent models of neuropathic and inflammatory pain, researchers discovered an enzyme GT cyclohydrolase (GCH) to be involved in nociceptive sensitivity and injury-induced hyperalgesia. When the impact of a haplotype of the *GCH1* gene was explored in humans, it was found to be associated with lower levels of persistent pain following lumbar surgery for disc herniation (Tegeder et al, 2006, 2008). The presence of this pain-protective haplotype also correlated with lower sensitivity to EIP in two separate groups of healthy individuals in which thermal, pressure, and ischemic pain along with mechanical hyperalgesia were used. However, a separate group of researchers using cold and heat pain found no such correlation. This discrepancy could be secondary to the use of different stimuli.

The *TRPV1* is known to encode the capsaicin heat receptor. Kim et al (2004) initially reported an association of the ile585val SNP of *TRPV1* with cold-pain ratings, but only among females. However, a subsequent study did not find any association of *TRPV1* with cold or heat pain (Kim et al, 2006). Likewise, although they initially reported an association of *OPRD1*, the delta-opioid receptor gene, with heat pain ratings among males (Kim et al, 2004), the findings were not replicated in a subsequent study.

In summary, genetics appear to account for about 50% of the variability in EIP. *COMT, OPRM1, GCH1, TRPV1,* and *OPRD1* are among the most commonly considered candidate genes linked to variability in individual experience of EIP. Failure to replicate the findings from one study to another is common. The reasons vary widely and include the use of different pain models. Subtle differences (e.g., population stratification) even among otherwise healthy individuals may be another factor. Dispositional characteristics such as gender, race and ethnicity, personality, and age have been associated with varying pain responses, as have situational variables, such as mood state and stress.

Furthermore, the mechanism by which these candidate genes and SNPs exert their effect is unknown. There may be a network of intricate interactions triggered by some as-yet unidentified gene, SNP, or molecule, as might be expected of a complex adaptive system. The almost overwhelming complexity of this issue is highlighted by the documented association of *COMT* polymorphism with phenotypes related to schizophrenia. A study by Levesque et al (2012) determined that schizophrenics tend to have heightened pain sensitivity to acute pain but reduced sensitivity to prolonged pain. The authors concluded that the nociceptive processing was intact and that the effect had to be supraspinal. Therefore, the point at which genetic variations exert their effect, through transduction, transmission, perception, or a combination of these processes, remains unclear.

Figure 12.1 presents a summary, arranged by Foulkes and Wood (2008), of the genetic contributions to transduction, transmission, conduction, and modulation. Many of the genes identified have been discussed here and some will be referred to later in the chapter. It would be difficult to give adequate attention to each of the

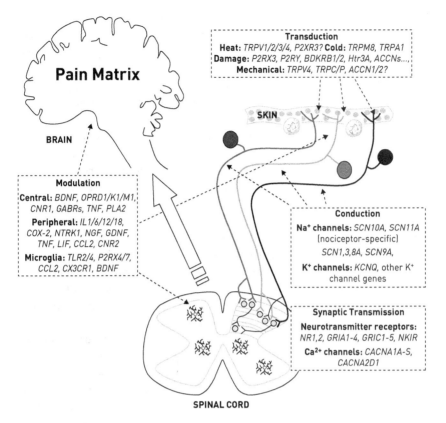

Pain Matrix

BRAIN

Transduction
Heat: *TRPV1/2/3/4, P2XR3?* **Cold:** *TRPM8, TRPA1*
Damage: *P2RX3, P2RY, BDKRB1/2, Htr3A, ACCNs...,*
Mechanical: *TRPV4, TRPC/P, ACCN1/2?*

SKIN

Modulation
Central: *BDNF, OPRD1/K1/M1, CNR1, GABRs, TNF, PLA2*
Peripheral: *IL1/6/12/18, COX-2, NTRK1, NGF, GDNF, TNF, LIF, CCL2, CNR2*
Microglia: *TLR2/4, P2RX4/7, CCL2, CX3CR1, BDNF*

Conduction
Na⁺ channels: *SCN10A, SCN11A* (nociceptor-specific)
SCN1,3,8A, SCN9A,
K⁺ channels: *KCNQ, other K⁺* channel genes

Synaptic Transmission
Neurotransmitter receptors: *NR1,2, GRIA1-4, GRIC1-5, NKIR*
Ca²⁺ channels: *CACNA1A-S, CACNA2D1*

SPINAL CORD

FIGURE 12.1

Genes involved in pain perception and modulation. Nociceptors are commonly divided into three groups: peptidergic (blue, NGF-responsive) and nonpeptidergic (black, GDNF-responsive) unmyelinated C-fibers, and myelinated Ad-fibers (red, NGF-responsive). Gene expression profiles differ between these groups, with functional distinctions. TRP channels appear to be involved in transduction of several stimulus modalities. Synaptic transmission occurs through NMDA, AMPA, and kainate receptors, in addition to neuropeptide and proton-mediated transmission. Neurotransmitter release is controlled by voltage-gated Ca^{2+} channels in the presynaptic membrane. Microglia in the spinal cord respond to damage or inflammation by releasing growth factors and cytokines that alter the excitability of spinal neurons. In certain cases, this can lead to the ongoing activation of pain pathways. Brain-derived neurotrophic factor (BDNF), fractalkine, and chemokines have been invoked as important mediators. Pain pathways in the central nervous system are modulated by endogenous opioid peptides and arachidonic acid metabolites, acting through G-protein-coupled receptors (opioid receptors and cannabinoid receptors) to limit neuronal excitability. GABAergic pathways also act to regulate the excitability of neuronal circuits involved in pain perception. From Foulkes T, Wood JN. Pain genes. *PLoS Genetics.* 2008;4(7):1–9. www.plosgenetics.org. Reprinted with permission.

elements indicated. The figure is presented to emphasize the organization and complexity of the genetic system related to nociceptive processing.

GENETICS AND PAIN: CLINICAL PAIN STATES

Another means of exploring genetic influences on the experience of pain is by examining different clinical conditions thought to represent pain phenotypes, such as LBP,

TMD, and fibromyalgia. Broader categories of clinical pain might include postoperative pain or neuropathic pain. Neuropathic pain is often explored under laboratory conditions, though these results may differ from real-world experiences. In any case, it is important to differentiate the genetic contribution to the disease state (e.g., arthritis gene involved in joint degradation) from genes involved in pain processing. Admittedly, these groupings can be very heterogeneous. Very specific and stringent inclusion criteria are needed if the results are to be useful.

Genetic links to postsurgical pain have been explored in German, Chinese, Korean, Jewish, Taiwanese, Asian, Caucasian, and African-American populations. The types of surgery in relation to pain have included oral and abdominal surgery, gastrectomy, hysterectomy, cesarean, tonsillectomy, and knee surgery. Four studies reported no association between the genotype and postoperative pain intensity or analgesic consumption. The *CYP2D6* genotype was associated with increased use of tramadol in three separate investigations. One study found that IL1R influenced morphine consumption, and four studies reported *OPRM1* variations to have a similar effect.

Mamie et al (2009) examined the postoperative, orthoscopic, or abdominal pain response of children 4 to 16 years of age. They found that P-glycoprotein 1 (MDR1) influenced the transportation of opioids such that an impairment of MDR1 could result in increased concentration of opioids in the brain. MDR1 activity can be altered by any one of 100 known *ABCB1* polymorphisms. They were able to identify that an SNP 3435C/T of the *ABCB1* gene, which occurs in about 50% of Caucasians, significantly altered MDR1 activity, thereby influencing pain intensity. Those with the T/T genotype reported 70% less pain, with the C/C 30% more pain, and with the C/T genotype a level in between. They concluded that the *ABCB1* 3435C/T SNP may well predict postoperative pain in children, potentially leading to a more patient-specific approach to postoperative pain management.

Kim and colleagues (2004) reviewed some 313 research articles dating from November 2003 to November 2008 that reported on investigation of chronic pain conditions. A variety of nationalities and ethnicities were involved. The types of disorders and pain locations studied included the following: LBP complex regional pain syndrome (CRPS); orofacial pain; angina (vasospastic and microvascular); sickle cell anemia; migraines or headache, with and without drug abuse; discogenic sciatica; neuropathic or musculoskeletal pain; fibromyalgia; osteoarthritis; TMJ pain; spinous process surgical discectomy; postherpetic neuralgia (PHN); arthralgia; hemochromatosis; juvenile idiopathic arthritis; pelvic or abdominal pain; atherosclerosis; and McArdle syndrome. *COMT* was the most frequently examined genotype; others included *ACE* and SNPs of *BCL11A, CHRM1, DRD2, GABA,* and *CNR1.* Phenotypes explored included pain intensity, movement scores, psychological factors, genotype, and allele distribution. These were compared within the clinical group and to controls. MRI findings, disc herniations, haplotype distribution, pain crisis rate, and opioid consumption were also examined.

Of the 34 studies that examined allele or genotype distribution, 15 reported an association and 19 reported no association. Three studies on pain crisis rates in patients with sickle cell anemia found Hbf-associated SNPs to be related to rate of pain crisis. Nine of the 13 studies that investigated pain intensity and movement scores found no association. One project studied patients with juvenile idiopathic arthritis and another, patients with LBP, using visual analogue scale (VAS) intensity ratings. Both found some association with the IL-6 and IL-1 genotypes, respectively. GABA-A beta-1 subunit was linked to increased movement in one study and thought to function like a muscle relaxant. Finally, *OPRM 118 G* was not associated with pain intensity or opioid consumption. However, the G-allele was less common in patients with chronic pain who required higher opioid doses. One study found a relationship with a haplotype for mechanical leg pain but not for thermal or ischemic leg pain in patients with chronic pain post-discectomy.

Genetics may help us to unravel some of the more seemingly mysterious chronic pain conditions, such as chronic fatigue syndrome (CFS) (Carmell et al, 2006; Kerr et al, 2008). CFS is characterized by debilitating fatigue and chronic widespread pain (CWP) of the type found in fibromyalgia syndrome (FMS). Genetics-based research has, in fact, identified biomarkers using gene expression to isolate as many as seven subtypes of CFS. There is evidence that these disorders are a consequence of dysregulation of the sympathetic nervous system (SNS) and the immune system (see Chapter 7). The human leukocyte antigen (HLA) has been implicated in at least one study (Burda et al, 1986). Variants of HLA have been identified as influencing the interaction between the body's response to trauma and the development of CRPS (van de Beck et al, 2003). Importantly, psychological factors and family environment did not emerge as relevant factors in studies examining familial clustering of fibromyalgia.

Light et al (2009) explored molecular receptors known to detect metabolites associated with muscle pain and fatigue. These molecular receptors included acid-sensing ion channel (ASIC3), puringergic type 2x receptors, and TRPV1. These molecular receptors are found on human leukocytes in addition to SNS and immune system genes. The effect of moderate exercise on gene expression in a group of CFS patients was compared to that on normal individuals. Increased expression was found in the mRNA for the metabolite detecting receptors ASIC3 and purinergic type 2x, SNS receptors alpha-2A, beta-1, and beta-2, IMS genes for IL10 and TLR4, and COMT, compared to expression in normal individuals. This increase in mRNA gene expression in the metabolic, adrenergic, and immune systems in response to exercise may represent objective biomarkers of CFS.

One of the most fruitful areas of genetic research regarding pain has been migraine headache. Heritability estimates of pain conditions such as migraine are higher than those for pain intensity. Gene variants can affect pain in three ways: (1) directly on the nociceptive pathway, (2) through a physiological pathway affecting disease susceptibility, and (3) through a psychological pathway, secondarily affecting the likelihood of experiencing chronic pain.

Mutations in the *ATPIA2* and *CACNA1A* genes are found in familial hemiplegic migraine. These genes may regulate ion homeostasis and could play a role in the initiation and pain phases of migraine headache. SNPs in the insulin receptor (INSR) have also been associated with migraine. A 50% heritability rate was reported for migraines with and without aura. Shared family environment was not a predictor. A Swedish report (Larsson et al, 1995) demonstrated a genetic association for tension headache in adults and children. A Finish twin register study examined widespread musculoskeletal pain in 11-year-olds (Mikkelsson et al, 2001). Shared family environment accounted for about 35% tendency toward pain in boys and 56% in girls.

Even the common LBP has been linked to polymorphisms in the IL-1 gene; an SNP at a specific position has been found to correlate with the presence of pain, days in pain, and degree of pain-related disability. MacGregor and his group (2004) conducted a twin study using patients with LBP or neck pain and concluded that genetics was more influential than shared environmental factors. However, a large part of the genetic variance was left unexplained. They also uncovered a strong correlation between an overall sense of well-being and neck and low back pain. It was proposed that perhaps there was a common genetic determinant for psychological well-being and neck and low back pain.

Several candidate genes have been examined for association with TMD, including the serotonin transporter gene (SLC6A4); COMT, the gene that encodes catechol-O-methyltransferase, an enzyme involved in catecholamine metabolism; β_2-adrenergic receptor gene (ADRB2), and estrogen receptor alpha. Ojima et al (2007) reported a significant association between the serotonin transporter gene polymorphism and TMD, with patients showing greater frequency of the long allele relative to controls in a Japanese population. Diatchenko et al (2005) examined five SNPs of the COMT gene among 202 healthy young women. They constructed three haplotypes, termed low-pain sensitive (LPS), average-pain sensitive (APS), and high-pain sensitive (HPS) on the basis of their associations with measures of experimental pain sensitivity. The authors followed individuals prospectively to determine new-onset cases of TMD. The results indicated that individuals with at least one LPS haplotype were less than half as likely to develop TMD compared to those without any LPS haplotypes.

Based on previous findings of decreased concentrations of serotonin (5-HT) and norepinephrine (NE) metabolites in the cerebrospinal fluid of patients with fibromyalgia (Russell et al, 1992), several studies have examined genetic polymorphisms in serotonin, dopamine, and catecholamine systems in fibromyalgia. These studies have found significant associations with fibromyalgia of promoter regions of the 5-HT transporter gene (5-HTT) (Offenbaecher et al, 1999) as well as 5-HT2A receptor gene, located on the long arm of chromosome 13 (Bondy et al, 1999; Cohen et al, 2002). In addition, several gene polymorphisms of serotonin receptor (HTR) subunits, including HTR3A and HTR3B, have been associated with fibromyalgia (Frank et al, 2004). Another polymorphism of considerable interest is related to the involvement of the COMT gene in patients with fibromyalgia. One study reported significant differences in allele frequencies of a COMT SNP (G1947A) among patients with fibromyalgia and controls (Gursoy et al, 2003). Also, a possible genetic association with fibromyalgia has been detected for the TACR1 gene, which encodes the neurokinin 1 (NK1) receptor, the target for substance P (SP) (Ablin, 2005).

Most of the research conducted on patients with cancer has been carried out among Caucasians or African Americans, females and males, with various types of cancer (Klepstad et al, 2011). Some studies have examined the patient's response to opioids, others have focused on interindividual differences in pain intensity. Most have found some influence of COMT and OPRM on opioid responsivity. One study showed a relationship to medication side effects but not pain intensity. Cytokine genes (i.e., IL-8) were associated with pain intensity in Caucasians with lung cancer but none in a group of African Americas with mixed types of cancer.

Fink and colleagues (Fink, 2008; Fink et al 2011; Glorioso et al, 2003, 2009) explored the use of gene therapy in an attempt to find a way of obtaining pain relief without the problems of tolerance, constipation, confusion, respiratory suppression, lethargy, and potential abuse and addiction issues. Nonreplicating gene transfer vectors created from the herpes simplex virus type 1 (HSV-1) was used to transfer the required genes into the primary sensory afferents in the DRG. The goal was to target the first synapse between the primary nociceptor and secondary nociceptive neuron in the dorsal horn of the spinal cord. The HSV-based vector was designed to express proenkepha-lin. When injected, the HSV is incapable of replication. It is taken up from the skin by sensory nerve terminals and transported to the DRG where the genome is estab-lished. Evidence for the release of vector-mediated encephalin (VME) was confirmed by noting that it could be reversed by administering antagonists such as naloxone and naltrexone.

The effect of VME expression has been shown to last for weeks and reoccurs with repeated injections. The VME is additive to systemic morphine and has been effective in animals tolerant to morphine. HSV-VME seems to prevent increased expression of $Na_v1.7$ in the DRG typically found in diabetic peripheral neuropathic pain (DPNP), characterized by an enhanced pain response to cold, heat, and mechanical stimuli. Activation of presynaptic delta opioid receptor by enkephalin prevents the increase in neuronal $Na_v1.7$ in DRG through inhibition of protein kinase C (PKC) and p38 mitogen-activated protein (MAP). The preproenkephalin gene transfer may be more effective with inflammatory than neuropathic pain. The use of a GAD-expressing vector interfered with the usual reduction in GABA found in neuropathic pain states, which has the effect of rendering the organism more sensitive to mechanical and ther-mal stimulation. (This effect has been demonstrated using T9 spinal cord hemisec-tioned, spinal nerve ligation (SNL), and diabetic animal models of neuropathic pain). Others have used HSV vectors to reduce the expression of voltage-gated channels or the neurotransmitter calcitonin gene-related peptide (CGRP) in primary sensory afferents to produce analgesia.

Phase 1 safety and dosing studies have been carried out in terminal cancer patients with pain, under U.S. Food and Drug Administration (FDA) guidance (Wolfe et al, 2009). Fink and his group have produced some promising results clinically, and some preliminary findings suggest potential effects on pain severity.

CONGENITAL INSENSITIVITY TO PAIN

Congenital insensitivity to pain (CIP) is a term applied to individuals with an impaired ability to perceive type, intensity, and quality of noxious stimuli (Indo, 2004). Hereditary sensory and autonomic neuropathies (HSAN) are marked by the absence of primary sensory and autonomic neurons necessary to the perception of pain. This may result from a failure of these structures to emerge during the developmental pro-cess, atrophy of the structures after they had emerged, or degeneration. Five types of HSAN have been described. Type I (HSAN-I; MIM [Mendelian Inheritance in Man] 162400) predominantly affects the distal portion of the lower extremities and has been associated with mutations in the *SPTLC1* gene. The loss of peripheral sensory modalities characterizes type II (HSAN-II) and is also referred to as congenital sen-sory neuropathy (MIM 201300). The sensory loss is found in all of the extremities, occasionally in the torso, and includes the modalities of cold, heat touch, vibration, pressure, and nociception. Patients so afflicted began showing symptoms and signs as early as infancy. Ulcerations of the fingers and toes, autoamputation of distal digits, and joint deterioration without pain are common.

Type III, HSAN-III, is defined by diffuse peripheral autonomic and sensory nerve dysfunction. Poor feeding, failure to thrive, vomiting, corneal insensitivity, and insen-sitivity to pain are observed early on and are frequently associated with early death.

The *DYS* gene is thought to be responsible for HSAN-III. There is an ethnic bias with an estimated 1 in 30 Ashkenazi Jews being carriers and an occurrence rate of 1 in 36,000 births.

HSAN-IV is thought to be a variant of HSAN-V. It is also referred to as congenital insensitivity to pain with anhidrosis (CIPA). HSAN-IV is somewhat unique among the HSANs as it appears to be a result of apoptosis of NGF-dependent neurons.

HSAN-V patients are rare. These individuals demonstrate insensitivity to noxious stimuli but normal reactions to other sensory modalities. They approach having an average number of peripheral sensory neurons with normal autonomic sudomotor functions and average cognitive functions. Mutation in the *TRKA* gene has been linked to HSAN-V. It is also noteworthy that NGF-TRKA regulates both nociceptive and sympathetic neuronal activity during embryonic development and thereafter.

The following text, an excerpt from Yasuhiro Indo's chapter in *The Genetics of Pain*, edited by Mogil (2004), gives a graphic description of what these unfortunate children go through.

Initially, impaired pain perception may not be apparent, but parents may recall that their children did not cry during blood sampling. Biting of the tongue or lip starts after the first teeth erupt and can result in bifid or absent tongue. Self-mutilation...is frequent. Bruises, cuts and burns do not elicit normal reactions and often go unrecognized. Accidental injuries such as a fall or burns lead to multiple scars, and bone or joint fractures can be complicated by deep infections....[L]arge weight-bearing joints appear particularly susceptible to repeated trauma, frequently developing neurogenic arthropathy [Charcot joints], and osteomyelitis. Amputation of fingers or limbs is common....Twenty-percent of affected children succumb to hyperpyrexia [temperature of 106°F] within the first 3 years of life....[S]ome CIPA children remain incontinent of urine and feces [and] local and systemic infections may lead to death from sepsis....Most children with CIPA are mentally retarded [and] there can be severe learning problems....Hyperactivity and emotional liability are common. Recurrent febrile convulsions are also observed. (pp. 175–176, references cited by Indo are not included here)

This description leaves no doubt as to the system-wide impact a genetic variation can have.

Individuals with congenital absences of a sense of pain are very rare, even more so than those with the absence of vision or hearing. Congenital indifference to pain (Landrieu et, 1990), also known as autosomal recessive congenital analgesia (OMIM 243000), congenital insensitivity to pain, or hereditary sensory and autonomic neuropathy type 5 (OMIM 608654), can be distinguished, as the latter is characterized by the presence of a neuropathy. Cox et al (2006) identified three families in northern Pakistan manifesting the absence of a pain phenotype. The case that attracted their attention was that of a 10-year-old boy performing all manner of unusual feats, such as driving knives through his arms and walking on hot coals without any apparent pain. Such cases are not to be confused with those able via altered mental states, such as those through meditation or self-hypnosis, to withstand such insults. Unfortunately, this young boy died at the age of 13 from injuries sustained after jumping off a house; he was never aware of his injuries because he could not feel pain.

Six other similar cases have been found and studied. These six children came from three consanguineous families and were described as never having felt pain anywhere on their bodies, at any time in their life. Injuries to their lips and tongue, with some having bitten off the distal third in their tongue in their younger years, were common. Bruises, cuts, fractures, and osteomyelitis, diagnosed only as a result of a painless limp or decreased use of the limb, had been recorded in their medical histories. All children were considered of normal intelligence. Surprisingly, their neurological examination was intact in that they could perceive touch, heat, cold, warmth, position (proprioception), and tickle. They had normal reflexes and taste and could detect hot from cold food and drink. Studies of nerve function and nerve biopsies were unremarkable.

Mapping for the mutated gene in these six children revealed a different mutation in each of the three families. A sequence analysis found distinct mutations in *SCN9A*. The authors note that "SCN9A encodes for, the Na$_v$1.7 alpha subunit of a tetrodotoxin-sensitive voltage-gated sodium channel that is expressed at high levels in peripheral sensory neurons, most notable in nociceptive small-diameter dorsal root ganglia (DRG) neurons" (Cox et al, 2006, p. 896). Thus, they called this new syndrome *channelopathy-associated insensitivity*. Na$_v$1.7 appears to be necessary for the generation of an action potential in DRG neurons. Genetic mutations causing the Na$_v$1.7 dysfunction was related to the loss of pain perception. Whether the absence of pain perception is related to a defect in peripheral transmission, activity in the spinal cord, or brain remains in question as *SCN9A* has been found to be expressed in all three areas. Mutations in *SCN9A* have also been likened to the autosomal-dominant pain disorder primary erythermalgia (Waxman and Dib-Hajj, 2005) characterized by burning pain in the extremities that is associated with exposure to warm or moderate exercise. Given the complexity of the pain processing system, it seems remarkable that a defect in a single gene would be responsible for the absence of nociceptive activity.

Bowsher et al (2009) included a group of 15 researchers that investigated two unrelated adults manifesting CIP associated with remarkable hyperhidrosis. By comparison, most patients with HSAN have anhidrosis (reduced sweat response) along with impaired pain, touch, and temperature perception. Both of the adults were of average intelligence and led fairly productive lives despite their apparent inability to experience pain from broken bones, burns, and severe cold. Indeed, one additional patient suffered hypothermia when working in cold water and was unable to detect thermal pain at non-damaging intensities. This patient died in 1968 without undergoing genetic studies.

Their examination and testing data noted that their threshold for detecting several modalities including noxious stimuli was at least 2 standard deviations above the norm. Their sweat response was 3 to 8 times greater. Biopsies revealed a significant reduction in myelinated and unmyelinated fibers. One of the patients had normal innervations of vasculature and sweat glands, but all types of cutaneous C, A-delta, and A-beta fiber were absent. One unique finding was cholinergic arterial innervations. No genetic variations were identified in *SCN9A, SCN10A, SCN11A, NGFB, TRKA, NRTN,* and *GFRA2*. The authors put forth three hypotheses to explain their findings: (1) that development or maintenance of sensory innervations to cutaneous vasculature and sweat glands may be under separate genetic control from that of all other cutaneous sensory innervation, (2) the latter innervation is preferentially vulnerable to some environmental factors, and (3) vascular and sweat gland afferents may contribute to conscious cutaneous perception.

LESCH-NYHAN SYNDROME (LNS)

Lesch-Nyhan syndrome (LNS) is somewhat unique in that patients engage in remarkably destructive self-mutilation despite an apparent appreciation for pain (Casas-Bruge et al, 1985). Although formally described in 1964 by a Michael Lesch and Bill Nyhan, LNS may have been recognized as early as 1267. Despite the absence of neurological abnormalities at birth, LNS is characterized by neurological deficits, progressive encephalopathy, hyperreflexia, seizures, behavioral disturbances, and, less consistently, mental retardation. Uncontrolled self-mutilation beginning by the second year of life and becoming increasingly compulsive and severe is a hallmark of the syndrome. Head and leg banging; nose gouging; biting of the tongue, lips, and fingers; and loss of vision from eye rubbing are not uncommon.

In a profile article appearing in the *New Yorker*, Richard Preston (2007) gave this account of a Lesch-Nyhan patient:

> He was a gregarious child, whose hands seemed to hate him. Over time, his fingers had got inside his mouth and nose and broken out and removed the bones of his upper palate and parts of his sinuses, leaving a cavern in his face. He had also bitten off several fingers. A Lesch-Nyhan person may be fine for days, until suddenly the hands jump into his mouth with the suddenness of a cobra strike, and he cries for help. People with Lesch-Nyhan feel pain as acutely as anyone else does, and they are horrified by the idea of their fingers or lips being severed. They feel as if their hands and mouth don't belong to them and are under the control of something else. Some Lesch-Nyhan people have bitten off their tongues, and some have a record of self-enucleation—they have pulled out their eye or stabbed it with a sharp object.

LNS appears to be caused by a mutation in the *HPRT* gene, which results in a deficiency in the enzyme HGPRT (hypoxanthine-guanine phosphoribosyltransferase). Deficits in the HGPRT enzyme can lead to a buildup of uric acid throughout the bodily fluids because of decreased degradation and excretion. Furthermore, diminished HGPRT may also produce a nucleotide deficiency in guanosine triphosphate (GTP). GTP is known to be involved in the regulation of dopamine receptor activity. GTP decreases the effects of dopamine agonists by reducing their binding affinity to the postsynaptic dopamine receptors. Therefore, a deficiency in GTP would result in an increase in the responsiveness of dopamine receptors to dopamine agonists. These events effectively create a "dopamine supersensitivity" primarily involving the D1 receptors found in several areas of the brain, including the prefrontal cortex. This so-called functional denervation of the D1 receptor may underlie the self-mutilation behavior.

Goldstein et al (1985) compared the effects of fluphenazine (Prolixin®), a selective D1-recptor antagonist, to that of a placebo in treating individuals with LNS. They reported that fluphenazine effectively suppressed self-mutilation in LNS. Furthermore, haloperidol (Haldol®), a selective D2-antagonist, proved to be ineffective. Experimental studies using animal models have demonstrated increased autotomy following administration of a dopaminergic agonist, and a decrease after using an antagonist, providing further support for the dopamine supersensitivity hypothesis.

In addition to this supersensitivity phenomenon, the functional denervation of the D1 receptor could cause a disruption in the normal dopamine–adenosine relationship.

This relationship contributes heavily to a balance between the activating and inhibiting pathways in the basal ganglia. The basal ganglia serve to regulate the expression of bodily movements, affective behavior, and certain cognitive processes by integrating widespread inputs from the cerebral cortex and modulating the activity of relevant thalamic relay nuclei. The excitatory–inhibitory imbalance could lead to inadequate modulation of the thalamic activity. It is the thalamus that processes information regarding bodily representations as part of the somatosensory system. This abnormal thalamic activity may leave the patient being unaware of parts of their own body (anosognosia), which could contribute to self-mutilation.

Pellicer et al (1998) hypothesized that this dopaminergic dysfunction results in a disruption of the functional relationship between the genetic body and real body formed in the neuromatrix, as outlined by Melzack (see Chapter 5). Processing of information regarding the real body involves the thalamus and somatosensory cortex. The genetic body is wired into the system, as it were, and processes information in parallel with the real body. The supersensitivity created in the D1 receptors may alter the neuromatrix "codification" of the genetic body. This, in turn, contributes to the development of anosognosia (denial of the existence or awareness, in this case, of certain body parts). Pellicer et al, therefore, posited self-mutilation to be "pain consciousness" problem.

Data from animal studies confirm the presence of self-mutilation (autotomy) following the denervation of limbs (Coderre et al, 1986). The animal appears to be attempting to remove this unfelt and useless appendage. Whether this self-mutilation represents a form of autotomy is unclear. Another intriguing finding is the notable reduction in myelinated nerve fibers, while the unmyelinated fibers are preserved. The etiology of this remains unknown. The condition does not seem to be directly related to sensory loss and is thought to be caused by damage to higher level neurocognitive functions involved in integrating sensory information with processes that support spatial or bodily representations.

PHARMACOGENETICS

The terms *pharamacogenetics* and *pharmacogenomics* (Desmeules et al, 2004) are often used interchangeably. Some differentiate the two terms by defining pharmacogenetics as the study of genetic influence on differing responses to drugs, and pharmacogenomics (Kalow, 2004) as the process of drug discovery. The interest in pharmacogenetics is driven in part by the broad variation in individual responses to a particular drug, especially analgesics such as opioids (Smith, 2009; Vuilleumier et al, 2012). The study of a drug's action involves its pharmacodynamics (what the drug does to the body and how it does it) and its pharmacokinetics (what happens to the drug while it is in the body). Typically, these processes are examined at the cellular and molecular levels.

Drug safety has taken on greater importance, as some 5–7% of hospital admissions and over two million deaths can be attributed to adverse drug reactions (ADRs) (Meyer, 2000; Stamer and Stüber, 2007a). Both ADR and the efficacy of the drug can be affected by alteration in drug metabolism caused by genetic-based variations (polymorphisms) in the metabolizing enzymes. Developing a cost-effective and efficient means of early identification of these genetic variations could improve drug therapy, save lives, and significantly reduce medical expenditures.

One of the primary limiting factors in the pharmacological treatment of pain, particularly with non-steroidal anti-inflammatory drugs (NSAIDs) and opioids, is that of ADRs. Depending on the study and the drug, as many as 25% or more of patients discontinue their use of an otherwise effective drug because of one or more ADRs. The most common ADRs include nausea, gastrointestinal distress, pruritus (itching), constipation, sedation, hormonal changes, and respiratory depression. For example, there is evidence linking the altered coagulation and gastrointestinal bleeding found with NSAIDs to the *CYP2C8/9* genotype (Agundez et al, 2009), and ABCB1 polymorphisms to respiratory depression associated with opioid use (Park et al, 2007). The use of other agents such as laxatives, stimulants, or hormone replacement therapies to counteract these side effects adds substantially to the cost of the drug therapy, and these drugs may have ADRs of their own.

Absorption, distribution, metabolism, and excretion represent the four main processes involved in drug pharmacology. Many drugs are absorbed through the intestine and taken up into the bloodstream and transported to their target cells. Chemical stability, solubility, transit time, and gastric emptying time can each affect the rate and degree of absorption. Distribution relates to the movement of the drug from one part or compartment of the body to another. This is usually reversible. Drugs metabolism involves the breaking down or degradation of the compound, often in the liver, by various enzymes, such as cytochrome P450. Metabolism can cause an activation or deactivation of the drug. This process also creates metabolites, which may be pharmacologically active or inactive (inert). Drugs and their metabolites are typically excreted in the urine via the kidneys or in feces. Incomplete excretion may result in an accumulation of metabolites that can negatively affect the metabolic process or cause a toxic reaction. In short, once ingested, drugs are metabolized into their various ingredients, are transported to their respective receptor where they bind and create an effect, then must be excreted to avoid an accumulation.

Genetic variations can influence the efficacy of analgesic agents as well as nociception and susceptibility to painful conditions. Significant individual variations in opioid requirements for treating postoperative, cancer, and non-cancer-related chronic pain have been reported.

Pharmacotherapeutics has focused on multiple areas, including receptor polymorphisms, transport systems, and drug-metabolizing enzymes. That is, how sensitive are the receptors to a particular agent? How easily and efficiently does the drug get to its target? And, how well is it broken down and utilized?

Several candidate genes have been selected for investigation because of their likely link to pain processing (Max and Stewart, 2008). The mu-opioid receptor mutations (*OPRM1*) are of special interest because of their allelic frequency and their potential impact on opioid therapy including ADR. The A118G polymorphism accounts for 10–15% of the allelic frequency in Caucasians. There is a significant decrease in response to morphine-6-glucuronide (M6G), the major active metabolite of morphine, in carriers of two G118 alleles instead of one. For example, 2–4 times more alfentanil is required to produce the same analgesic response to EIP, and 10–12 times higher concentrations are needed to produce the same degree of respiratory depression. Carriers of the G-allele appear to be protected against ADRs including the risk of toxicity and opioid-induced vomiting. Clinically based studies using patients with cancer, those who underwent elective abdominal hysterectomy, and those receiving total knee replacements also discovered that carriers of variants of *OPMR1* required higher doses of morphine.

COMT metabolizes biogenic amines such as catecholamines including dopamine and norepinephrine (NE), thus affecting the pain neurotransmission system (Gursoy et al, 2003; Zubieta et al, 2003) One common COMT polymorphism, G472A, aka COMTVal158Met, substitutes one amino acid for another, effectively reducing COMT activity by a factor of 3–4 times. This polymorphism has been associated with increased sensory and affective pain ratings and reduced endogenous opioid system activity in response to EIP. Furthermore, postmortem brain tissue analysis found what appears to be a compensatory up-regulation in opioid receptor expression.

Variations in COMT haplotypes have also been associated with high, medium, and low pain sensitivity. Heightened levels of NE and epinephrine in response to reduced COMT activity resulted in higher pain. Catecholamines, serotonin, and nitric oxide are regulated in part by tetrahydrobiopterin (TTHB). Guanosine triphosphate cyclo-hydrolase (GCH1), often referred to as the "protective gene," is an enzyme that influences the rate at which TTHB is synthesized and is found in about 15% of studied populations. Alterations in this particular pathway have been associated with neurological disorders including dystonia, and cognitive dysfunction. Injections of TTHB increased the pain behavior in rat models of neuropathic and inflammatory pain, while inhibition of the TTHB synthesis pathway resulted in reduced pain behaviors. In humans, a GCH1 haplotype was associated with reduced pain sensitivity to EIP and improved long-term (1 year) response in leg pain following surgery in patients with LBP (Tegeder et al, 2006, 2008).

Of the three opioid receptor types, mu, delta, and kappa ( ), k-agonists such as pentazocine (Talwin®) and nalbuphine (Nubain®) tend to be differentially effective with women compared to men. The melanocortin-1 receptor (MC1R) was found to mediate the sensitivity of the k-opioid receptor in mice. In humans, variants of MC1R tend to be associated with pale skin and red-headed phenotypes. Indeed, red-headed women tend to be more sensitive to experimentally induced thermal pain and in one study required 19% more analgesic in response to painful electrical stimulation (see Gear et al, 1996; Mogil et al, 2003). However, Mogil et al (2003) directly examined *MC1R* genotypes and found that red-headed women with two variant *MC1R* alleles demonstrated greater analgesic responses to pentazocine than their non-red-headed counterparts. This "gender-specific" pain modulation appears to only involve the k-opioid system.

Another vital area of pharmacogenetic research has focused on drug metabolism. One class of enzymes known to metabolize a variety of drugs and thus impact efficacy and toxicity is the polymorphic cytochrome P450 (CYP, P450), which is a very large and diverse superfamily (Day et al, 1996; Marez et al, 1997). The term *cytochrome* reflects the fact that these are colored ("chrome") cellular ("cyto") proteins. The enzyme P4502D6 or CYP2D6, for example, metabolizes codeine, tramadol, and oxycodone. There are some known 100 allelic variants for the *CYP2D6* gene. Depending on the genotype and particular alleles present, a patient could be classified as an extensive, ultrarapid, poor, or intermediate metabolizer. Poor metabolizers are at a much greater risk for ADRs secondary to drug accumulation leading to a possible drug overdose. Furthermore, the therapeutic effect of the drug is significantly compromised by failure of the prodrug to be metabolized into its active metabolite, that is, codeine to morphine. For example, mutations in the gene that encodes for this enzyme would produce a poor metabolizer of codeine and render the person relatively insensitive to codeine's potential analgesic effects. Even after a four-fold increase, poor metabolizers of tramadol manifesting the *CYP2D6* genotype reported inadequate analgesia.

Extensive metabolizers have a high degree of CYP2D6 activity, and intermediate metabolizers are somewhere in between. The ultrarapid metabolizer will likely have multiple copies of the *CYP2D6* gene expressed and thus greater than normal CYP2D6 function. These patients may metabolize the drug up to 30% fast than the extensive group and thus demonstrate subtherapeutic blood levels of the drug because of the increased rate of metabolism. Clinically, they will not respond to conventional dosages and could require a 10- to 50-fold increase in the drug to obtain the desired effect. However, a study by Andreassen et al (2012) involving 450 patients with cancer pain receiving oxycodone found a lack of correlation between CYP2D6 metabolizer status and the degree of analgesia as well as cognitive functioning, suggesting a more complicated relationship.

Similarly, the metabolism of NSAIDs is influenced by the CYP2C9 substrate. An estimated 1–3% of Caucasians demonstrate a decrease in their ability to metabolize NSAIDs. It is estimated that 3–5% of Caucasians are ultrarapid metabolizes, as are 0.5% of Asains and up to 29% of Saudi Arabians and Ethiopians.

Many substances can increase or inhibit CYP activity. This can lead to adverse drug interactions. For example, if drug A inhibits the CYP-induced metabolism of drug B, drug B could accumulate in the body, causing a toxic reaction or overdose. Therefore, caution is required when using two or more drugs, to avoid those that affect the CYP system. This becomes even more important if one drug is critical to the patient or when there is a small therapeutic window. In the latter case, even a small variation in metabolism could negate the drug's effect.

CYP activity can also be affected by some naturally occurring products. Grapefruit juice, for example, contains certain bioactive compounds known to inhibit CYP3A4-induced metabolism. Avoidance of grapefruit and grapefruit juice is recommended when taking opioid drugs such as codeine, tramadol, oxycodone, and methadone; benzodiazepines, including alprazolam and midazolam; antidepressants such as trazodone; and sleep aids such as zolpidem. Likewise, smoking induces CYP2A6 activity, influencing the metabolism of some antipsychotic drugs, including clonazapine and olanzapine. The common herbal compound St. John's wort can affect many CYP substrates, including CYP3A4 and CYP2D6, thus affecting the metabolism of some antidepressants and opioids, respectively.

Individual variation in pain sensitivity and in response to opioids significantly complicates pharmacological treatment. The mu-opioid receptor (MOR) is a major site of action for opioids and as such is the source of great interest (Lötsch et al, 2006). The MOR is coded by the *OPRM1* gene. One of the more common SNP or allelic variants of the MOR gene is the substitution of adenine (A) for guanine (G) at the 118 location, or what is referred to as the A118G SNP. This change produces intracellular and extracellular events that influence opioid responsivity. The role of the A118G SNP in postoperative opioid requirements has been examined (Janicki et al, 2006). SNP genotyping has been used to identify the presence or absence of A118 and the G118 MOR allele in the whole blood. The A118 MOR is considered the "major" allele of the A118G SNP, and its variant, G118 MOR, a "minor" allele. The presence of the A11G MOR polymorphism did not have an impact on pain scores or opioid needs in the postoperative patients. G118 MOR was found much less often in the patients with chronic pain than in the opioid-naive surgical group. Carriers of the A118 major allele required more opioid than those with the G118 minor allele, with the chronic pain patients requiring the highest amount of opioid.

The interpretation of such data is not easy. It is tantalizing to theorize that the relative absence of the G118 MOR minor allele of the A118G SNP for the MOR gene gives it some type of protective function against chronic pain and modifies the patient's responsiveness to opioids. This hypothesis is bolstered by noting that the presence of the A118 major allele was associated with resistance to or the requirement for higher opioid doses. Furthermore, the A118G SNP has been associated with substance abuse disorders involving alcohol, methamphetamine, and heroine. So might the A118G SNP of the MOR function as a "general-risk gene" for substance abuse rather than for chronic pain or opioid resistance? This was suggested by Janicki et al (2006). However, they were quick to point out that related studies' findings conflict and that the mechanisms by which these polymorphisms exert their effect remain elusive.

Preclinical studies heralded the association of the *OPRM1* 118G allele with decreased opioid requirements and decreased opioid effectiveness. Enthusiasm over the obvious clinical implications seemed unbridled. To date, however, these expectations appear to be unfulfilled. Walter and Lötsch (2009) undertook a meta-analysis of the relevant data. By combining the results of several studies, a meta-analysis makes use of a statistical procedure called *meta-regression*. The meta-regression produces overall averages while controlling for important study characteristics. The resulting meta-effect is a more powerful estimate of the true effect size than can be derived from a single study. Using a PubMed database, the authors obtained 174 hits. However, only 23 of the studies were relevant and only 8 of these met the criteria for inclusion in the meta-analysis. The overall sample size included 677 carriers of at least one minor 118G allele. The clinical populations incorporated cancer pain, non-cancer pain, and postoperative pain patients, as well as women in labor. Opioid requirements, pain relief, and ADRs were examined. Studies of postoperative (Sadhasivam and Chidambaran, 2012) and cancer pain patients tended to report higher opioid use and less pain relief among those with the *OPRM1* 118G allele. However, studies with chronic pain patients and those receiving opioids for labor pain showed no association. In the end, *OPRM1* 118A>G could explain only 7% of the variance and thus was considered of questionable clinical relevance. It did, however, seem to afford some protection against opioid-induced nausea.

CONCLUSION

Pain genetics is in its infancy; the nuances and complexities are significant. Technological advances have allowed for the scanning of millions of genes and gene variants along with thousands of molecules. The interpretation of the findings remains unclear. Generalizing from one species to another is compromised by differences in the way pain is processed and experienced (Lascelles and Flecknell, 2010). The interaction of various transmission, amplification, and suppression systems involves an untold number of molecules and an inestimable number of genes. Even changes at the molecular-genetic level are susceptible to influences of gender, ethnicity, and psychological states, adding to the dynamic and complex nature of pain genetics (Belfer et al, 2013).

Genetic variations may play a complex role in psychological states and the response to trauma. For example, the presence of one or more G-alleles of the A118G SNP has been associated with reduced pain immediately after sexual assault and 6 weeks post-assault (Ballina et al, 2013). This implicates involvement of the endogenous opioid system. Similar findings have been reported from examining symptom severity in acute stress disorders and posttraumatic stress disorder. This could represent a variant of stress-induced hyperalgesia, also implicating the role of the endogenous opioid system. These observations emphasize the complexity of the system (individual) and potential impact of any genetic manipulation not only within but also outside the arena of pain.

The probability of a chance relationship or false-positive finding is not insignificant. Indeed, the replication rate for association studies is only about 30%. This point was highlighted by the European Pharmacogenetic Opioid Study (EPOS; Klepsted et al, 2011). This study represents the largest opioid response genetic association study to date, including nearly 2,300 cancer patients and 112 SNPs in 25 genes. It failed to identify any association between the SNPs tested and oral opioid requirements. Confirmatory results from systematic replication and specificity of the findings in conjunction with in vitro data demonstrating that the candidate polymorphism does, indeed, alter the expression or function of a particular protein are required.

The technology for bedside genotyping to identify sensitivities exists. However, given the gene–gene and gene–environment interactions, the goal of personalized pain control and personalized opioid prescribing is far from certain (Branford et al, 2012); according to Mogil (2009), incorporating genotyping into clinical pain practice is premature, at best. We must be careful that the fascination with "gadgets" does not betray sound sense.

The relatively low rate of replication raises questions as to the reliaiblity of research methodolgy and findings to date. Also lacking are guidelines for determining when genetic testing should be performed. How should the proposed treatment be adjusted? How available should the information be? And, finally, how sure are we that a genetic-based treatment modification will affect the intended target, and only the intended target, and not trigger a cascade of unanticipated actions and reactions? It is clear that relatively small variations in the genotype can have system-wide effects. The downstream consequences for the individual and offspring have yet to be systematically evaluated.

There is still much to be done in understanding the mechanism by which genetic variations express themselves. Possible targets for future study include proteins, cytokines, and neurotransmitters involved in pain and pain control. Also requiring further study are genes known or thought to change their expression in response to damage or injury, thus propagating or enhancing nociceptive processing and the experience of pain.

The profound untold consequences of even a single substitution must be uncovered. Furthermore, not all changes are known to have a functional consequence. Why is this so? Perhaps much like "silent nociceptors" these variations await a particular set of circumstances to trigger their activity. Indeed, the effect may be indirect through influencing other genetic activity. In addition, while many have been captivated by genetic research and its possibilities, its interaction with psychological and environmental variables is undeniable and requires further clarification. This interaction disallows the notion of genetic determinism and mandates that the patient and pain be understood from the perspective of a complex adaptive system.

REFERENCES

Ablin IN. Possible association between fibromyalgia and a novel 1354G>C polymorphism in the *TACR1* (substance P receptor) gene in Ashkenazi patients. *Arthritis Rheum.* 2005;52:S269.

Abrahamsen B, Zhao J, Asante CO, et al. The cell and molecular basis of mechanical, cold, and inflammatory pain. *Science.* 2008;321:702–705.

Agundez JA, Garcia-Martin E, Martinez C. Genetically based impairment in CYP2C8- and CYP2C9-dependent metabolism as a risk factor for gastrointestinal bleeding: is a combination of pharmacogenetics and metabolomics required to improve personalized medicine? *Expert Opin Drug Metab Toxicol.* 2009;5:607–620.

Altshuler David, Daly MJ, Lander ES. Genetic mapping in human disease. *Science.* 2008;322:881–888.

Andreassen TN, Eftedal I, Klepstad P, et al. Do *CYP2D6* genotypes reflect oxycodone requirements for cancer patients treated for cancer pain? A cross-sectional multicentre study. *Eur J Clin Pharmacol.* 2012;68(1):55–64.

Ballina LE, Ulirsch JC, Soward AC, et al. Mu-opioid receptor gene A118G polymorphism predicts pain recovery after sexual assault. *J Pain.* 2013;14(2):165–171.

Belfer I, Segall SK, Lariviere LR, et al. Pain modality- and sex-specific effects of *COMT* genetic functional variants. *Pain.* 2013;154(8):1368–1376.

Bondy B, Spaeth M, Offenbaecher M, et al. The T102C polymorphism of the 5-HT2A-receeptor gene in fibromyalgia. *Neurobiol Dis.* 1999;6:433–439.

Bowsher D, Woods CG, Nicholas AK, et al. Absence of pain with hyperhidrosis: a new syndrome where vascular afferents may mediate cutaneous sensation. *Pain.* 2009;147(1):287–298.

Brand P, Yancey P. *Pain: The Gift No One Wants.* Grand Rapids, MI: Zondervan Press. 1993.

Branford R, Droney J, Ross JR. Opioid genetics: the key to personalized pain control? *Clin Genet.* 2012;82:301–310.

Burda CD, Cox FR, Osborne P. Histocompatibility antigens in the fibrositis (fibromyalgia) syndrome. *Clin Exp Rheumatol.* 1986;4:355–358.

Carmel L, Efroni S, White PD, Aslakson E, Vollmer-Conna U, Rajeevan MS. Gene expression profile of empirically delineated classes of unexplained chronic fatigue. *Pharmacogenomics.* 2006;7:375–386.

Casas-Bruge M, Almenar G, Grau IM, Jane J, Harrera-Marschitz M, Ungerstedt U. Dopaminergic receptor supersensitivity in self-mutilatory behaviors of Lesch-Nyhan disease. *Lancet.* 1985; April: 991–992.

Chesler EJ, Wilson SG, Lariviere WR, Rodriguez-Zas SL, Mogil JS. Identification and ranking of genetic and laboratory environment factors influencing a behavioral trait, thermal nociception, via computational analysis of a large data archive. *Neurosci Biobehav Rev.* 2002;26:907–923.

Coderre TJ, Grimes RW, Melzack R. Deafferentation and chronic pain in animals: an evaluation of evidence suggesting autotomy is related to pain. *Pain.* 1986;26:61–84.

Coghill RC, McHaffie JG, Yen YF. Neural correlates of interindividual differences in the subjective experience of pain. *Proc Natl Acad Sci U S A.* 2003;100:8538–8542.

Cohen H, Buskila D, Neumann L, Ebstein RP. Confirmation of an association between fibromyalgia and serotonin transporter promoter region (5-HTTLPR) polymorphism, and relationship to anxiety related personality traits. *Arthritis Rheum.* 2002;46:845–847.

Cox JJ, Reimann F, Nicholas AK, et al. An *SCN9A* channelopathy causes congenital inability to experience pain. *Nature.* 2006;444:894–898.

Day AK, Brockmoller J, Broly F, et al. Nomenclature for human CYP2D6 alleles. *Pharmacogenetics.* 1966;6(3):193–201.

Desmeules JA, Piguet V, Ehret GB, Dayer P. Pharmacogenetics, pharmacokinetics, and analgesia. In Mogil JS, ed. *The Genetics of Pain: Progress in Pain Research and Management*, Vol. 2. Seattle: IASP Press; 2004:211–237.

Diatchenko L, Nackley AG, Slade GD, Fillingim RB, Maixner W. Idiopathic pain disorders—pathways of vulnerability. *Pain.* 2006;123:226–230.

Diatchenko L, Slade GD, Nackley AG, et al. Genetic basis for individual variations in pain perception and the development of a chronic pain condition. *Hum Mol Genet.* 2005;14:135–143.

Diatchenko L, Slade GD, Nackley AG, et al. Genetic architecture of human pain perception. *Trends Genet.* 2007;23(12):605–613.

Edwards RR. Individual difference in endogenous pain modulation as a risk factor for chronic pain. *Neurology.* 2005;65:437–443.

Fillingim RB. Social and environmental influences on pain: Implications of pain genetics. Mogil JS, ed. *The Genetics of Pain.* Seattle: IASP Press, 2004:283–303.

Fillingim RB, Kaplan L, Staud R, et al. The A118G single nucleotide polymorphism of the mu-opioid receptor gene (*OPRM1*) is associated with pressure pain sensitivity in humans. *J Pain.* 2005;6:159–167.

Fillingim RB, Wallace MR, Herbstman DM, Riberiro-Dasilva M, Staud R. Genetic contributions to pain: a review of findings in humans. *Oral Dis.* 2008;14:673–682.

Fink DJ. Applications of gene therapy to the treatment of chronic pain. *Curr Gene Ther.* 2008;8(1):42–48.

Fink DJ, Wechuck J, Mata M, et al. Gene therapy for pain: results of a phase I clinical trial. *Ann Neurol.* 2011;70(2):217–212.

Foulkes T, Wood JN. Pain genes. *PLoS Genet.* 2008;4(7):1–9.

Frank B, Niesler B, Bondy B, et al. Mutational analysis of serotonin receptor genes: *HTR3A* and *HTR3B* in fibromyalgia patients. *Clin Rheumatol.* 2004;23(4):338–344.

Gear RW, Miaskowski C, Gordon NC, Paul SM, Heller PH, Levine JD. Kappa-opioids produce significantly greater analgesia in women than in men. *Nat Med.* 1996;2:1248–1250.

George SZ, Dover GC, Wallace MR, et al. Biopsychosocial influence on exercise-induced delayed onset muscle soreness at the shoulder: pain catastrophizing and catechol-O-methyltransferase (COMT) diplotype predict pain ratings. *Clin J Pain.* 2008;24(9):793–801.

Glorioso JC, Fink DJ. Herpes vector-mediated gene transfer in the treatment of chronic pain. *Mol Ther.* 2009;17(1):13–18.

Glorioso JC, Mata M, Fink DJ. Therapeutic gene transfer to the nervous system using viral vectors. *J Neurovirol.* 2003;9:165–172.

Goldstein M, Anderson LT, Reuden R, Dancis J. Self-mutilation in Lesch-Nyhan disease is caused by dopaminergic denervation. *Lancet.* 1985;1:338–339.

Gursoy S, Erdal E, Herken H, Madenci E, Alasehirli B, Erdal N. Significance of catechol-O-methyltransferase gene polymorphism in fibromyalgia syndrome. *Rheumatol Int.* 2003;23:104–107.

Hunt SP, Mantyh PW. The molecular dynamics of pain control. *Nat Rev Neurosci.* 2001;2:83–91.

Indo Y. Congenital insensitivity to pain. In Mogil JS, ed. *The Genetics of Pain: Progress in Pain Research and Management*, Vol. 2. Seattle: IASP Press; 2004:171–191.

Introduction to genetics. http://en.wikipedia.org/wik/Introduction-to-genetics

Janiciki P, Schuler G, Francis D, et al. A genetic association study of the functional A118G polymorphism of the human mu-opioid receptor gene in patients with acute and chronic pain. *Anesth Analg.* 2006;103:1011–1016.

Kalow W. Human pharmacogenomics: the development of a science. *Hum Genomics.* 2004;1(5):375–380.

Kerr JR, Petty R, Burke B, et al. Gene expression subtypes in patients with chronic fatigue syndrome/myalgic encephalomyelitis. *J Infect Dis.* 2008;197:1171–1184.

Kim H, Clark D, Dionne RA. Genetic contributions to clinical pain and analgesia: avoiding pitfalls in genetic research. *J Pain.* 2009;10:663–693.

Kim H, Dionne RA. Genetics, pain, and analgesia. *Pain: Clinical Updates.* 2005;13(3):1–4.

Kim H, Mittal DP, Iadarola MJ, Dionne RA. Genetic predictors for acute experimental cold and heat pain sensitivity in humans. *J Med Genet.* 2006;43:1–8.

Kim H, Neubert JK, Miguel AS, et al. Genetic influences in variability in human acute experimental pain sensitivity associated with gender, ethnicity, and psychological temperament. *Pain.* 2004;109:488–496.

Klepstad P, Fladvad T, Skorpen F, et al. Influence from genetic variability on opioid use for cancer pain: a European genetic association study of 2294 cancer pain patients. *Pain.* 2011;152(5):1139–1145.

Kumar V, Mahal BA. NGF—the TrkA to successful pain treatment. *J Pain Res.* 2012;2(5):279–287.

Landrieu P, Said G, Allaire C. Dominantly transmitted congenital indifference to pain. *Ann Neurol.* 1990;27:574–578.

Larsson B, Billie B, Pendersen NL. Genetic influence in headache: a Swedish twin study. *Headache.* 1995;35:70–78.

Lascelles BD, Flecknell PA. Do animal models tell us about human pain? *Pain: Clinical Updates.* 2010;18(5):1–6.

Levesques M, Potvin S, Marchand S, et al. Pain perception in schizophrenia: evidence of a specific pain response profile. *Pain Med.* 2012;13(12):1571–1579.

Light AR, White AT, Hughen RW, Light KC. Moderate exercise increases expression for sensory, adrenergic, and immune genes in chronic fatigue syndrome patients but not in normal subjects. *J Pain.* 2009;10:1099–1112.

Lötsch J, Stuck B, Hummel T. The human mu-opioid receptor gene polymorphism 118A>G decreases cortical activation in response to specific nociceptive stimulation. *Behav Neurosci.* 2006;120:1218–1224.

MacGregor AJ, Andrew T, Sambrook PN, Spector TD. Structural, psychological, and genetic influences on low back and neck pain: a study of adult female twins. *Arthritis Rheum.* 2004;51:160–167.

MacGregor AJ, Griffiths GO, Baker J, Spector TD. Determinants of pressure pain threshold in adult twins: evidence that shared environmental influences predominate. *Pain.* 1997;73:253–257.

Mamie C, Rebsamen M, Morris MA, Morabia A. *ABCB1* gene modulates the intensity of postoperative pain in children. *Proceedings of the Annual Meeting of the American Society Anesthesiologists.* 2009; Abstract A1597.

Marez D, Legrand M, Sabbagh N, et al. Polymorphism of the cytochrome P450 *CYP2D6* gene in a European population: characterization of 48 mutations and 53 alleles, their frequencies and evolution. *Pharmacogenetics.* 1997;7:193–202.

Max MB, Stewart WF. The molecular epidemiology of pain: a new discipline for drug discovery. *Nat Rev.* 2008;7:647–658.

Meyer UA. Pharmacogenetics and adverse drug reactions. *Lancet.* 2000;356:1667–1671.

Mikkelsson M, Kaprio J, Salminen JJ, Pulkkinen L, Rose RJ. Widespread pain among 11-year-old Finnish twins. *Arthritis Rheum.* 2001;44(2):481–485.

Mogil JS. The genetic mediation of individual differences in sensitivity to pain and its inhibition. *Proc Natl Acad Sci U S A.* 1999;96(14):7774–7751.

Mogil JS, ed. *The Genetics of Pain.* Seattle: IASP Press; 2004.

Mogil, JS. The nature and nurture of pain: the role of genetics and environmental issues in the experience of pain. In Mahajan G, Fishmen SM, eds. *Plenary Proceedings of the 24th Annual Meeting of the American Academy of Pain Medicine, AAPM*, Glenview, IL. 2008:81–94.

Mogil JS. Are we getting anywhere in human pain genetics? *Pain.* 2009;146:231–232.

Mogil JS, Sorge RE, LaCroix-Fralish ML, et al. Pain sensitivity and vasopressin analgesia are mediated by a gene–sex–environment interaction. *Nat Neurosci.* 2011;14(12):1569–1573.

Mogil JS, Wilson SG, Bon K, et al. Heritability of nociception I: responses of 11 inbred mouse strains on 12 measures of nociception. *Pain.* 1999;80(1-2):67–82.

Mogil JS, Wilson SG, Chesler EJ, et al. The melanocortin-1 receptor gene mediates female-specific mechanisms of analgesia in mice and humans. *Proc Natl Acad Sci U S A.* 2003;100(8):4867–4872.

Mogil JS, Yu L, Basbaum AI. Pain genes? Natural variation and transgenic mutants. *Annu Rev Neurosci.* 2000;23:777–811.

Nielsen CS, Staud R, Price DD. Individual differences in pain sensitivity: measurement, causation and consequences. *J Pain.* 2009;10:231–237.

Nielsen CS, Stubhaug A, Price DD, Vassend O, Czajkowski N, Harris JR. Individual differences in pain sensitivity: genetic and environmental contributions. *Pain.* 2008;136:21–29.

Norbury TA, MacGregor AJ, Urwin J, Spector TD, McMahon SB. Heritability of responses to painful stimuli in women: a classical twin study. *Brain.* 2007;130:3041–3049.

Offenbaecher M, Bondy B, de Jonge S, et al. Possible association of fibromyalgia with a polymorphism in the serotonin transporter gene regulatory region. *Arthritis Rheum.* 1999;42:2482–2488.

Ojima K, Watanabe N, Narita N, Narita M. Temporomandibular disorder is associated with a serotonin transporter gene polymorphism in the Japanese population. *Biopsychosoc Med.* 2007;1:1–3.

Park HJ, Shinn HK, Ryu SH, Lee HS, Park CS, Kang JH. Genetic polymorphisms in the *ABCB1* gene and the effects of fentanyl in Koreans. *Clin Pharmacol Ther.* 2007;81:539–546.

Patsopoulos NA, Tatsioni A, Ioannidis JP. Claims of sex differences: an empirical assessment in genetic associations. *JAMA.* 2007;298:880–893.

Pellicer F, Buendia-Roldan L, Pallares-Trujilloa VC. Self-mutilation in the Lesch-Nyhan syndrome: a corporal consciousness problem? A new hypothesis. *Med Hypotheses.* 1998;50(1):43–47.

Pollard KS. What makes us human? *Sci Am.* 2009; May: 44–49.

Preston R. An error in the code: what can a rare disorder tell us about human behavior? *New Yorker,* August 13, 2007. http://www.newyorker.com/reporting/2007/08/13/070813fa_fact_preston#ixzz2LfDImRqF. Accessed February 22, 2013.

Roses AD. Pharmacogenetics and the practice of medicine. *Nature.* 2000;405(6788):857–865.

Russell IJ, Vaeroy H, Javors M, Nyberg F. Cerebrospinal fluid biogenic amine metabolites in fibromyalgia/fibrositis syndrome and rheumatoid arthritis. *Arthritis Rheum.* 1992;35:550–556.

Sadhasivam S, Chidambaran V. Pharmacogenomics of opioids and perioperative pain management. *Pharmacogenomics.* 2012;13(15):1719–1740.

Smith HS. Opioid metabolism. *Mayo Clin Proc.* 2009;84(7):613–624.

Stamer UM, Stüber F. Genetic factors in pain and its treatment. *Curr Opin Anesthesiol.* 2007a;20:478–484.

Stamer UM, Stüber F. The pharmacogenetics of analgesia. *Expert Opin Pharmacother.* 2007b;8(14):2235–2245.

Tegeder I, Adolph J, Schmidt H, Woolf CJ, Geisslinger G, Lötsch J. Reduced hyperalgesia in homozygous carriers of a GTP cyclohydrolase 1 haplotype. *Eur J Pain.* 2008;12(8):1069–1077.

Tegeder I, Costigan M, Griffin RS, et al. GTP cyclohydrolase and tetrahydrobiopterin regulate pain sensitivity and persistence. *Nat Med.* 2006;12:1269–1277.

Temple LKF, McLeod RS, Gallinger S, Wright JG. Defining disease in the genomics era. *Science.* 2001;293:807–808.

Uhl GR, Sora I, Wang Z. The mu opiate receptor as a candidate gene for pain: polymorphisms, variations in expression, nociception, and opiate responses. *Proc Natl Acad Sci U S A.* 1999;96:7752–7755.

van de Beck WJ, Roep BO, van der Slik Giphart MJ, van Hilten BJ. Susceptibility loci for complex regional pain syndrome. *Pain.* 2003;103:93–97.

Vuilleumier PH, Stamer UH, Landau R. Pharmacological considerations in opioid analgesia. *Pharmacogenomics Pers Med.* 2012;5:73–87.

Walter C, Lötsch J. Meta-analysis of the relevance of the *OPRM1* 118A>G genetic variant for pain treatment. *Pain.* 2009;146:270–275.

Waxman SG, Dib-Hajj SD. Erythromelalgia: a hereditary pain syndrome enters the molecular era. *Ann Neurol.* 2005:52:758–788.

Wolfe D, Wechuck J, Kirsky D, Mata M, Fink DJ. Clinical trial of gene therapy for chronic pain. *Pain Med.* 2009;10:1325–1330.

Zubieta JK, Heitzeg MM, Smith YR, et al. *COMT* val158met genotype affects mu-opioid neurotransmitter responses to a pain stressor. *Science.* 2003;299:1240–1243.

13 Pain and Consciousness

Thus, if it is held that pains have no physical effects, then one must say either (i) pains do not cause beliefs that one is in pain, or (ii) beliefs that one is in pain are epiphenomenal. For, if pains caused beliefs that one is in pain, and the latter had physical effects, then pains would, after all, have effects in the physical (albeit indirectly).
–W. Robinson (2012, p. 1)

INTRODUCTION

The International Association for the Study of Pain (IASP) definition of pain describes it as a sensory and emotional experience. It is clear that the phenomenological experience of pain represents more than a one-time single-sensory-input encounter. It is formed and refined over time. It would also imply a level of conscious awareness. Indeed, Chapman and Nakamura (1999b) describe pain as a consciousness-dependent experience. Devor (2008) asserts that the pain experience, like all experience, requires consciousness. To the extent that consciousness implies a certain degree of awareness or attention, what happens to the pain when one is not consciously aware of it? Does pain require an observer, in the quantum theory sense of the term? Does consciousness serve the function of the observer? Does pain reside in some type of superposition until it is attended to?

Previous chapters have described the neurochemical, anatomical, and neurophysiological aspects of pain. There is a vast array of activity at the cellular and molecular level. Electrical impulses are transmitted with great efficiency throughout the peripheral and central nervous systems. Networks of neurons are created along with complex and dynamic patterns of interactions among various parts of the brain. The hard question, as Chalmers (1995) puts it, is how does our conscious or subjective experience arise (emerge) from this amalgamation of physical processes? In particular, how does pain become a conscious experience, and does pain exist at a nonconscious (subconscious) level?

DEFINITION OF CONSCIOUSNESS

The study of consciousness in humans and animals has faced a number of obstacles, not the least of which is that of definitions. For example, Tamietto and de Gelder (2010) have recommended using the term *nonconscious* to represent the "experimental psychology tradition and indicates a perceptual state in which the subject does not report the presence of a stimulus or one of its attributes (for example, its emotional content) even though there is evidence (behavioral, psychophysiological or neuro-physiological) that the stimulus has in fact been processed" (p. 698). They preserve the term *unconscious* for the psychoanalytical tradition of postulating "the existence of an active mechanism of psychodynamic suppression of conscious information." They also differentiate sensory unawareness from attentional unawareness. *Sensory unawareness* occurs when a stimulus is not perceived because it is too weak or too short, while *attentional unawareness* is the absence of awareness resulting from attentional selection.

The word *consciousness* itself comes from the Latin root *conscio*, which is a combination of *cum* meaning "with" and *scio* meaning "know." According to Zeman (2001), in the Latin sense of the word it referred to the sharing of some special, often shameful, knowledge, the source of which was one's bad *conscientia* (conscience). The term *conscious* or *consciousness* as used in the more contemporary sense did not emerge until the 1700s. A common definition of consciousness since then has been "a subjective experience (qualia), or awareness, or wakefulness, or the executive control system of the mind" (Zeman, 2001, p. 1265); a mental state of awareness of internal and external stimuli.

Operationally this awareness could include a localized response to a noxious stimulus. Depending on the quantitative or qualitative degree of awareness, Lindahl (1997) notes that consciousness can be described as existing in a primary state or an extended state. *Primary consciousness* is the ability to generate a mental scene in which diverse information is integrated for the purpose of directing behaviour of self (Edelman and Tononi, 2000). *Extended consciousness* is thought to involve higher order, advanced cognitive abilities such as a linguistic capability or self-consciousness as self-knowledge (Zeman, 2001). For Damasio (2003), extended consciousness represents the system of memories that are consciously accessible to the organism (both of the past and of the future). He speculates that it (a) may be uniquely human, (b) involves working memory, (c) represents an awareness of one's actions on one's self and others, and (d) is the ability to change reality.

In addition to his three principle meanings of consciousness as (a) a waking state, (b) a subjective experience (qualia), and (c) mind, Zeman (2001) also provides five meanings of the term *self-conscious*: (a) self-detection, (b) awareness of awareness (theory of mind; see Chapter 11), (c) self-knowledge, (d) self-recognition, and (e) proneness to embarrassment. The aspects of consciousness referring to a state of mind (awareness) and self-consciousness as self-detection (perceptual awareness) will be used in the discussion here. In this regard, it is important to distinguish sensation from perception. In the most simplistic terms, *sensation* refers to how physical energy is detected and encoded as neural signals, and *perception* to the manner in which information is organized and interpreted.

There are various levels of consciousness or altered consciousness, including (a) normal consciousness, (b) confusion, (c) delirium, (d) somnolence, (e) obtunded consciousness, (f) stupor, and (g) coma. Usually, an adequate noxious stimulus can advance a person from a lower to a higher level of alertness or consciousness. Three major states are considered to be permanently unconscious. A *persistent vegetative state* (PVS) exists when the patient demonstrate an eyes-opened nonconsciousness. During periods of normal wakefulness the eyes are occasionally open, and they have sleep–wake cycles. Such patients may demonstrate reflexive but not purposeful behaviors. They are awake, but not aware. In general, their cortex has been damaged but the brainstem is intact and functional. *Coma* is an eye-closed nonconsciousness—unarousable unresponsiveness. The brainstem is damaged and the patient is considered to be terminally ill with a life expectancy of a few weeks or months. The final category is *anencephalic infants*. In this condition the unfortunate infant has a congenital condition marked by the absence of a cortex but with varying amounts of a functioning brainstem.

Minimally conscious patients are unable to communicate but show inconsistent nonreflexive behaviors that may give the appearance of being aware of one's self or the environment. In the locked-in syndrome, commonly caused by a stroke, patients are awake and conscious but have no means of communicating by speech, limb, or facial movements due to complete paralysis of nearly all voluntary muscles except for the eyes. For purposes of this chapter, the term *consciousness* will be used in the most common and general sense, as an awareness of one's self and the environment (internal and external).

NEURAL CORRELATES OF CONSCIOUSNESS

The search for the neural correlates of consciousness (NCC) is ongoing. The ability of sleepwalkers to successfully navigate their environment absent any subsequent recall of their behavior illustrates how the customary relationship between motor control, perception, and memory can be disrupted. Despite their outward appearance, many patients exhibiting symptoms of a vegetative state are, in fact, thought to be aware of their surroundings. The study of consciousness often differentiates between explicit and implicit neural processes. Implicit neural processes give rise to conscious awareness while the explicit ones are carried out without any apparent awareness. *Awareness* in this case refers to the individual's ability to relate his or her experience.

It would be natural to assume that pain, and probably consciousness itself, requires higher level involvement. The upper brainstem reticular formation and thalamocortical structures appear to play significant roles in consciousness. However, Devor (1999, 2008) questioned the assumption that the cortex is a major cite for pain and conscious experience. It appears that stimulation of the cortex, including aspects considered to be part of the pain matrix, do not occasion the experience of pain, unlike non-pain areas such as those associated with vision, smell, and hearing. Although widespread stimulation, such as that found during epileptic seizures, arouses a sense of smell, tingling, lights, and odors, less than 4% of patients report pain as part of their aura.

Furthermore, focal lesions in the pain matrix do not eliminate pain but may in fact produce a central pain syndrome.

Based on these observations, Devor has suggested that subcortical structures may play a major role in the pain experience. He does not reject the role of cortical activation but proposes that this is in response to the transmission of subcortical messages to the cortex. If this is true and subcortical networks are indeed "sufficient to subserve (real) pain," then perhaps consciousness itself can be sustained in subcortical networks, thus rendering it independent of cortical functioning. Indeed, after performing substantial cortical excisions and radical hemispherectomy, and following the study of hundreds of intractable epileptics, in 1954 Penfield and Jasper concluded that "the highest integrative functions of the brain are not completed at the cortical level, but in a system of highly convergent subcortical structures supplying the key mechanism of consciousness" (cited in Anand and Clancy, 2006, p. 2).

Experientially, events that are not consciously perceived can affect our experience, thoughts, and actions—for example, blindsight. In this condition the individual is blind on one side of their visual field (a blind spot) due to a lesion or damage in the primary visual cortex. However, under controlled conditions, when asked to guess when or if a stimulus was presented in their blind spot, subjects respond with a high degree of accuracy. This better-than-chance performance occurs despite the fact that the subject reports no awareness of the stimulus having been presented. Zeman (2001) explains this by appealing to (a) subthreshold stimulation of systems that sometimes subserves consciousness and (b) systems that invariably operate in the absence of consciousness.

Fetal Pain and Consciousness

The issue of pain and consciousness is not likely to be debated with more fervor than when applied to the fetus, neonate, and infant (see Chapter 9). This debate also begs the question of the origin or beginning of human consciousness. In a review of the literature on fetal pain, Lee et al (2005) noted that

pain is a subjective sensory and emotional experience that requires the presence of consciousness to permit recognition of a stimulus as unpleasant....[P]ain is fundamentally a psychological construct that may exist even in the absence of physical stimuli....Because pain is a psychological construct with emotional content, the experience of pain is modulated by changing emotional input and may need to be learned through life experience....[T]he psychological nature of pain presupposes the presence of functional thalamocortical circuitry required for conscious perception. (p. 948)

Thalamocortical pathways judged to be necessary for the conscious perception of pain appear and become functional at about 29 to 30 weeks' gestational age. Therefore, Lee et al hypothesize that conscious perception of pain does not begin before the third trimester.

Burgess and Tawia (1996) explored the beginnings of human consciousness and concluded that "the fetus become conscious at 30 to 35 weeks after conception" (p. 1). They defined consciousness, as experienced in adults, as "a multi-dimensional continuous stream of events and states of which the subject is (more or less) aware"

(p. 4). However, they note that sensation precedes conceptualized thought and emotions, as well as consciously object-direct feelings and emotions, and therefore limit the conscious experiences of the fetus to those having only sensational (sensory) content. In carefully tracking the development of a functional nervous system they speak of it as an evolution rather than birth. The latter term would suggest a sudden emergence rather than a gradual development. They consider the capacity to experience pain and suffering as a minimal prerequisite to being considered sentient.

Lowery et al (2007) expressed concern over requiring functional thalamocortical cortical connections and activation as a criterion for pain and consciousness. They fear that fetal reactions to noxious stimuli will garner less concern if they are thought to be lacking any conscious awareness. They note that the stress response (activation of the hypothalamus–pituitary–adrenal [HPA] axis) is often interpreted as a sign of pain. However, activation of the HPA axis does not require cortical activation and has been observed prior to the maturation of thalamocortical connections, which customarily occurs at 24 weeks, although other connections to the subplate neurons do exist. Developmentally, the thalamus emerges much earlier than the sensory cortex in the fetus. Consistent with Craig's (2003a,b) notion of pain as a homeostatic emotion, in which the thalamus plays a central role, Lowery et al argue against the necessity of functional cortical, in particular sensory cortex, activity to the experience of pain.

However, regardless of whether or not one accepts the response of the pre-30- to 35-week-old fetus to a noxious stimulus as a proxy for a conscious experience, repeated activation of the stress response can produce permanent changes in the system. Lowery et al (2007) state:

Strong and recurring stimuli may result in the formation of abnormal synapses; once formed, these aberrant connections may remain and result in hyperactive responses to stimuli. The plasticity of the developing brain can lead to an alteration of the pain response center, which may make these infants at risk for stress disorders and anxiety-mediated adult behavior. (p. 280).

These data also illustrate that the human organism functions as a complex adaptive system almost from conception.

Derbyshire (1999) rejects the notion of pain as a physical sensation resulting from a noxious stimulus or disease, describing it as "a conscious experience which may be modulated by mental, emotional and sensory mechanisms and includes both sensory and emotional components" (p. 4). Furthermore, he feels the "conscious appreciation of pain" cannot be explained by the activation of a pain center but involves a "neuromatrix of regions incorporating structures…which show(s) a plasticity with learning and development….Parallel interacting areas, many of which are in a dynamic relationship with experience, each of which adds a component to the experience of pain but none of which define it in its entirety, make it impossible to infer pain on the basis of a single active 'center'" (p. 15).

Although the 30-week-old fetus may have a well-developed projection system from the periphery to the CNS, Derbyshire notes that the real explosion of events in the cortex occurs from 3 to 6 months postnatally. Thus, despite the presence of the basic connections, it is the subsequent neuronal development that gives rise to a sophisticated nervous system. He further asserts that the identification of neurological and neurohormonal activity and responses is not sufficient to explain

the phenomenological experience of "pain." These phenomena may exist independently of conscious experience.... [T]he key to understanding consciousness lies in the relationship of the individual to the world in which he exists rather than within biology per se. Conceptual and symbolic abilities along with purposive, directed awareness are suggested as the core components of consciousness. Conscious growth is here suggested as being contingent upon biological development within a social world that exchanges thoughts and ideas through common language (in whatever form). (pp. 22, 23)

Relying on the premises put forth by Dennet (1996) in *Kinds of Minds: Towards an Understanding of Consciousness*, Derbyshire (1999) essentially cautions against assuming that the mind of a nonverbal (non-language) organism, human or otherwise, is like that of a verbal organism; adding a language changes things. One must be careful about assuming that the fetus thinks or has thoughts at all. To know this at all would require the fetus to tell us. However, a brain capable of doing so could no longer be considered the brain of a fetus.

Conceptual abilities, symbolic abilities, and purposive directed awareness are given as the core components of consciousness. The growth of consciousness is seen as contingent upon "biological development within a social world," or biosociohistorical. This notion ties consciousness to biology and would seem to eliminate the possibility of a conscious machine, no matter the degree of complexity or sophistication. As consciousness emerges it forces our instinctual, biological reflexes into submission and thus reaches beyond biological determinism.

Derbyshire supports Greenfield's (1996) theory of consciousness in which he equates it to "a dimmer switch, gradually moving from fully off to fully on." Figure 13.1 presents the model formed from combining Leventhal and Scherer's (1987) theory of how pain development is associated with child development with that of Greenfield. Leventhal and Scherer suggest that "pain is elaborated through the development of innate expressive-motor mechanisms into schematic processing and finishing with a conscious abstract conceptual system" (p. 26). The transitioning from one level to another occurs in the context of increased complexification. Obviously, the system continues to develop and expand consistent with its experiences and learning beyond the 40 months shown in the figure.

THEORIES OF CONSCIOUSNESS

Theories of consciousness can be conveniently divided into neurobiological, informational processing, and social. Some adhere to the concept of functionalism (mental states are logically linked to behavior, but they are not reducible to it), others to representationalism (accounting for a conscious state's phenomenal character in terms of its representational content). The interested reader is referred to summaries by Zeman (2001), Kriegel (2006), and Block (2009). This chapter will sample theories from a number of different perspectives, including neurobiological, systems theory, and quantum theory. Special attention will be given to the dynamic core hypothesis (DCH) of Tononi and Edelman (1998), as it closely approximates the ongoing emphasis on the role of complexity.

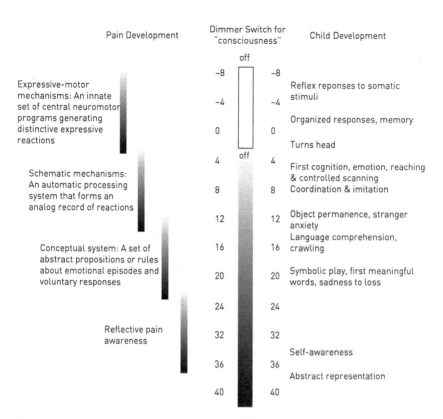

Pain Development	Dimmer Switch for "consciousness"	Child Development

off

Expressive-motor mechanisms: An innate set of central neuromotor programs generating distinctive expressive reactions

-8   -8
-4   -4   Reflex reponses to somatic stimuli
0   0   Organized responses, memory
off
4   4   Turns head

Schematic mechanisms: An automatic processing system that forms an analog record of reactions

4   4   First cognition, emotion, reaching & controlled scanning
8   8   Coordination & imitation
12   12   Object permanence, stranger anxiety

Conceptual system: A set of abstract propositions or rules about emotional episodes and voluntary responses

16   16   Language comprehension, crawling
20   20   Symbolic play, first meaningful words, sadness to loss
24   24

Reflective pain awareness

32   32
36   36   Self-awareness
40   40   Abstract representation

FIGURE 13.1

The dimmer switch, shown on the left, is the hierarchical development of pain as described by Leventhal (1984). Expressive-motor and schematic mechanisms are both considered preconscious, however, the main consciousness switch is activated from 4 months of age. On the right is the corresponding cognitive development deemed necessary for the increasing complexity of Leventhal's pain hierarchy. The numbers represent age in months; the first "off" is conception and "0" is birth. From Derbyshire SWG. Locating the beginnings of pain. *Bioethics*. 1999;13(1):26. Reprinted with permission.

Any discussion of pain and consciousness requires mention of the contributions of René Descartes (1596–1650). Descartes is thought by many to be the father of modern philosophy and analytical geometry. He rejected the Aristotelian reliance on sensation as the source of knowledge, and the emphasis on final cause as a scientific explanation. He favored a more modern mechanistic model. In *Passions of the Soul* (1649) and *The Description of the Human Body* (1648), Descartes described the human as working much like a machine and thus following the physical laws. The mind or soul were nonmaterial in nature and thus not subject to these physical laws. The body and the mind were said to interact in the pineal gland. Although he agreed with his predecessors that the rational mind controlled the body, Descartes also noted that the body could influence the mind, as in the case when one acts in response to heightened emotions. Furthermore, Descartes identified the mind with consciousness and self-awareness, whereas the brain was thought of as the seat of intelligence. This apparent mind–body or Cartesian (*Cartesius* is Latin for Descartes) dualism influenced thinkers into the 21st century.

Descartes may be best known for his statement, "Cogito ergo sum"—translated "I think, therefore I am," or "I am thinking, therefore I exist." Thoughts exist and cannot be separated from the thinker and are thus the one thing that ensures that we, in fact, do exist. Information provided via the senses can be unreliable. Thinking was considered to be the essence of being human, and thought for Descartes is defined by what one is conscious of. Descartes drew a very definite distinction between the outer world and the inner world of the mind, which formed the basis of the principle of Cartesian dualism. Although he recognized that animals, like humans, have a pineal gland, he believed that only humans possessed a mind. Therefore, animals could not feel pain. Thus, he linked pain to the concept of mind.

Quantum Mind Theories

The theory of relativity and quantum theory were developed in the early 1900s. A strict mechanical view of nature, the objectivity of the scientist, and the theory-making process were questioned. It became apparent that in order to understand events at the atomic, subatomic, and cosmological level, the existing mechanical paradigm had to be abandoned and replaced with one that emphasized interconnectedness and wholeness. Like Einstein's theory of relativity, quantum physics saw the universe as a single gigantic field of energy in which matter is merely a form of slowed-down energy. Quantum physics, however, transcends Einstein's theory by describing the universe as an undivided whole which is in a perpetual state of dynamic flux. Rather than matter and energy existing in definite places at a given time, they were discovered to show tendencies to exist. Key concepts in quantum theory include the observer effect, the uncertainty principle, nonlocality, entanglement, and coherence (see Chapter 1).

The principle of nonlocality asserts that events on one side of the universe can instantly affect matter on the other side of the universe. Nonlocality is said to be a fact of nature. The universe contains nonlocal connections (once two particles have interacted they will continue to interact; their wave functions are entangled forever). Hebb's cell assemblies, Tononi and Edelman's functional clusters (see later discussion) and the notion of synchronization may be examples of cortical events that manifest nonlocality. It appears difficult to explain how two particles separated by half a universe (or areas of the brain separated by cortical tissue) can be viewed as connected such that they interact as though they were right on top of each other. Using a computer simulation as an analogy, the question becomes, "How can two pictures at the far corners of the screen be viewed as connected such that the distance between them is irrelevant?" And, in fact, the measured distance between any two pixels (dots) on the computer monitor's display turns out to be entirely irrelevant, since both are merely the products of calculations carried out in the bowels of the computer as directed by the programming.

It was only natural that quantum theory would find its way into explorations of brain functions including the mind and consciousness. In 1997, Mae-Wan Ho published her notion of quantum theory and consciousness, which she felt rested on the concept of quantum coherence. Ho believed there was a need for a conceptual framework for understanding how the organism functions as an "integrated whole…where global and local are mutually entangled, and every part is as much in control as it is sensitive and responsive." In particular, the brain and its functions were viewed as a coherent whole, and not a collection of cells, separate circuits, and structures, similar to Tononi and Edelmen's (1998) dynamic core hypothesis (discussed later in this chapter). Likewise, the functioning of the brain as a coherent whole cannot be separated from the functioning of the body as a coherent whole. In the ideal, the organism is a quantum superposition of coherent activities, with instantaneous (nonlocal), noiseless intercommunication throughout the system. The primary function of the brain may well involve the mediation of "coherent coupling of all subsystems." Therefore, the more highly differentiated and complex the subsystems are, the larger the brain is.

Ho proposed the existence of a body-consciousness, thought to precede the nervous system in evolution. This body-consciousness functions in tandem with, yet is independent from, the brain-consciousness (the nervous system). The body-consciousness is considered to be the basis of sentience—the prerequisite for conscious experience that involves the intercommunicating whole. Instantaneous coordination of body functions is mediated, not by the nervous system, but by the body-consciousness. For example, if one examines brain activity during locomotion, the patterns of activity in the motor centers of the brain are coordinated with those of the limbs. "The reason macroscopic organs such as the four limbs can be coordinated is that each is individually a coherent whole, so that a definite phase relationship can be maintained among them" (Ho, 1997, p. 268).

The extraordinary hand–eye coordination of an accomplished pianist provides a second example. Ho asserts the need for some inherent coherence of participating subsystems enabling instantaneous intercommunication. She notes that there is insufficient time for information to be sent to the brain, integrated, and coordinated, with the outputs being sent back to the hands. Consciousness is said to be distributed throughout the entire body. Therefore, brain-consciousness is embedded in body-consciousness, and brain- and body-consciousness mutually inform and condition each other.

Ho further believes that we perceive ourselves as a singular "I" intuitively, despite the extremely diverse multiplicity of tissues, cells, and molecules constituting our being.

Quantum coherence entails a plurality that is singular, a multiplicity that is a unity. The "self" is the domain of coherence, a pure state or pure duration that permeates the whole of our being. It is because we perceive ourselves as a singular whole that we perceive the real world as colour, sound, texture and smell, as a unity all at once. Sounds presented in linear sequences are recognized as speech or music, much as objects in motion are recognized as such, rather than as disconnected configurations of light and shadow. (Ho, 1997, p. 269)

As Ho puts it, there is a grandmother cell that integrates these separate features. Several studies have revealed that oscillations in brain activity to be simultaneous, uniform, and coherent (see Chapter 4). These oscillations occur in separate areas of the brain and are synchronous in phase and frequency. The absence of a common source for these synchronized oscillations implicates that coherence already exists. If so, then a "genuine nonlocal simultaneity may be involved"; apparent communication is instantaneous, and synchrony can be established with no delay.

For Ho, it seems clear that quantum coherent systems can bind and segment simultaneously and nonlocally. Circulation, metabolism, and muscular and nervous activities go on simultaneously and independently, yet cohere into a whole. A multitude of bound and segmented simultaneities are created in the act of experiencing, which define the here and now. These simultaneities are nonlocal and heterogeneous.

Systems Theory Approach

Chapman (Chapman and Nakamura, 1999a,b) does not define consciousness but shows the relationship between nonconscious process, awareness, and pain within a systems theory approach. Chapman describes pain as a conscious-dependent phenomenon (Chapman and Nakamura, 1999a). He feels that to the extent that consciousness is considered an emergent property of brain activity, pain may also be an emergent property of brain activity. *Emergence* in this context means that combining elements (sensory, affective, cognitive) at a given level of a complex system produces an outcome whose properties are not found in the individual elements and could not be wholly predicted on the basis of knowledge of the individual elements. The emergent phenomenon does not exist in any of the component parts. That is, simply having information regarding transduction, transmission, modulation, and perception relating to nociceptive impulses would not be adequate to predict the resultant pain. Chapman and Nakamura suggest that the neural systems involved in nociception and pain perception, and the cognitive processes resulting in flexible behavior, probably evolved as an interactive dynamic system within the central nervous system.

Chapman rejects the notion of pain perception in humans as a type of reflexive response. Rather than being a passive recipient and respondent to sensory (nociceptive) input, the central nervous system, in particular the brain, is an active participant in the organization and interpretation of the incoming neural information. Nociception occasions arousal in the subcortical autonomic nervous system. This reaction is seen as critical in creating the psychological experience of pain. Furthermore, this system is not a functionally separate entity in humans. Rather, it is part of a complex system characterized by multiple and complicated communication patterns: "Human brains are complex, dynamical systems that exist in relationships of continuous adaptation to the bodies they inhabit, the external environment, and other brains. They exhibit autopoiesis and have as a feature an observer" (Chapman and Nakamura, 1999a, p. 115).

For Chapman, a system is represented by a group of interacting parts that function as a whole and is distinguishable from its surroundings by recognizable boundaries. Dynamical systems are deterministic in that their behavior at one point in time is related in some fashion to a previous state. Dynamical systems tend to be nonlinear and are often characterized by sudden or abrupt transitions from one phase (state) to another. Experimentally induced pain in controlled conditions may yield what appears to be a type of linear relationship between the magnitude of the stimulus and intensity of the pain. However, this relationship rarely exists in the clinical setting. There appear to be rapid, unpredictable, and spontaneous changes (phase or state transitions), making chronic pain far different from and not just an extension of acute pain (see Chapter 8). Chronic pain as an extension of acute pain is unintentionally perpetuated when time, customarily 3 to 6 months, is the only or the most distinguishing characteristic.

Self-organization is a property of complex systems and refers to the spontaneous emergence of new forms or order. With self-organization, that there is no external agent that designs, constructs, or maintains the system. Chapman uses sleeping nociceptors, dorsal-horn modulation, and opioid tolerance as examples self-organizing systems. The evidence for self-organization in the brain seems all but overwhelming. Given the ongoing processing and organizing of information and the tendency for small perturbations to result in large consequences, it would seem to fit the description of a nonlinear dynamical system. Incoming nociceptive information appears to unleash a series of complex patterns of processing in which many components of the brain participate simultaneously (nonlocal effect).

The term *autopoietic* is used to refer to any system that renews itself and regulates the renewal process in such a way that its overall structure is preserved. Autopoietic systems are a type of self-organizing system and must produce their own components in addition to conserving their organization. Complex-adaptive systems are open, self-organizing systems that have the added capacity to conserve and process high levels of information. They live, as it were, on the edge of chaos, where the system maintains enough structure to process information but fluctuates enough that new information (in the form of new patterns and structures) is always being created.

At any given point in time, a dynamical system has a state that can be represented by a point in the appropriate state space. Injured tissues have two states—on or off. However, when one considers the large number of neurons, injured and uninjured, the number of possible states expands exponentially. Indeed, Sweedler (Lanni et al, 2012) has pioneered technology that will enable scientists to analyze miniscule amounts of material in a single brain cell. The amounts are referred to as nanoliters and are so small that it would take 335 billion of them to fill a 12-ounce glass. The number of total states existing in one cell is all but incomprehensible.

A *phase transition* is a form of bifurcation, a change from one state to another. This particular kind of bifurcation (precipice), however, is one in which the fundamental properties of the material or system change. Systems tend to move about and transition from a larger to a smaller phase or state space. This smaller space is referred to as an *attractor*. An attractor is a preferred position for the system. It evolves over time in accordance with the dictates of the dynamical system. If disturbed, the system will continue to transition until it arrives at the attractor, where it remains until disturbed again. Some attractors are point-attractors that achieve a state of equilibrium; others are periodic attractors represented by episodic oscillations, and yet others are described as strange attractors. Strange attractors tend to typify chaotic systems

Chapman describes pain schemata which exist as dynamic entities in the brain, not unlike visual and auditory schemata. Schemas are nonconscious patterns of concepts and associations that reflect a person's past experience, as well as expectations for the present and future—"fuzzy, preconscious, and dynamical functional entities (implicit rather than explicit) roughly related to neural network patterns" (Chapman and Nakamura, 1999a, p. 119). Schemas are not discrete brain circuits. They represent a basin of attraction in the state-space of a complex adaptive system. Schemas associate with one another, forming assemblages of schemas. The brain stores images and motor patterns associated with somatosensory and visceral sensory awareness. The brain constantly produces revised drafts of awareness, mixing old with newer sensory, affective, and cognitive representations without particular regard to time (Dennett and Kinsbourne, 1992; multiple-drafts concept). Past and present schemata compete. Schemata emerge from nonconscious processing into awareness. Chaotic brain processes create and organize the knowledge that receptor input shapes. Such processes can never capture the actualities of the matter and energy that impinge on receptors.

Complexity Theory: Dynamic Core Hypothesis (DCH)

Tononi and Edelman (1998) define a *dynamic core* as "a large cluster of neuronal groups that together constitute, on a time scale of hundreds of milliseconds, a unified neural process of high complexity.... The term dynamic core deliberately does not refer to a unique, invariant set of brain areas ... and the core may change in composition over time" (pp. 1849–1850). Rather than a set of neural regions, a dynamic core is a functional interaction involving distributed groups of neurons whose makeup can changes over time. The dynamic core must also have high complexity; its global activity patterns must be selected within less than a second out of a very large repertoire. In a very real sense, the nervous system has the potential to generate consciousness. Therefore, consciousness can be considered to be an emergent phenomenon.

Increased coherence among separated brain regions is associated with awareness of a given event. Weak stimuli are not likely to activate this neural activity to a strength sufficient enough to trigger these rapid, often involving only hundreds of milliseconds, distributed interactions and thus become part of perception without awareness. Attention, however, can enhance the strength of the stimulus, thus facilitating the neural response and corresponding neural interactions. The establishment of synchronous activity among cortical structures and between the thalamus and cortex is referred to functional clustering. The number of states that can occur as a result of the interaction of the neural structures is a reflection of its complexity.

The consciousness experience is seen as both integrated and highly differentiated. Although the distributed neural activity is primarily in the thalamocortical system, consciousness involves activation of widely dispersed brain areas. When the task is novel, the distribution is more widespread than when it is automatic or habitual. Once the stimulus becomes habitual, it evokes neural activity almost exclusively in the sensory pathways and involves little or no consciousness. Indeed, this set of circuits becomes functionally insulated, which enhances speed and precision but at the cost of context sensitivity, flexibility, and accessibility. This is not unlike the distinction between declarative and procedural memory. Declarative memory (aka explicit memory) entails memories taht can be consciously recalled, for example, facts and knowledge. Procedural or nondeclarative memory involves unconscious memories such as skills, for example, learning to ride a bicycle.

The rapid integration of neural groups in the thalamocortical systems is achieved by a process Tononi and Edelman call reentry. Re-entry is

the ongoing, recursive, highly parallel signaling within and among brain areas ... [R]eentry can achieve the rapid integration or "binding" of distributed, functionally specialized neuronal groups, dynamically, that is, in a unified neural process rather than in a single place.... [I]ntegration of distributed neuronal populations through reentrant interactions is required for conscious experience. (Tononi and Edelman, 1998, p. 1847)

The brain is structured in such a fashion that many of the areas of the brain are connected via widespread parallel reciprocal connections (connectivity). The process of reentry involves transmission of signals passing back and forth along these connections. There is no single or fixed feedback loop. In order to account for the enormous variability among individuals in terms of qualities of consciousness, they hypothesize that the patterns or maps generated by populations of neurons must be constantly changing.

The DCH emphasizes rapidly shifting functional interactions and connectivity among distributed neuronal groups, rather than their anatomical proximity. As part of a functional cluster or dynamic core, the participating neuronal groups are much more strongly interactive among themselves than with the rest of the brain. However, the same group of neurons could, at one time, constitute part of the dynamic core and participate in creating a conscious experience and at another time be part of the nonconscious process. In essence, the dynamic core is a process and not a thing or a location. As an example, Tononi and Edelman note the quality of red to be a state of the dynamic core incorporating input from several cortical structures involving sensory areas, internal bodily states, past experience, and areas signaling the significance of the experience. A key notion of the DCH is that consciousness is generated by a neural process and cannot, therefore, be characterized as a specific thing or in a particular location. Furthermore, it cannot be understood or explained by an analysis of the structure and function of its individual constituent parts.

Neurophysiological Theories

Some neuroscientists believe that the material basis of consciousness can be clarified without recourse to new properties of matter or to quantum physics. Consciousness is viewed as a subjective experience, awareness, wakefulness, or the executive control system of the mind. Data extrapolated from brain-imaging studies, attention and working memory studies, the neuropsychological functioning of brain-injured patients, and awareness–unawareness dissociation research, among others, have formed the basis of these theories. The formation of a type of neural assembly is considered to be the fundamental mechanisms of consciousness.

Casey (1999), for example, states that "the neural mechanism of pain, as experienced in the normal conscious human, can ultimately be understood in physical, mechanistic terms" (p. 125). He subscribes to William James' notion that "consciousness is the personal and private experience that accompanies the act of distinguishing self from non-self"—"self-awareness" (Casey, 1999, p. 125). A prerequisite for achieving consciousness is a brain in a aroused state as defined by low-voltage and high-frequency activity: "The aroused state establishes the potential for using sensory and motor information to achieve consciousness" (Casey, 1999, p. 125). In some cases, as with locked-in patients, the issue may be one of communication rather than consciousness. Casey notes the presence of a withdrawal response resembling aversion to a particular stimulus without the usual affective response, as well as the occurrence of expressions of painful grimacing and vocalization without any withdrawal behavior in patients recovering from a large hemispheric stroke. This suggests that at some level of impaired consciousness and arousal a nociceptive stimulus can evoke an unpleasant experience. This may be some primitive fear response mediated by subcortical mechanisms. Because it is possible for pain to be absent in the fully conscious human and for a pain-like aversive experience to occur in states of grossly impaired consciousness, Casey claims that the two phenomena, pain and consciousness, are likely to have different neural mechanisms.

James-Lange Theory

Antonio Damasio (1994) and A.D. Craig (2009a) have outlined differing theories regarding consciousness and pain. Both Damasio and Craig drew on the often overlooked James-Lange theory of emotions. Working independently, in the 19th century, psychologist William James and neurologist Carl Lange proposed similar theories of emotion. The two theories were eventually combined into the James-Lange theory of emotion. The role of and interaction among cortical structures, physiological responses, and cognitive awareness and interpretation are main features of their theory. Previously, and consistent with a common-sense notion, conscious-emotional experience was thought to be the trigger for emotional responses; for example, you fear bears, therefore, your heart starts to pound when you see one, and you run. James and Lange, however, reasoned that an emotional eliciting event must first be perceived by the sensory portion of the brain. Next, the autonomic nervous system stimulates a variety of motor and physiological responses (muscular tension, increased heart rate, increased perspiration, and dryness of the mouth) driven by certain output areas of the brain, based on predispositions and learning. Finally, there is a behavioral response.

For example, consider being suddenly confronted with a rattle snake, large black bear, a loud crash, or a physical assault. By virtue of one's disposition and learning history, these events are known to be frightening. Chemicals such as adrenaline surge into the body, causing a myriad of physiological reactions, including increased heart rate and muscles tension. The James-Lange theory postulates that the brain will recognize, albeit at a nonconscious level, these physiological changes as ones that happen in response to a frightening (threatening) event and consequently will activate, at the conscious level, the emotion we know as fear or fright. This notion is not as far-fetched as it may seem when considering that the sound of someone snapping their fingers is processed more rapidly than the visual stimuli, yet the two are perceived as occurring simultaneously.

The emotion, then, is the becoming aware of, or the feeling of, bodily changes that follow the perception of an exciting event. Thus, fleeing from the bear is not caused by fear. Rather, fear is a consequence of running away. As stated by James:

> My theory . . . is that the bodily changes follow directly the perception of the exciting fact, and that our feeling of the same changes as they occur is the emotion. Common sense says, we lose our fortune, are sorry and weep; we meet a bear, are frightened and run; we are insulted by a rival, are angry and strike. The hypothesis here to be defended says that this order of sequence is incorrect . . . and that the more rational statement is that we feel sorry because we cry, angry because we strike, afraid because we tremble. . . . Without the bodily states following on the perception, the latter would be purely cognitive in form, pale, colorless, destitute of emotional warmth. We might then see the bear, and judge it best to run, receive the insult and deem it right to strike, but we should not actually feel afraid or angry. (quoted in Ellsworth, 1994, p. 224)

To many the theory seemed then, and still does to this day, counterintuitive. However, evidence shows that when the thalamus is stimulated by high-frequency stimuli, sensory detection without awareness occurs within 150 ms, yet it requires some 500 ms for the production of a conscious sensory experience. Furthermore, a single conscious decision requires a few hundreds of milliseconds, referred to as the "psychological refractory period" by Pashler (1994). These types of observations have given the James-Lange theory new vitality.

For James, attention is the sentry at the gate of consciousness, and consciousness involves the entire brain. He noted that one's experience is what one agrees to attend to. Consciousness is not a thing or a place but a process or stream that is changing on a time scale of fractions of seconds. This stream of consciousness is highly unified and integrated (Tononi and Edelman, 1998). Most of the neurophysiological theories work from the premise that the neural correlates of consciousness will prove to be a neuronal cell-assembly of some kind. Hebb defined the cell assembly as "a diffuse structure comprising cell in the cortex and diencephalon...capable of acting as a closed system, delivering facilitation to other such systems" (Hebb, 1949; quoted in Zeman, 2001, p. 1279).

Damasio's Theory

The relationship between sensory, perception, autonomic reactions, awareness/feeling, and emotion as presented in the James-Lange theory is central to the contemporary neurophysiological theories of Damasio and Craig relating to pain, self-awareness, and consciousness. Damasio used the visual system as a model for his theory. In short, he noted that external environmental stimuli cause the activation of a pattern of retinal receptive cell activity. These patterns are processed serially and in parallel in the brain. The processing of these patterns results in the extracting of the visual aspects of our environment that we perceive. Likewise, he noted there to be patterns of nerve-cell activity in the brain, which he refers to as *cognitive representations*, that correspond to patterns in the external world.

He reasoned that, in the same way that our sense of vision, hearing, touch, taste, and smell (nociception could have easily been included in this list) operate by activating patterns of nerve-cell activity in the brain representing the state of the external world, emotions are nerve-cell activation patterns representing the state of our internal world. Therefore, when we feel fear (threat), the brain records this as a body state (phase state in systems theory) represented by a particular nerve-cell activation pattern derived via feedback from other neural and hormonal systems. If, for example, upon engaging a situation perceived as threatening (pain), based on previous experiences, the internal environment immediately changes. Activation of the sympathetic nervous system results in muscular and hormonal changes, creating a body state corresponding to the emotion we recognize as fear (threat), and activation of certain nerve-cell patterns in the brain.

Thus, emotions are viewed as cognitive representations of body states. These body states are part of a homeostatic mechanism by which the internal world is monitored and controlled, and by which this internal world influences the behavior of the whole organism. They are a product of input to the brain from the internal body environment, just as olfactory, auditory, or visual information is a product of inputs to the brain from the external environment. The brain, in a sense, functions as an organ for homeostasis—collecting, collating, and providing feedback on body states for the purpose of maintaining consistency in the internal world.

In the process of interacting with the external world, events and stimuli associated with positive (pleasant) or negative (unpleasant) consequences are encountered. An association is thus created between the event and a particular physiological affective state. For example, situations associated with damage or injury (pain) to our person become linked to a physiological state, which includes increased blood pressure, flushing, increased heart rate (fear). These types of associations are stored, probably in the ventromedial prefrontal cortex (VMPFC), as somatic markers. These somatic markers are reinstated when encountering the same or similar events in the future and thus are capable of influencing decision-making processes regarding the manner in which the event is responded to—for example, approach or avoid, fight or flight. In the case of a very complex situation involving multiple and perhaps ambiguous or unfamiliar stimuli (pain associated with a reward), somatic markers from all previous encounters are summed to produce a net somatic state that guides or biases our actions. This processing may occur consciously or nonconsciously (without awareness or in the cognitive unconscious; Kihlstrom, 1987), yielding what is frequently called a gut reaction. Occasionally, these somatic makers direct us away from the most detrimental or unfavorable actions, thereby simplifying the decision-making process. The amygdala, orbitofrontal cortex (OFC), orbitomedial (OM), and VMPFC appear to be involved in the establishment, processing, storage, and retrieval of these somatic markers.

Exposure to a dangerous or potentially punishing (aversive, noxious, painful) situation is usually associated with heightened arousal and increased sympathetic nervous system activity. The latter can be measured by changes in the galvanic skin or sweet response. The neurologically intact person quickly learns to avoid potentially dangerous and threatening situations ("Fool me once, shame on you; fool me twice shame of me"). The planning of future action requires two events. The brain needs to create a cognitive representation containing (a) the external perceptual information (the dangerous or threatening event) and (b) the internal emotional information (fear or apprehension). Those with certain types of brain injury do not appear to profit from experience. Patients with OFC damage or dysfunction do not show the customary physiological changes and will often perseverate on an unfavorable response, appearing not to learn from their experience. Likewise, patients with pain asymboli respond with indifference to nociceptive input that would otherwise produce painful reaction. This apparent ambivalence is due in part to the absence of any somatic marker cueing the presence of a harmful stimulus, thus prompting a corrective, or homeostatically oriented, response.

The somatic marker mechanism (SMM) is the manner in which the cognitive representations of the internal world interact with those of the external world (where perceptions interact with emotions). Unlike animals, which clearly show an awareness of the external environment, humans also have an awareness of "self" which forms the basis for consciousness. Damasio sees consciousness as the awareness of the somatic milieu or inner states. This awareness allows for the use these somatic states, such as emotions, to mark and thus evaluate perceptual information from the external world. It is thought that the interaction of these various cognitive representations occurs in the working memory, believed to be localized in the dorsolateral prefrontal cortex (DLPF). Ironically, this is one of the areas of the brain reportedly affected, at least in terms of volume, in patients with chronic pain (see Chapter 4).

The self is viewed as a process rather than a thing, for which there is a neural basis that involves the neural mapping of one's own body. Some parts of the brain are free to roam and respond to the external world, as occurs when we are distracted or willingly turn our attention from one event to another and back again. Other structures are designated to monitor the structure and internal state(s) and thus map only the internal body. This then, represents the source of the "continuous being" and, as such, anchors the mental self (Damasio, 2003, p. 227). The neural machinery, as Damasio puts it, necessary for this function includes pathways that transmit information about the internal status of the organism to various structures in the brain. Within the brain there are dedicated pathways that pass on this body-related information to areas in the thalamus and insular cortex (IC). The information is then integrated, generating composite and dynamic moment-to-moment maps of the body's state. Continuous updating of these maps is required for the brain to regulate life.

In Damasio's somatic marker theory of consciousness, the subjective process of feeling emotion requires the involvement of the same areas of the brain that participate in homeostasis (self-regulation). These areas, especially the anterior insular cotex (AIC), continuously map and regulate our ever-changing internal states. These internal feelings direct our quality-of-life- and survival-related behaviors. These feelings also produce what he refers to as a "perceptual landscape," which "represents the emotional significance of specific stimuli being experienced or of a future action by means of a further 'as-if-body-loop' mechanism" (Craig, 2002, p. 663). These feelings also discriminate the outer-world (exteroceptive) from inner-world (interoceptive) events, "allowing the brain" to create a "meta-representational model" of the relationship between the two worlds. The representational image of the body's state enables a distinction between self and non-self. The re-representations of this image provide a basis for projecting the consequences of possible actions and interactions with other outer-world events onto the state of the body. The degrees of conscious awareness, according to Damasio, are products of upgrades in the self-representational maps that occur as a result of our ongoing interactions and experiences.

Craig's Model of Consciousness

Craig's (2003a) model of pain and its portrayal as a homeostatic emotion was discussed earlier (Chapter 5). To summarize, Craig noted that in nonhumans the ascending lamina I input is integrated in several brainstem sites. However, there is a direct thalamocortical homeostatic afferent pathway to the IC in humans. Subjective emotions, in addition to other sensations, including sadness, disgust, anger, anticipated anxiety, pain, panic, sexual arousal, gut reactions, trustworthiness, and positive and negative emotional responses to music, are each associated with activation of the IC. The middle and right (nondominant) AIC are identified as the location for this interoceptive cortical image, which provides a meta-representation of the state of the body by incorporating all emotionally salient inputs from all sensory modalities as well as from subcortical homeostatic control regions (hypothalamus and amygdala). This interoceptive cortical image constitutes a basic emotional state, which Craig likens to Damasio's somatic marker, and is thought to be crucial to the motivation to make appropriate decisions that affect our survival and quality of life. The right and left anterior insula are considered to be crucial components of a network that engenders human awareness.

Craig (2009b) proposes that the left and right AIC interact in an opponent fashion: the right AIC subserves sympathetic, energy-consuming emotions and negative feelings, while the left AIC subserves parasympathetic, energy-enriching emotions and positive feelings. The left AIC is predominantly involved in monitoring, rather than generating, behaviors. The right side tends to lead and the left side to follow. Normally, both sides are coactivated, suggesting an opponent process. Thus, there may be a neural basis for one feeling "of two minds" when considering a complex situation. Importantly, a remapping of the interoceptive cortex in the right AIC of humans appears to be linked to the emotional awareness of the "material me." This self-awareness (consciousness) is based on a mental image of the homeostatic condition of the body, or as Craig puts it, "how you feel."

Craig suggests that the AIC contains a representation of the "self" at each moment in time and acts as a comparator between these points in time. He also suggests that this may be interpreted phenomenologically as the "Cartesian theatre" and that the role of the AIC in predictions may explain the effect that emotions such as anxiety might have on predictions. Craig hypothesizes the existence progressively more sophisticated processing from the posterior insular cortex (PIC) through to the AIC, the latter being the phylogenetically most recent area. Furthermore, he proposes the existence of a meta-representation of a global-emotional moment near the junction of the frontal operculum and the AIC, where a subjective awareness of self is generated and is able to compare feelings of the past, present, and future.

Activation of the AIC is seen in tests where the organism recognizes an image of itself. Studies involving the "feeling of knowing," which is the level of the individual's confidence in his or her ability to recall certain information, have identified activation in the AIC, ACC, and inferior frontal gyrus correlating with the subjects' degree of confidence (intensity of feelings). Time perception and mental-durational tasks have also been found to involve coactivation of the AIC and ACC.

In addition to the AIC forming the basis for subjective awareness, it, in combination with the ACC, forms a volitional agency. This volitional agency allows for the discretionary switching of cognitive processing types, such as between object-oriented and self-reflective. It has been proposed that the unique population of von Economo or spindle neurons found in the AIC and ACC functions to enhance the communication between these two areas. Furthermore, the largest concentration of these neurons is found in humans, with lesser amounts in gorillas and chimps, respectively, once again, supporting the uniqueness of humans. Finally, lesions in the AIC have been associated with various psychological and dissociative disorders.

A key feature of Craig's theory is the concept of a global-emotional moment. A global-emotional moment is defined as "the realization of a coherent representation of all salient conditions across all relevant systems at each immediate moment of time" and is considered as the sentient self at each moment of time. The AIC incorporates all the emotionally salient activity from other limbic cortical regions (ACC, OFC), as well as cortical regions involved in contextual planning such as the dorsolateral prefrontal cortex. The ability of the human IC to generate sequential re-representations provides a foundation for the integration of the homeostatic condition of the body with the sensory environment, the internal autonomic state, motivational, and social conditions. This unified representation of all salient conditions, encoded as "feelings," is in effect a representation of the entirety of the individual, or Craig's "the sentient self"; Sherrington's (1953) "the material me," and Damasio's "neural self." The essential ingredient of this model of a sentient self is the neural construct for a feeling, which represents a homeostatic sensory condition in the body that guides energy utilization or energy acquisition.

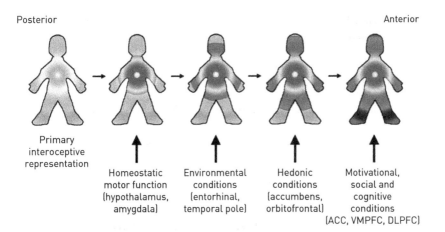

Primary
interoceptive
representation

| Homeostatic motor function (hypothalamus, amygdala) | Environmental conditions (entorhinal, temporal pole) | Hedonic conditions (accumbens, orbitofrontal) | Motivational, social and cognitive conditions (ACC, VMPFC, DLPFC) |

FIGURE 13.2

This view (of consciousness) suggests that the representation of all possible feelings in elements that one refers to as "global emotional moments" in the anterior insula depends on a functional ability to shift interconnections hierarchically with all cortical networks at each moment. In this model, feelings represent not only the state of the body and the environment but also the state of the brain, which includes in particular the activity of the motivational agent or agents that one suggests are represented in the anterior cingulate. If the anterior insula can represent the activity of the controllers, then the illusion that such feelings actually cause the behavior could easily be instantiated by the near-simultaneity of the action and the feeling. ACC, anterior cingulate cortex; DLPFC, dorsolateral prefrontal cortex; VMPFC, ventromedial prefrontal cortex. From Craig AD. Emotional moments across time: a possible neural basis for time perception in the anterior insula. *Philos Trans R Soc Ser B Biol.* 2009;364:1933-1942. Reprinted with permission.

Craig believes feelings to be the common currency of awareness (consciousness). Other salient features of a particular event are incorporated via interaction with other cortical structures, including temporal poles, nucleus accumbens, orbitofrontal cortex, ventromedial cortex, dorsolateral cortex, and the anterior cingulate cortex. (Figure 13.2) A global-emotional moment is formed in the AIC and is the holistic representation of the totality of all the feeling for an individual at a precise moment in time. Awareness emerges with the sequencing, updating, and processing of each global-emotional moment in the AIC.

Craig (2009a) proposes a cinemascopic model of awareness or consciousness. The existence of a series of global-emotional moments provides the basis for time-shifting of representations of the sentient self. His view of consciousness is elucidated through his homeostatic model of awareness. Awareness is essentially the continuous mental instantiation of one's own existence. Interoceptive (physiological condition of the tissues of the body) information is transmitted via homeostatic afferents from lamina I of the spinal cord dorsal horn. Information is then carried by spinal thalimocortical pathways to the PIC. These "feelings of the body" are then re-represented sequentially from the posterior to anterior insula in accordance with their behavioral complexity. All feelings, he argues, are related to homeostatic needs and behavioral motivation critical to the maintenance of the body image, and thus are endowed with homeostatic primacy. The interoceptive state of the organism is re-represented cortically and provides "the basis for subjective awareness of the feelings of the body" and thus self-awareness and consciousness (Craig, 2002, p. 657). According to Craig, this meta-representation of the state of the body is associated with subjective awareness of the material self as a feeling (sentient) entity, that is, emotional awareness, consistent with the ideas of James and Damasio.

A Proposed Model of Pain and Consciousness

Given what we have discussed thus far, Figure 13.3 represents a model for conceptualizing the experience of pain.

Presenting the model in this fashion should not be taken to imply that these aspects are linear and always occur in the same sequence. Rather, the model emphasizes that nociceptive input, from the periphery or internal organs, is certainly sufficient for the experience of pain, but not necessary. The patients described by Melzack et al (1997) with phantom pain in a congenitally absent limb represent one example of pain in the absence of activation of peripheral nociceptors. In addition, psychological processes such hypnosis, and mood states (depression) have been found to stimulate the experience of pain. In the presence of nociceptive input the system must recognize, attend to, or be consciousness, although processing of this input is likely to be at a nonconscious level.

This nonconscious processing may be part of what Raichle (2010) refers to as the brain's "dark energy." This "dark energy" represents part of the brain's intrinsic activity (ongoing neural and metabolic activity that is not directly associated with subjects' performance of a task) and is reflected in slow cortical potentials (SCPs), which can be found in the default mode network. He suggests that "these signals coordinate access that each brain system requires to the vast storehouse of memories and other information needed for survival in a complex, ever-changing world. The SCPs ensure that the right computations occur in a coordinated fashion at exactly the correct moment" (p. 48).

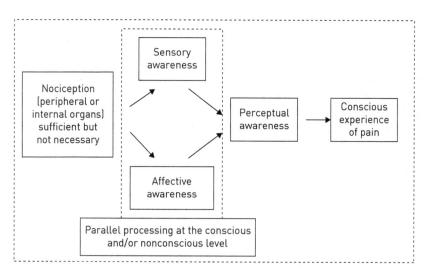

FIGURE 13.3

Oversimplified version of a developing model for conceptualizing the processing of pain. The figure illustrates the essential components of the model. There no doubt will ultimately be multiple systems and subsystems nested under each component. The systems and subsystems would form networks that would interact and interconnect. Communication may be carried out at the cellular level via microtubules, consistent with Stuart Hameroff's theory (Frank, 1998). The connectionist view of memory and processing, distrusted over the concept of modules and their networks, is adopted here.

Another approach to this intrinsic activity in the brain is Friston's (2010, 2012) notion of "free energy." Indeed, he presents his free-energy model as a unified brain theory. Free energy can be thought of as the amount of prediction error that occurs following the application of the brain's hierarchical models to predict sensory input. Neuronal activity, including synaptic connections, tries to minimize this prediction error (free energy). Free energy is thus a measure of "surprise" or uncertainty. The free-energy principle states that systems change to decrease their free energy: the more precise the processing, the more accurate the predictions, and the less uncertainty (free energy) there is. Any adaptive changes in the brain are thought to minimize "free energy." The less this free energy, the more recalcitrant the system is to any tendency toward disorder.

Krahé et al (2013) used a "free-energy framework" to account for socially mediated pain. A key aspect of their theory is that

the perception of salient interpersonal interactions may enhance the precision of predictive signals regarding the salience of a noxious stimulus in a given environment, thus ultimately affecting the perceptual and active inferential processes that lead to pain perception and related motivated actions. Specifically, interpersonal exchanges affect precision or salience by socially signaling the safety or threat of the impending stimulus itself or the environment in which the stimulus occurs. (p. 17)

Thus, there is parallel as well as hierarchical processing of information from the environment (sensory input) and interpersonal and social (affective) context. As regards the present discussion, this free-energy model is yet another approach to understanding the complex and dynamic nature of the nonconscious processing of affective and sensory information which precedes any perceptual awareness or experience of pain. Also, there is the recurrent emphasis on the importance of salience (see discussion of threat detection system in Chapter 11).

The meaning, aversiveness, and threatening nature (salience) of the stimulus to the self are all part of "affective awareness." Patients with pain asymbolia or certain types of neurological injuries or deficits, and those having had a cingulotomy, may express an awareness of the sensory input but do not demonstrate the emotional, physiological, and behavioral characteristics that define chronic pain. Fitzgibbon et al's (2012) notion of mirror-pain synesthesia (see Chapter 11) resulting in enhanced activity in the otherwise normal and nonconscious somatosensory mirror system lends support to the supposition of significant nonconscious processing of affective and sensory information. The implication, of course, is that in the absence of an affective (emotional) response, sensory input, including that involving the peripheral nociceptive system, would not be considered as "pain" any more than seeing a picture or hearing a sound would be considered as pain.

Finally, perceptual awareness (akin to the observer effect) reflects the highest level of consciousness wherein the patient is clearly responding to, demonstrating, and reporting the emotional, physiological, and behavioral features of the experience of pain. In this sense, pain, especially in the chronic setting, is an emergent phenomenon. The complex adaptive system (the brain) continuously re-represents the state of the organism. There is continual transitioning from one phase state to another, not unlike as in Chapman and Nakamura's model. A type of bifurcation can occur such that a system can no longer return to a previous state. The analogy might be that of a fork in the road vs. a precipice: one can choose to go left or right at the fork. If nonproductive, one can return to the fork and choose the other direction. However, when at a precipice, going over the edge may represent a point of no return. There has been a fundamental shift in the system. Clinically this may be seen in a patient whose pain is now recalcitrant to any form of the treatment, as it has embedded itself, as it were, deep into the system.

This notion is similar to Chapman's when he noted that chronic pain was not a single entity. Rather, it is a dynamical entity (system-state, attractor):

In some chronic pain patients large assemblies of interactive neuronal populations can fall into the basin of a low-dimensional strange attractor, creating a stereotypic neuronal activity pattern from which the brain cannot easily escape. This helps to explain how chronic pain, once developed, is difficult of 'undo' by the standard interventions that work well with acute pain. (Chapman and Nakamura, 1999a, p. 118)

Chapman's constructivist (Pfah and Wolters, 1997) view suggests that the brain builds and constantly revises (Craig's global-emotional moment; Damasio's somatic marker mechanism) a dynamical representation of its own reality. It dynamically distributes processing in large-scale networks, probably operating in parallel, and integrates and synthesizes noxious signaling and other products of central processing to construct pain. Signals from injured nerves are only a minor feature of the stream of neuronal signals that reach the brain, yet they are the ones that affect consciousness.

CONCLUSION

It seems ironic that pain appears to require consciousness for its existence, yet depending on its intensity, pain is capable of inducing a state of nonconsciousness or used to arouse one from a reduced state of consciousness (lethargy or stupor). Loeser and Melzack (1999) declared, "It is not the duration of pan that distinguishes acute from chronic pain, but more importantly, the inability of the body to restore its physiological functions to normal homeostatic levels" (p. 1609). Chapman and his colleagues (2008) described pain and a complex interaction among the endocrine, immune, and nervous systems. When combined with Craig's notion of pain in humans as a "homeostatic emotion...represented by the forebrain integration of both specific labeled lines and convergent somatic activity in a well-organized hierarchical system that subserves homeostasis...one aspect of the representation of the physiological condition of the body (interception)" (Craig, 2003b, p. 1), there appears to be a major paradigm shift in the conceptualization of pain. Furthermore, there are aspects of the neuroanatomy and neurophysiology of pain and pain processing that are distinctly human, thus limiting the degree to which animal data may be applicable.

Chalmers (1995) draws a distinction between the easy and hard problems in the study of consciousness. The easy problems relate to how humans discriminate and react to sensory stimuli; how the brain integrates multisensory information; how we can verbalize internal states. The hard problem is how our subjective experience emerges from physical processes. Sir John Eccles (1994) wrote, "We have to recognize that we are spiritual beings with souls existing in a spiritual world as well as material beings with bodies and brains existing in a material world" (p. 241). According to Eccles, we have a nonmaterial mind or self which acts upon, and is influenced by, our material brains; there is a mental world in addition to the physical world, and the two interact.

The foundations of science were laid down by Aristotle, Plato, and Socrates. The principles and methods of science and philosophy were refined by Newton and Descartes. The discoveries and theories of Einstein and Hawking have added a new dimension. Our brains possess the capacity to go beyond mere facts and entertain the possibility of the unimaginable. Although systems theory, complexity theory, and quantum theory may not hold all the answers regarding pain as well as consciousness, strict adherence to a Newtonian physics imposes unnecessary and artificial boundaries. There can be little doubt regarding the potential benefits of expanding the paradigm through which pain is viewed. The ultimate definitions of pain and consciousness are yet to be realized. The nature of the research and theory-building will influence the specifics of the definitions. However, the notion of pain already appears to be taking on the characteristics of a process vs. outcome, a construct vs. an event.

REFERENCES

Anand KJS, Clancy B. Fetal pain? *Pain: Clinical Updates.* 2006;14(2):1–4.

Block N. Comparing the major theories of consciousness. In Gazzaniga MS, ed. *The Cognitive Neurosciences IV.* Cambridge, MA: MIT Press; 2009:1111–1122.

Burgess JA, Tawia SA. When did you first begin to feel it?—Locating the beginning of human consciousness. *Bioethics.* 1996;10(1):1–26.

Casey KL. A neurologist's perspective on pain and consciousness. *Pain Forum.* 1999;8(3): 124–126.

Chalmers D. Facing up to the problems of consciousness. *J Consciousness Studies.* 1995;2(3): 200–219.

Chapman CR, Nakamura Y. Pain and consciousness: a constructivist approach. *Pain Forum.* 1999a;8(3):113–123.

Chapman CR, Nakamura Y. A passion of the soul: an introduction to pain for consciousness researchers. *Conscious Cogn.* 1999b;8:391–422.

Chapman CR, Tuckett RP, Song CW. Pain and stress in a systems perspective: reciprocal neural, endocrine, and immune interactions. *J Pain.* 2008;9(2):122–145.

Craig AD. How do you feel? Interoception: the sense of the physiological condition of the body. *Nat Rev Neurosci.* 2002;3(8):655–666.

Craig AD. A new view of pain as a homeostatic emotion. *Trends Neurosci.* 2003a;26(6):303–307.

Craig AD. Pain mechanisms: labeled lines versus convergence in central processing. *Annu Rev Neurosci.* 2003b;26:1–30.

Craig AD. Emotional moments across time: a possible neural basis for time perception in the anterior insula. *Philos Trans R Soc B.* 2009a;364:1933–1942.

Craig AD. How do you feel—now? The anterior insula and human awareness. *Nat Rev Neurosci.* 2009b;10:59–70.

Damasio AR. *Descartes' Error: Emotion, Reason, and the Human Brain.* New York: Grosset/ Putnam; 1994.

Damasio AR. The person within. *Nature.* 2003;423:227.

Dennett DC. *Kinds of Minds: Towards an Understanding of Consciousness.* New York: Basic Books; 1996.

Dennett DC, Kinsbourne M. Time and the observer: the where and when of consciousness in the brain. *Behav Brain Sci.* 1992;15:183–247.

Derbyshire SWG. Locating the beginnings of pain. *Bioethics.* 1999;13(1):1–31.

Descartes R. *Description du corps humain*. In *Oeuvres de Descartes*. Vol. 11. Paris: J. Vrin; 1648/1896.

Descartes R. *Les passions de l'âme*. Amsterdam: Lodewijk Elsevier; 1649.

Devor M. Avenues to the future of pain research. *e-News for Somatosensory Rehabilitation*. Ronald Melzack special issue. 1999 (June).

Devor M. Consciousness and pain. In Bushnell KC, Basbaum AI, eds. *The Senses: A Comprehensive Reference*. St. Louis: Elsevier; 2008:961–969.

Eccles JC. *How the Self Controls its Brain*. New York: Springer-Verlag; 1994.

Edelman G, Tononi G. *A Universe of Consciousness: How Matter Becomes Imagination*. New York: Basic Books; 2000.

Ellsworth PC. William James and emotion: Is a century of fame worth a century of misunderstanding? *Psychol Rev*. 1994;101(2):222–229.

Fitzgibbon BM, Enticott PG, Rich AN, Giummarra MJ, Georgiou-Karistianis N, Bradshaw JL. Mirror-sensory synaesthesia: exploring "shared" sensory experiences as synaesthesia. *Neurosci Biobehav Rev*. 2012;36(1):645–657.

Frank K. Stuart Hameroff's theories regarding microtubules as the seat of consciousness. *Rolf Lines*. 1998;(Nov):38–40.

Friston K. The free-energy principle: a unified brain theory? *Nat Rev Neurosci*. 2010;11(2):127–138.

Friston K. A free energy principle for biological systems. *Entropy*. 2012;14:2100–2121.

Greenfield SA. *Toward a Science of Consciousness: Journey to the Centers of the Mind*. New York: W.H. Freeman & Company; 1996.

Ho M-W. Quantum coherence and conscious experience. *Kybernetes*. 1997;26(3):265–276.

Kihlstrom JF. Cognitive unconscious. *Science*. 1987;237:1445–1452.

Krahé C, Springer A, Weinman JA, Fotopoulou A. Social modulation of pain: others as predictive signals of salience—a systematic review. *Front Hum Neurosci*. 2013;7 (article 386):1–20.

Kriegel U. Consciousness, theories of. *Philosophy Compass*. 2006;1(1):58–64.

Lanni EJ, Rubakhin SS, Sweedler JV. Mass spectrometry imaging and profiling of single cells. *J Proteomics*. 2012;75:5036–5051.

Lee SJ, Ralston HJP, Drey EA, Partridge JC, Rosen MA. Fetal pain: a systematic multidisciplinary review of the evidence. *JAMA*. 2005;294(8):947–954.

Leventhal H. A perceptual-motor theory of emotion. *Adv Exp Soc Psychol*. 1984;17:117–175.

Leventhal H, Scherer K. The relationship of emotion to cognition: a functional approach to a semantic controversy. *Cogn Emot*. 1987;1:3–28.

Lindahl B. Consciousness and biological evolution. *J Theor Biol*. 1997;187:613–629.

Loeser JD, Melzack R. Pain: an overview. *Lancet*. 1999;53:1607–1609.

Lowery CL, Hardman MP, Manning N, Hall RW, Anand JKS. Neurodevelopmental changes of fetal pain. *Semin Perinatol*. 2007;31:275–282.

Melzack R, Israel R, Lacroix R, Schultz G. Phantom limbs in people with congenital limb deficiency or amputation in early childhood. *Brain*. 1997;120:1603–1620.

Pashler H. Dual-task interference in simple tasks: data and theory. *Psychol Bull*. 1994;116:220–244.

Penfield W, Jasper HH. *Epilepsy and the Functional Anatomy of the Human Brain*. Boston: Little, Brown; 1954.

Phaf RH, Wolters G. A constructivist and connectionist view on conscious and nonconscious processes. *Philos Psychol*. 1997;10(3):287–307.

Raichle ME. Neuroscience: the brain's dark energy. *Sci Am*. 2010;302(3):44–49.

Robinson W. Epiphenomenalism. In Zalta EN, ed. *The Stanford Encyclopedia of Philosophy* (Summer 2012 ed.). http://plato.stanford.edu/archives/sum2012/entries/epiphenom-enalism/>. Accessed October 20, 2013.

Sherrington C. *Man and His Nautre*. Cambridge, UK: Cambridge University Press; 1953.

Tamietto M, de Gelder B. Neural bases of the non-conscious perception of emotional signals. *Nat Rev Neurosci.* 2010;11:697–709.

Tononi G, Edelman GM. Consciousness and complexity. *Science.* 1998;282:1846–1851.

Zeman A. Consciousness. *Brain.* 2001;124:1263–1289.

14 Pain: Present and Future Considerations

The important thing in science is not so much to obtain new facts as to discover new ways of thinking about them.
–Sir William Lawrence Bragg

INTRODUCTION

Technological advancement is a frequent precursor to the acquisition of new scientific information. This is no truer than when one examines the data generated by modern neuroimaging techniques in the arena of pain. However, the context in which this information is interpreted may enhance or limit it usefulness. Perpetuating existing philosophical predilections and models may artificially restrict expanding into and the exploration of novel hypotheses about the nature of pain, especially clinical pain. Throughout this book there has been an emphasis on broadening the view of pain by incorporating some concepts from systems theory and quantum mechanics. This final chapter will (a) consider the potential effect of an expanded view of pain on its treatment, (b) revisit the impact of recent data on the existing notion of a pain matrix, and (c) highlight some areas for future exploration.

SYSTEMS APPROACH TO TREATMENT

Conceptualized as an emergent phenomenon, pain, especially chronic pain, is an entity greater than the sum of its parts and not reducible to its individual nociceptive mechanisms. Therefore, treatments would need to extend beyond that which focuses solely on the hypothesized pain generator. Understanding the patient and their pain as a complex-adaptive system requires a treatment algorithm with flexibility. Chapman et al (2008; see Chapter 8) have gone to great lengths to outline a supersystem, its nested subsystems, and the various types of dysfunction and dysregulation that can occur. Within this model there is some urgency about introducing effective treatments to prevent the patient from going over the precipice and the system transitioning to a state of decomplexification.

Chen et al (2013) provided an example of this type of systems-focused approach using a group of patients with temporomandibular disorders (TMD). They selected 25 markers, such as circulating cytokines, pain sensitivity, somatic awareness, and resting heart rate, from four regulatory domains: sensory, autonomic, inflammatory, and psychological. They described these regulatory domains as "interconnected and...integrated in the central nervous system (CNS) to maintain homeostasis. Because of this interconnectivity between different regulatory domains and the parallel multisystem modulation within the CNS, multiple compensatory systems contribute to pain processing and modulation" (p. 984). The presence and magnitude of these markers were assessed and totaled for each domain (system). A higher score reflected a greater degree of impairment and disability (system dysregulation). The combined score represented a multisystem dysregulation index (MDI). Using the MDIs they identified the presence of several subgroups of patients, prompting them to suggest that heterogeneous multisystem dysregulation may exist in the TMD population. The degree of functional connectivity among these markers and domains has yet to be studied but could be determined by the manner in which altering one marker or domain would affect the others.

With careful history-taking and examination, one often can identify those at risk for heart attack, diabetes, and hypertension, and preventative measures can be taken. Sometimes the disease can be prevented or the degree to which it manifests itself can be altered. It is theoretically possible that combining the approaches and information such as that from Borsook et al (2011a,b), Chapman et al (2008), and Chen et al (2013) may ultimately lead to the identification of markers/biomarkers and domains, including neurochemical, neurophysiological, hormonal, and psychosocial variables that render an individual vulnerable to the emergence of chronic pain (see Epigenetics and Endophenotypes section later in this chapter). Targeted screening could reveal the signs of potential or already existing evidence of system dysfunction and dysregulation and prompt the introduction of preventative or modulatory interventions.

As a hypothetical construct, pain becomes a euphemism for a complex and dynamic interaction among a variety of symptoms. Nociceptive input, mood, disability behavior, personality, coping, acceptance, pharmacological use, readiness for change, dependence of the medical system, subjective pain rating, and activity engagement may each play a role. At any given time the constellation of variables that assume prominence can vary. From this perspective, treating chronic pain would demand a multidisciplinary, multifactorial, and flexible approach. The therapeutic target or targets could vary from patient to patient and within the same patient over time. Outcome measures would favor goal achievement within the individual rather than assuming the same goal—a reduction in subjective pain rating—to be equally relevant and enduring across time for each patient. Tinetti and Fried (2004) believe this type of integrated, individually tailored model should replace the existing disease-oriented model in which the disease rather than the patient is the focus of treatment.

The management of pain, like that of diabetes and hypertension, becomes an ongoing process and not a single event or intervention. Changing one aspect of a dynamic system can provoke a cascade of other changes—hopefully adaptive, but possibly not. Thus there is the need for ongoing assessment. The patient's role is critical given our understanding of the importance of the mind and brain. The term *self-directed neuroplasticity* (Schwartz et al, 2005) becomes very descriptive and meaningful regarding the patient's involvement.

Surgical correction of anatomical deformities and removal of tumors and diseased organs will continue to be part of treating pain. Advances in technology have made some surgeries less destructive and minimally invasive. The use of interventional and minimally invasive therapies and surgery is growing rapidly (Alo et al, 2011). The term *minimally invasive* applies only insofar as it relates to the amount of dissection and structural damage that occurs as a consequence of the procedure. Implantable devices are finding new applications, including stimulation of specific areas of the brain. Radiation oncologists are currently using very sophisticated instruments, such as stereotactic devices, linear accelerators, the gamma knife, and laser beams, to irradiate tumors. The use of such technology to target areas of the pain processing matrix, such as the anterior cingulate cortex (ACC) (cingulotomy), is under way.

However, the destruction of cortical structures carries with it many inherent dangers. One alternative to destructive procedures may be the use of intracranial stimulation to enhance the activity of pain-competitive or pain-suppressive areas of the brain, much the same as one does with counterstimulation in the periphery. What changes these procedures are likely to provoke at the molecular and system level are yet to be determined. Such medically oriented treatments may facilitate the development of dysfunction or dysregulation, making it more difficult for the system to adapt and approach a state of normal homeostasis or homeodynamics.

Psychological and behavioral treatments aimed at altering the system and influencing network connectivity should be considered over more destructive interventions that may introduce further uncertainty and functional anomalies interfering with the normal homeostatic and homeodynamic activity of the system. Jensen (2010) has linked various psychological symptoms to certain cortical regions and matched these to one or more psychological treatments known to affect these behaviors or symptoms. Presumably, if successfully implemented, there would be an adaptive change in the particular part of the brain targeted. For example, maladaptive pain-related cognitions involving the prefrontal cortex are addressed by cognitive and acceptance-based therapies; heightened pain sensitivity involving the sensory cortex is approached with self-hypnosis and relaxation training; elevated affective component involving the ACC is treated with operant-conditioning, motivation interviewing, and acceptance-based therapies. This self-directed neuroplasticity may occur at the conscious and nonconscious level, affecting the affective and perceptive components of the conscious experience of pain.

Pain memories are a product of peripheral sensitization, central sensitization, and cortical reorganization. Alterations in the production, availability, and activity of neurochemicals associated with nociception and pain processing, and changes in neurophysiological processing and cortical plasticity contribute to the establishment of these "memories." Song and Carr (1999) and Flor (2002) have provided convincing arguments for the contribution of these memories to chronic pain. The use of GABA and NMDA antagonists along with sensory discrimination training and psychological treatments may prevent or reverse these pain memories. Early, aggressive, and more comprehensive treatments of this type may minimize the need for more destructive procedures.

Advances in pharmacodynamics and pharmacokinetics will lead to the development of more effective drugs and patient selection. Studies involving the melanocortin-1 receptor gene (*MC1R*) have already found it to be nonfunctional in natural redheads with fair skin. This gene is linked to the activity of the kappa-opioid receptor. Pentazocine is a well-known kappa-opioid antagonist. Red-headed females demonstrating a nonfunctional MC1R receptor reported much higher levels of pain relief than that in similar groups with a functional MC1R receptor (Gear et al, 1996; Mogil, 2008). Certain genotypes appear to respond differentially to different opioids. In addition, Nagi and Piñeyro (2011) have identified the cellular and molecular basis for developing and antiopioid-tolerance system. The idea of point-of-care genotyping to determine at-risk patients and for implementing a pain-prevention or pain-relief treatment is attractive. At present, however appealing this personalized pain medicine seems, additional work is needed to overcome the low rate of replication among genetic association studies and therefore ensure the accuracy and validity of the findings (Muralidharan and Smith, 2011).

Future treatment may focus on restoration of normal structure and function via transplantation instead of compensating for a dysfunctional or defective system. For example, Braz et al (2012) have transplanted immature GABAergic interneurons form the embryonic rat medial ganglionic eminence (MEG) into the spinal cord of animals with neuropathic pain caused by an experimentally induced sciatic nerve injury. The results showed that MGE cells become neurons and formed functional circuits in the dorsal horn, thereby almost completely reversing the mechanical hypersensitivity. In a sense, this represents a disease-modifying approach to treatment in which the integrity of the system is restored rather than attempting to compensate for the dysfunction or dysregulation.

The current understanding of persistent pain begins with activation of peripheral nociceptors, resulting in peripheral sensitization. With continued input, central sensitization occurs at the level of the spinal cord and, ultimately, functional and structural changes at the cortical level (neuroplasticity). However, "there is no simple leftward shift in the stimulus response curve in the areas of the pain neuromatrix induced by a spinal gain in the transmission of nociceptive signaling" (Seifert and Maihofner, 2011, p. 517); this process is nonlinear but also nonrandom.

Attempts to identify a mechanism to prevent or reverse sensitization as a treatment approach are ongoing. Some evidence from hip replacement studies suggests that when the pain is eliminated, there is a reversal of the loss of cortical gray matter (Rodriguez-Raeche et al, 2013). The precise causes of this loss and whether or not there is a time period beyond which recovery will not occur are unknown. Clearly, removing the presumed nociceptive generator is not always effective, as shown with phantom limb pain following amputation. From a systems perspective there may be a point where a phase transition occurs such that altering nociceptive input will not be sufficient to reverse the newly formed maladaptive connectivity or network. Perhaps the resilience of lower back pain following discectomy could represent a "phantom disc" phenomenon secondary to a presurgical phase transition.

Nanotechnology (manipulating matter on an atomic and molecular level) is a reality. Nanotechnology deals with structures sized between 1 and 100 nanometers; a nanometer represents one-billionth of a meter. Nanoprobes may provide the opportunity to visualize previously unimagined physiological and molecular processes. The potential to alter activity at the receptor level, thus influencing nociceptive transmission, is emerging and may allow one to directly impact the course of neurogensis and neuroplasticity. This technology could render most contemporary pain therapies obsolete. However, in the search to relive pain, the dangers of eliminating it must not be overlooked (see Chapter 12). Cautioned must be exercised when using any approach that completely alters the very nature of the system.

One important distinguishing characteristics of the human system, compared to others, is the mind. Whether the mind is seen as what the brain does, as part of consciousness, some ethereal phenomenon, or part of a universal oneness in the quantum sense, if not unique to humans, it is surely qualitatively and quantitatively different from other species. The undeniable involvement of the mind in pain may render the experience of pain in humans different and potentially incomparable. As part of the system, the mind is affected by many factors but also exerts an enormous "top-down" influence. It may be the ultimate therapeutic target.

MEASURING PAIN

There is a certain amount of philosophical irony that in the midst of the struggle to find a means to measure the experience of pain (see Chapter 6) an agreed-upon definition of pain continues to evolve and remains unsettled, even within the pain research community. A similar degree of uncertainty surrounds the manner in which the outcomes of pain therapies should be evaluated (Younger et al, 2009). The meaning of statistically derived significance and its relationship to clinical significance is a core concern (Farrar et al, 2003; Todd, 1996). Researchers and clinicians alike remain skeptical and uneasy about the reliability and validly of self-report measures and continue to search for an objective measure (biomarker) of pain.

Physiologically based methodology (Brown et al, 2011) represents one approach to the search for an objective measure of pain. Machine-learning algorithms based on fMRI data are used to identify and predict the presence and intensity of pain. Presumably, this eliminates the concerns over the subjective nature of self-reports measures and could benefit those with significant cognitive or communicative disabilities. Marquand et al (2010) applied this approach to examining whole-brain rather than regional-brain activity. Brown et al (2011) and Wager et al (2013) provide other examples of attempts to identify a neurologically or brain-based signature of pain. fMRI data from experimentally induced thermal pain, nonpainful warmth, socially mediated stimuli, and response to short-acting analgesics are collected. Machine-learning algorithms are generated and designed to identify the fMRI images reflecting the presence of pain and its intensity. Accuracy measures approaching 94% have been reported depending on the experimental conditions.

The data obtained from fMRI can be analyzed in a number of ways (Brodersen et al, 2012). Images can be evaluated at the level of the individual voxel, single anatomical region, combination of brain regions, or whole-brain activity. Which of these, if any, will be judged to be the most useful or accurate measure continues to be explored. Similarly, the information can be approached using a univariate or multivariate analysis. The use of a multivariate analysis examining the dependencies between voxels compared to a univariate analysis revealed that the significance assigned to a specific brain region via univariate analysis was not equivalent to its contribution in the context of the whole-brain view. This observation appears to support the notion of the whole being greater than the sum of its parts.

Brown et al (2011) discussed the need to determine if these support vector machine (SVM) models will differentiate physical pain from anticipatory pain, pain empathy, imagined pain, and pain secondary to social exclusion. A note of caution is needed regarding the separation of "physical" pain from that presumed to be more affectively based. Intended or not, this could re-energize the psychogenic pain, mind–body, and "real" vs. "unreal" pain controversy. Alternatively, the experience of pain could be addressed as an emergent phenomenon (hypothetical construct; see earlier discussion) consisting of multiple components (physical and affective) interacting in a complex and dynamic fashion. Linear-based physiological methodologies may or may not be capable of detecting the essence of the experience. It is worth considering how one would approach the patient whose neurological signature differs significantly from the self-report data. Does one treat the brain or the person?

This area of exploration and the manner in which the results are interpreted could have a profound effect on the paradigm through which pain is viewed. The development of therapeutic approaches and targets and the manner in which treatment outcomes are evaluated will also be influenced (Younger et al, 2009). For example, the same neural networks appear to be involved in both opioid and placebo analgesia (Petrovic, 2005). Therefore, the effectiveness of a therapy may well be determined by its impact on the neural network associated with the experience of pain, regardless of the degree to which the therapy alters the presumed nociceptive mechanism (neuropathic, nociceptive, inflammatory). This could stimulate a greater interest in treatments that have fewer negative anatomical and physiological consequences.

Robinson et al (2013) have called into question any attempt to consider functional neuroimaging data as a proxy for the patient's self-report. Given that the brain is part of the individual (the self), perhaps neuroimaging data should be considered another form of self–report. The information on which machine vector learning algorithms are based arises from the patient's verbal self-report. Without the expression or acknowledgment of pain in some form or another, the meaning of neuroimaging data is open to speculation. The absence or disruption of the normal communicative or cognitive processes is likely to be associated with structural or functional alterations compared to the "normal" brain (Borsook, 2012; Cole et al, 2011). It therefore begs the question to assert that the neuroimaging data from a verbal and cognitively intact brain (patient) would be comparable to that from the nonverbal and cognitively altered brain (patient). There may be advantages to developing a multidimensional patient-specific pain profile within which the valence of the various components varies and changes over time.

THE PAIN MATRIX REVISITED

The pain matrix, generally consisting of S1 and S2 somatosensory cortices, insular, prefrontal cortex, and cingulate cortex, has been referred to frequently in this book. This network of brain regions is often considered to constitute a unique cortical signature for pain perception (a biomarker) and an objective measure of pain. The pain matrix has also been associated with the pain experienced as a result of empathy or social rejection. Melzack's notion of a neuromatrix was the forerunner of the pain matrix.

The present concept of the pain matrix, however, has been challenged. Some have suggested using the phrase "neuronal matrix" to reflect a more generic function; others encourage using the salience detection system (Cauda et al, 2012; Iannetti and Mouraux, 2010; Legrain et al, 2011; Mouraux et al, 2011). According to Iannetti and Mouraux (2010) the neuromatrix was proposed precisely because "spatially segregated cortical regions specifically devoted to the perception of pain" could not be identified. The function of the neuromatrix was not limited to the perception of pain. Indeed, the neuromatrix was described as a "widespread ensemble of neurons integrating various sources of input, both nociceptive and non-nociceptive." Therefore, it was not pain specific; "the neuromatrix, distributed throughout many areas of the brain, comprises a widespread network of neurons that generates patterns, processes information that flows through it and ultimately produces the pattern that is felt as a whole body possessing a sense of self" (Melzack, 2005; quoted from Iannetti and Mouraux, 2010, p. 3). The experience of pain was a product of the "transient binding of a widespread network of neurons" rather than the encoding of nociceptive-specific neurons located in spatially segregated regions of the brain.

Iannetti and Mouraux (2010) put forth a number of arguments for reconsidering the nature of the pain matrix. First, nociceptive-specific neurons are sparsely distributed in cortical regions making up the pain matrix. Although spatially segregated cortical areas devoted to the initial processing of thalamocortical sensory input have been identified for most sensory modalities, no cortical area devoted exclusively to the initial processing of thalamocortical nociceptive input (i.e., a primary nociceptive cortex) has ever been clearly identified. Therefore, nociception may not, in fact, represent a distinct sensory modality.

The second reason for reconsidering the nature of the pain matrix is that although some neuroimaging studies have demonstrated that the magnitude of the pain matrix response can predict the level of perceived pain, others have shown that the magnitude of the response can be entirely dissociated from the intensity of the nociceptive stimulus and the perceived pain.

A third reason is that the context, including the degree of stimulus uncertainty and novelty, in which the pain stimulus is presented influences the magnitude of the pain matrix's response. Fourth, there is strong EEG and fMRI evidence illustrating similar patterns of response to non-nociceptive and nociceptive somatosensory stimuli. In fact, evoked-response potential research has shown that the response to a nociceptive stimulus is a multimodal neuronal activity, including nociceptive, somatosensory, auditory, and visual.

Finally, although direct stimulation of aspects of the pain matrix can elicit a painful sensation, it appears to be rare. Indeed, Ostrowsky et al (2002) produced this effect in only 18.2% of stimulated sites and in only 32.5% of patients. Moreover, there was an overlap in areas in which stimulation was associated with painful and nonpainful responses. Not only are pain and nonpainful areas not spatially distinct, but stimulation of the ACC by Bancaud et al (1976) elicited an arousal or "urge-to-move" response rather than a painful sensation.

Iannetti and Mouraux (2010) suggest that the so-called pain matrix is in fact a multimodal network devoted to the detection of stimulus saliency and prioritizing its access to attentional and executive functions. They believe this concept more closely approximated Melzack's original neuromatrix. Saliency relates to the degree to which a stimulus is in contrast to the rest of the environment—internal or external—rather than any physical characteristic of the stimulus. Although not specific to nociceptive stimuli, such stimuli are considered to have intrinsically high saliency content. This notion is supported by research demonstrating that sudden changes in the sensory environment, independent of their sensory modality, elicit activity within a wide cortical network whose spatial distribution closely matches that of the pain matrix.

Furthermore, they propose a thalamic matrix that projects widely to all sensory and motor cortices, including the ACC. The activity of the thalamic matrix is driven by external inputs but also from widespread corticothalamic input and ascending reticular formation. Iannetti and Mouraux (2010) state: "These anatomical connections suggest a relationship to the orienting response that allows organisms to respond immediately to the occurrence of a change in its environment by triggering broad cortical activation following the detection of salient events, regardless of the sensory modality through which these events are conveyed" (p. 8). The idea of pain perception originating from thalamic rather than cortical neuronal activity dates back to 1911 and appears to have been echoed by Devor's (1999, 2008) emphasis on subcortical structures (see Chapter 13). Cauda et al (2012) interpreted the overlapping activity of pain-related networks with somatomotor-somatosensory and emotional-interoceptive networks as "the central part of an adaptive-control system involved in the processing and integration of salient information coming both from external and internal sources." In effect, the functional significance of the pain matrix becomes that of a "defensive system signaling potentially damaging threats for the body" and initiating appropriate action, rather than the nature of the painful sensation prompted by a noxious stimulus (see discussion of the threat detection system [TDS] in Chapter 11)

Apkarian et al (2009) have proposed a theory of chronic pain that is consistent with the notion of saliency detection. It is based on two fundamental hypotheses. First, "chronic, particularly neuropathic pain, in contrast to acute, subacute, and inflammatory pain states, involves distinct spinal cord nociceptive neurons with distinct supraspinal projections, resulting in distinct supraspinal modification of pain and hedonic circuitry." Second,

the transition from acute to chronic pain involves a time-dependent neural reorganization that initiates a series of events that potentiate one pathway at the cost of the other.... [I]njury-related reorganization and experience-related reorganization together shift the brain circuitry to distinct states in specific chronic pain conditions. This model...takes into consideration brain regions that have not been thought to be pain specific. The main conclusion...is that the transition from acute to chronic pain entails also a transition in the salience of pain, wherein the condition shifts from viewing a painful percept as a sign of external threat into an indication of an internalized disease state. (Apkarian et al, 2009, p. 94)

Chronicity is thus functionally determined, is dependent upon the type of pain, and is related to the reorganization of peripheral and central mechanism pertaining to each pain type.

In general, Apkarian et al differentiate input involving the sensory pathways (acute and inflammatory pain) from the more hedonic and affective pathways (neuropathic).

Inflammatory-type pain involves the peptonergic (substance-P) system with input predominately into lamina I. Encoding is carried out by the thalamus, primary and secondary somatosensory cortices (S1 and S2), insula parabrachial, ACC, and dorsolateral prefrontal cortex DLPFC. Neuropathic conditions involve non-peptide and sodium channel input to lamina II with projections to lamina V. Processing involves the hypothalamus, basal ganglia, amygdala, and medial prefrontal cortex (MPFC). The interaction among these components constitutes the emotional, motivational, and hedonic components, which Apkarian et al theorize to "influence the quality of perceived pain and also modulate nociceptive processing at the spinal cord level through descending pathways."

These authors have reportedly uncovered distinct cortical activation patterns for nociceptive (chronic low back pain [CLBP], osteoarthritis) and neuropathic (complex regional pain syndrome [CRPS], peripheral neuropathic) pain. However, these may not be as distinct as one might imagine. In clinical practice, it is most common to find pain disorders with mixed pathologies. Patients with CLBP are likely to have a neuropathic component. Patients with CRPS often have musculoskeletal and arthritic components. Perhaps, rather than distinct entities these represent modules (Meunier et al, 2012). Within each module would be various numbers of nodes and subnodes representing the multitude of chemical, physiological, and psychological characteristics. The connectivity among the nodes or subnodes within the module would be stronger than that between them. A change in any one node would influence the others in the module. This might help to explain why treating one component of the pain can have an overall beneficial effect.

CHRONIFICATION

In a sense, the real issue is not pain. In its acute form pain serves a necessary and desirable function. It is in its chronic (persistent) form that pain appears maladaptive and indicative of a system functioning far from equilibrium. As a progressive neurodegenerative disease (Apkarian and Scholz, 2006), chronic pain is far different from acute pain. The impact on the entire person (system) must be considered. The question remains, how does pain become chronic and why does this chronification of pain only happen to a minority (estimated 15–20%) of patients who experience acute pain? Are there measures that can be taken to help to prevent pain chronification?

The process of chronification is receiving greater attention. There are a variety of factors that contribute to this process, including genetics; behavioral, neurochemical, and physiological processing; and psychological factors and mood. Farmer et al (2012) have described chronification as the "dynamic interplay between anatomy and function as the brain progresses into persistent pain"—a "dynamic network perspective." They assert that the current perspective is that persistent (chronic) pain (a) is driven by ongoing afferent input, (b) sustained by a local reverberating circuit in the spinal cord, and (c) facilitated by descending pain modulation. Instead, they emphasize the role of mesolimbic circuitry and underlying learning mechanisms—emotional pain learning.

In their model, the cortex (brain) is viewed as a massive and "densely connected network of regions (network nodes)" that can be characterized as a "small-world network." There is a continuous and reciprocal flow of information among hierarchically arranged and functionally distinct entities connected across all scales (fractal or self-similarity). With continued nociceptive input from the periphery and ongoing central changes, the function and structure of the brain regions making up the nodes is altered. This is suggested by gray matter changes noted in fMRI studies and white matter alterations in DTI studies reflecting structural reorganization. Disruption of the underlying networks by disease, nociception, and brain injury can result in alterations of the strength of the existing pathways or degradation of network coherence through shifting connectivity. Farmer et al suggest that there is a shift from the sensory to the hedonic (mesolimbic) brain circuitry with ongoing nociception. Long-term memory traces emerge as a result of structural and functional changes at the synaptic level. Alterations in descending modulation enhance the already existing abnormal processing (central sensitization). It is the continued reinforcement and strengthening of these memory traces that maintain chronic pain.

EPIGENETICS

Epigenetics refers to functionally relevant modifications to the genome that lead to changes in gene function without any concomitant DNA sequence changes (Zhang and Meaney, 2010). There are several mechanisms capable of altering the fashion in which genes are expressed, including DNA methylation, chromatin remodeling, histone modification, and RNA interference (RNAi). The alterations can result in genetic overexpression, underexpression, or silencing. Epigenetic changes can be induced by factors internal or external to the organism and represent a very dynamic process. Nondevelopmental epigenetic changes can be triggered by environmental circumstances, nutrition, and stress. Survival of the system, especially central and peripheral neurons, depends on its ability to adapt to these factors. As DNA structure is inherently stable, this adaptiveness is probably a result of epigenetic regulation of gene expression.

Epigentic vulnerabilities have been found in various types of disorders, including headache, chronic bladder pain, endometriosis, inflammatory and neuropathic pain, low back pain, and the chronification of chronic pain states in general. While gene studies have uncovered some genetically linked pain states and phenotypes (see Chapter 12), understanding the development and treatment of chronic pain states will likely occur at the epigenomic level.

The epigenetic mechanisms referred to here have been summarized and described elsewhere (Buchheit et al, 2012; Denk and McMahon, 2012; Seo et al, 2013; Szyf and Meaney, 2008). Briefly, in chromatin remodeling, chromatin is a protein-based structure around which DNA is wrapped. Histone octamers and their surrounding DNA form a nucleosome, the fundamental building block of chromatin. The N-terminal tail of the histone extends from the nucleosome, rendering it susceptible to modification by acetylation, phosphorylation, and methylation. For example, acetylation adds an acetyl group, increasing gene expression, while deacetylation removes an acetyl group which suppresses gene expression. Likewise, DNA methylation generally "silences" gene expression by preventing the binding of transcription factors and has been associated with cancer, opioid addiction, intervertebral disc degeneration, and low back pain. Noncoding RNA (small interfering RNA [siRNA], micro-RNA [miRNA], short-hairpin RNA [shRNA]) molecules tend to silence gene expression by binding to mRNA, resulting in subsequent degradation of the direct gene product. These molecules may well have value in the treatment of chronic neuropathic pain conditions.

The International Human Epigenome Consortium is attempting to sequence and create maps of cell-specific DNA methylation and histone modifications. In addition, The U.S. National Institutes of Health Roadmap Epigenomics Mapping Consortium is tracking these potential epigenetic biomarkers through analyses at multiple time periods after the development of a disease in an attempt to determine the existence of a causal relationship.

The research investigating epigenetic mechanisms and pain has grown substantially in the last decade. Denk and McMahon (2012) and Crow, Denk, and Mahon (2013) identified three areas of research and summarized the findings: epigenetic regulation of peripheral inflammation, epigenetic gene regulation in pain processing, and epigenetic involvement in plasticity and cortical pain processing. Peripheral inflammatory mediators play a significant role in the development of conditions such as arthritis and colitis. Histone deacetylase (HDAC) inhibitors prevent the removal of acetyl groups from histones and have been shown to be effective in altering the arthritic and painful aspects of juvenile idiopathic arthritis. One advantage of epigenetic-based drugs such as HDAC inhibitors is that, unlike phenotypes based on genetic mutation, those caused by epigenetic processes can, theoretically, be chemically reversed.

Several epigenetic factors, such as histone acetylation and DNA methylation, have been found that can influence the expression of nociceptive genes, thus affecting pain processing in chronic pain states (Buchheit et al, 2012; Denk and McMahon, 2012; Seo et al, 2013). Both systemic and intrathecal administration of HDAC inhibitors proved to be analgesic in models of inflammatory pain. As might be expected, histone acetylation increased expression in pronociceptive genes producing a chronic pain state. DNA methylation produced an abnormal up-regulation in genes associated with inflammatory pain states. Reduced expression of the mu-opioid receptor in neuropathic conditions may be a contributing factor to its diminished responsiveness to opioids. Additionally, increased expression of BDNF could relate to the central hyperexcitability found in inflammatory conditions. Altered expression of potassium channel subunits and the down-reguation of postsynaptic genes may also contribute to nociceptor hyperexcitability.

The fact that postoperative development of chronic pain remains unchecked may be secondary to an inability to prevent epigenetic changes; an estimated 1,000 genes are activated in the dorsal root ganglion alone after injury. The transition from acute to chronic pain appears to be influenced by several epigenetic processes. First, immunological and inflammatory cytokine expression seem to be controlled by epigenetic mechanisms. Second, glucocorticoid receptor (GR) function affects pain sensitivity and inflammation. The onset of autoimmune disease is modulated by post-translational mechanisms and DNA methylation. GRs are protective against an excessive inflammatory response during injury, but GR dysfunction can be associated with fatigue, chronic pain states, and fibromyalgia. However, GR expression may be modified by maternal care, grooming, diet, and early-life stresses. Negative materially influenced expression patterns have been reversed in cross-fostering parent studies (Buchheit et al, 2012; Zhang and Meany, 2010). The third epigenetic process influencing the transition from acute to chronic pain is that genes which code for pain regulatory enzymes in the central nervous system are known to be hypoacetylated and down-regulated in inflammatory and neuropathic pain states. Finally, epigenetic modifications are involved in opioid receptor regulation and function, which suggests their active participation in endogenous pain modulation and pain severity (Buchheit et al, 2012).

The third area of study identified by Denk and McMahon is epigenetic involvement in plasticity and cortical pain processing. Day and Sweatt (2011) have provided a review of the literature on epigenetic processes in the regulation of memory and synaptic plasticity. HDAC2 overexpression affected spine density, synaptic function, and memory consolidation. Histone phosphorylation and methylation affected memory formation. In addition, learning processes, including the induction of long-term potentiation (LPT), could be altered by HDAC inhibitors. The encoding of noxious stimuli in the spinal cord and the brain involves neural plasticity. NDMA receptor function, protein kinase pathways, and BDNF release appear to play a role in this plasticity process. These signaling pathways seem to be epigenetically controlled in the hippocampus in a bidirectional fashion. Furthermore, cortical epigenetic processes are suspected to be involved in the altered connectivity in the ACC and amygdala-altered cortical representation of pain-related somatotopic areas, as well as in the dynamic changes in gray and white matter observed in chronic pain states.

Buchheit et al (2012) and Zhang and Meany (2010) have discussed a variety of opportunities for preventative or remedial strategies based on epigenetics. Early-life stresses are known to stimulate epigenetic processes and may be amenable to therapeutic interventions. As noted previously, HDAC inhibitors have been shown to be analgesic in inflammatory and neuropathic pain models. Glucosamine is one example of a substance that prevents DNA demethylation involving the IL-1beta gene promoter, reduces NF- B, and down-regulates inflammatory cytokine expression. RNAi-based gene-silencing therapies have relieved chronic neuropathic pain. siRNA abolished formalin-induced pain behavior in rats. Injections targeting a subunit of the NMDA receptor eliminated experimentally induced allodynia in mice. Finally, inflammatory hyperalgesia has been successfully prevented using RNAi and targeting TRPV1 channels. Much of this work has been accomplished without significant toxicity; human studies are sure to follow.

Telomeres represent another facet of epigenetic research. *Telomeres* are repetative single-strand DNA sequences that occupy regions at the end of chromosomes. Telomeres are essential for chomosomal stability. They also protect genes from degredation during the process of chromocome replication and from fusing with neighboring chromosomes. If cells were to divide without telomeres, the ends of the chromosomes and the information they contain would be lost. These telomeres, therefore, act as buffers blocking the ends of the chromosomes. They do not replicate fully during cell division and are ultimatley consumed. Therfore, their length may be an indication of aging. However, they are subsequently replenished by the telomerase reverse transciptase enzyme.

Telomere length (TL) has also been associated with psychosocial stressors such as childhood trauma. Indeed, shorter TL has been linked to pessimism in women and longer TL with moderated exercise. Sibille et al (2012) suggest that TL may well represent "a molecular indicator of the biological consequences of pain and stress" (p. 1792) and thus a measure of the overall burden on the "individual system." A study by Hassett et al (2012) found TL to be associated with widespread pain, age, pain sensitivity as measured by quantitative sensory testing, and cortical gray matter volume in a group of fibromyalgic patients compared to normal individuals. They concluded that chronic severe pain, especially with comorbid depression, may make a "unique contribution" to cellular aging.

One of the ironies of epigenetic alterations resides in the fact that DNA methylation, histone acetylation, and RNAi are necessary for normal tissue specialization and neurological development. Yet, each plays a significant role in the induction of chronic pain, especially following nerve injury. The manner in which complex adaptive systems adapt is not always beneficial to the organism. Fortunately, these epigenetically controlled changes have an element of reversibility, though it is unclear if there is an effective time period after which the system demonstrates aspects of decomplexification and enters a new phase state when the alteration can no longer be reversed.

Many questions regarding epigenetics in relation to pain and its treatment have yet to be answered (Seo et al, 2013). For example, what is the epigenetic basis for neuropathic pain and periphperal and central sensitization? How do experience, stress, and memory for pain affect patterns of gene expression in the brain, and are they reversable? Do "emotional" and "physical" pain manifest similar changes in genetic expression? Does pain relief follow the same epigenetic pathways as pain generation? All of these questions in one way or another address the issue of the chronification of pain. Denk and McMahon (2012) note that at the present time much of the data are correlational and a cause–effect relational awaits discovery. Furthermore, it is yet to be determined whether the effects are bidirectional. An understanding of complex and dynamic nature of epigenetic-induced changes in gene expression in complex chronic pain states is in its early stages.

ENDOPHENOTYPES

The search for pain endophenotypes (Tracey, 2011) represents a present and future endeavor. *Endophenotypes* "are measurable components (for example, biochemical, neuroanatomical or cognitive characteristics) of a disease or condition that have simpler links to genetic underpinnings than the disease syndrome itself. Pain endophenotypes could 'fill the gap' between pain behavior and the genes associated with the elusive processes that underlie the experience of pain … and could help to address the questions relating to the etiology of pain" (Tracey, 2011, p. 173). Because many endophenotypes are present before the disease onset and in individuals with heritable risk for disease such as unaffected family members, they can be used to help diagnose and search for causative genes or and the genes. To date, no unequivocal primary nociceptive or pain cortex has been identified. Furthermore, the mechanism by which the flow of neural impulses (information) is transformed into the experience of pain remains unknown. There is growing evidence that this does involve a dynamic multimodal network of brain regions. The search for pain endophenotypes is an attempt to identify biomarkers that may be precursors of pain and perhaps be used to identify those at risk for chronic pain, elucidate the
chronification process, and provide therapeutic targets.

Tracey (2011) reviewed a number of advanced technologies that may facilitate this search. The use of proton magnetic resonance spectroscopy (MRS) can help to unravel biochemical changes. For instance, MRS has shown elevations in glutamate compounds within the amygdala, insula, and thalamus of patients with fibromyalgia. This may represent a potential pain endophenotype. Investigations using proton MRS have also shown elevations in markers of microglia activity in the thalamus associated with inflammatory conditions. Quantitative arterial spin labeling uses magnetically labeled endogenous water in the brain to detect changes in perfusion during tonic, rather than the usual phasic, pain states and is thus more applicable to chronic pain. Spinal cord imaging, near-infrared spectroscopy, and optical imaging represent other possible tools.

Altered functioning in the prefrontal cortex (PFC), which is known to play a major role in pain modulation, has been noted in patients with chronic pain. Identification of the time course within which these alterations occur could represent an endophenotype of the chronification process. Maladaptive, neuroplastic, and volumetric changes in regions of the brain are well documented. PFC thickness is associated with levels of anxiety, depression, and fear extinction. Pre-injury PFC could be an endophenotype for an individual susceptible to developing chronic pain. This may also apply to what Tracey refers to the "endogenous chemical tone." That is, alterations in the release of opioids, dopamine, receptor expression of the chemicals, and polymorphisms in the catechol-O-methyltransferase (COMT) gene may also represent endophenotypes of chronic pain. A summary by Sachy (2010) is a reminder of the widespread involvement of the endogenous opioid system in various psychiatric and psychological conditions, adding further to Tracey's (2011) cautionary note on the interpretation of neuroimaging data.

HUMAN CONNECTOME

After 5 years of funding smaller ventures, the National Institutes of Health launched The Human Connectome Project (www.humanconnectomeprojects.org/) in 2010. The effort is to provide a detailed and complete map of the brain's neurocircuitry. One of the stated goals is to address the neural basis of chronic pain disorders. The enormity of the task is easily recognized given the billions of neurons and trillions of synapses. Sporns (2011; Sporns et al, 2005) presented an outline for approaching the connectome, noting at least two main challenges. First, the brain is highly complex and made up of a large number of structurally distinct and heterogeneous structures that are highly interconnected. Second, the basic structural elements will be difficult to define within a framework of network nodes and connections. Rather than being seen as an example of reductionism, the connectome project emphasizes the integrative aspects of multiple neural networks. It remains to be seen if evidence of nonlocality will be uncovered.

Investigation and analysis can occur at the microscale (single neuron and synapses), macroscale (anatomically distinct brain regions and interregional pathways), or mesoscale (neuronal groups and populations) level. Given the evidence that cognitive functions involve activity and coactivity in a large number of widely distributed neurons, they suggest that the macroscale level is the most appropriate and feasible level of investigation. The vast number of individual connections and rapidly changing dynamics render the microscale impractical if not impossible. Furthermore, some neuroinformatics regarding network characteristics such as clusters of brain regions, hierarchical organization, small-world attributes, distinct functional streams and motifs, and real contributions to global network measures already exist (Meunier et al, 2012). The use of diffusion tensor imaging (DTI) and tractography will play a large role. It is further suggested that cortical mini-columns, generally containing 80 to 100 neurons, serve as the basic function unit for the analysis at the mesoscale.

There will likely be significant individual variability, not unlike with the human genome. These variations may result from genetic differences, developmental and experiential history, gender differences, pathologies, or responses to injury. In addition, the connectome will be dynamic, undergoing changes over time and across developmental stages extending from the embryo to adolescence to adult. Incorporating and accounting for these individual differences will be challenging. Once connectivity networks are established (anatomical connectivity), there remains the task of determining the patterns of independence and dependence (functional connectivity), the causal effects of one neural network on another (effective connectivity), and the manner in which these are interrelated. Once known, the human connectome will contribute substantially to the understanding of brain damage, neurodegenerative processes (including chronic pain), and the manner by which network perturbation can cause dysfunction in the system. This understanding, in turn, will likely stimulate the development of prevention and recovery strategies.

CONCLUSION

Turk, Wilson, and Cahana (2011) presented some sobering results of an evidence-based review of the literature involving some 102 studies covering 16 different treatments for chronic pain, ranging from massage to surgery. They reported limited if any evidence to support the efficacy or effectiveness of any treatment for chronic pain. This despite the fact that a clinically meaningful outcome only requires a global overall improvement of 30%, a two-point reduction on an NRS, or a 35 mm reduction on the VAS (Younger et al, 2009). If true, this observation is both disappointing and discouraging. It is unclear if this represents a problem in the understanding of pain, the way it is treated, the difference between statistical significance so often emphasized in research and clinical significance, or the outcomes pursued. However, it does seem to support the need to carefully examine the prevailing concept of pain.

There are many levels at which pain can be analyzed, including cellular, molecular, nodal, modular, and network (systems neuroscience). The units participating in this system include individual neurons, neuronal populations, and anatomically segregated brain regions capable of forming three types of connectivity: anatomical, functional, and affective. The dynamic complexity of the system is highlighted by its developmental process and the potential for modular decompositions or dysmodularity. However unique pain may be among other human experiences, it does share component parts with other experiences, such as visual and auditory.

Technological advances have aided in efforts to unravel the complex and dynamic nature of pain. Much of the recent investigation has focused on cortical abnormalites. Sullivan et al (2013) have appropriately cautioned against considering pain a disease of the brain, potentially ignoring the person suffering from pain. Rather, pain is seen as a complex phenomenon arising from the individuals' physical and social environments.

The brain may indeed be the harbinger of the mind and consciousness, though some would argue that they exist throughout the body, and others that both are more ethereal. The brain should not be considered equal to the mind and consciousness. By considering whole brain activity and the brain as part of a system (person) influenced by and acting on the internal and external environments we can avoid the mereological fallacy of ascribing properties to the parts of a system that should only be ascribed to the whole (Bennett and Hacker, 2003). Furthermore, a preoccupation with technology can promote what William James referred to as medical materialism (reductionism), potentially reducing the experience of pain only to that which technology allows to be seen. The search for biomarkers of pain should continue, as it will no doubt enhance the appreciation for its complexity. However, it is hard to imagine that the experience of pain will be confined to the constraints of Newtonian physics.

Given the present information on pain, it would be difficult to conceptualize pain as anything other than an emergent phenomenon. Patrick Wall's 1995 comment that "it remains an act of faith to continue searching the brain and spinal cord for some still undiscovered nest of cells whose activity reliably triggers pain" (p. 741) seems even more prophetic. In like fashion, Sullivan et al (2013) assert that while pain involves the brain, it does not exist in the brain. Deeper exploration into the nature of the pain experience await a means of examining the functioning human behaving in a natural environment.

Formulating an understanding of the dynamic and complex nature of pain, the patient experiencing pain, and the society and culture in which it exists poses many challenges. By expanding the current view of pain beyond the focus of the nociceptive system of specific regions of interest in the brain we may gain a greater or at the very least different level of comprehension. Recognition of the complexity and dynamic nature of the system involved may redirect our attention and focus. Theorizing outside the boundaries of materialism and reductionism, without necessarily ignoring their contributions, could stimulate novel avenues of research and treatment. Efforts to uncover effective treatments that maintain the adaptiveness of the system should continue to be a priority and are in line with the changing perception of pain as involving a homeostatic and homeodynamic process.

REFERENCES

Alo K, Deer T, Levy R, Slavin K, eds. The evolving use of minimally invasive surgery for the treatment of pain. *J Neurosurg Rev.* 2011;1(S1):1–97.

Apkarian AV, Baliki MN, Geha PY. Towards a theory of chronic pain. *Prog Neurobiol.* 2009;87(2):81–97.

Apkarian WV, Scholz J. Shared mechanisms between chronic pain and neurodegenerative disease. *Disease Mechanisms.* 2006;3(3):319–326.

Bancaud J, Talairach J, Geier S, Bonis A, Trottier S, Manrique M. Behavioral manifestations induced by electric stimulation of the anterior cingulate gyrus in man. *Rev Neurol (Paris).* 1976;132:705–724.

Bennett M, Hacker P. *Philosophical Foundations of Neuroscience.* New York: Oxford University Press, 2003.

Borsook D. Neurological diseases and pain. *Brain.* 2012;135:320–344.

Borsook D, Becerra L, Hargreaves R. Biomarkers for chronic pain and analgesia: Part 1: The need, reality challenges, and solutions. *Discovery Med.* 2011a;11(58):197–207.

Borsook D, Becerra L, Hargreaves R. Biomarkers for chronic pain and analgesia: Part 2: How, where, and what to look for using functional imaging. *Discovery Med.* 2011b;11(58):209–219.

Bragg WL. http://quotationsbook.com/quote/20045

Braz JM, Sharif-Naeini R, Vogt D, Kriegstein A, Alvarez-Buylla A, Rubenstein JL, Basbaum AL. Forebrain GABAergic neuron precursors integrate into adult spinal cord and reduce injury-induced neuropathic pain. *Neuron.* 2012;74:663–675.

Brodersen KH, Wiech K, Lomakina EI, et al. Decoding the perception of pain from fMRI using multivariate pattern analysis. *Neuroimage.* 2012;63:1162–1170.

Brown JE, Chatterjee N, Younger J, Mackey S. Towards a physiology-based measure of pain: patterns of human brain activity distinguish painful from non-painful thermal stimulation. *PLoS ONE.* 2011;6(9):e24124, 1–8.

Buchheit T, Va de Ven T, Shaw A. Epigenetics and the transition from acute to chronic pain. *Pain Med.* 2012;13:1474–1490.

Cauda F, Torta DM-E, Sacco K, et al. Shared "core" areas between the pain and other task-related networks. *PLoS ONE.* 2012;7(8):e41929.

Chapman CR, Tuckett RP, Song CW. Pain and stress in a systems perspective reciprocal neural, endocrine and immune interactions. *J Pain.* 2008;9(2):122–145.

Chen H, Nackley A, Miller V, Diatchenko L, Maixner W. Multisystem dysregulation in painful temporomandibular disorders. *J Pain.* 2013;14(9):983–996.

Cole L, Gavrilescul M, Johnston LA, Gibson SJ, Farrekk MJ, Eagan GF. The impact of Alzheimer's disease on the functional connectivity between brain regions underlying pain perception. *Eur J Pain.* 2011;15(6):568.e1–568.e11.

Crow M, Denk F, McMahon SB. Genes and epigenetic precoesses as prospective pain targets. *Genome Med.* 2013;5:12.

Day JJ, Sweatt JD. Epigenetics mechanisms in cognition. *Neuron.* 2011;70:813–829.

Denk F, McMahon SB. Chronic pain: emerging evidence for the involvement of epigenetics. *Neuron.* 2012;73:435–444.

Devor M. Avenues to the future of pain research. *e-News for Somatosensory Rehabilitation.* Ronald Melzack special issue. 1999 (June).

Devor M. Consciousness and pain. In Bushnell KC, Basbaum AI, eds. *The Senses: A Comprehensive Reference.* New York: Elsevier, 2008:961–969.

Farmer MA, Baliki MN, Apkarian AV. A dynamic network perspective of chronic pain. *Neurosci Lett.* 2012;520:197–203.

Farrar JT, Berlin JA, Strom BL. Clinically important changes in acute pain outcome measures: a validation study. *J Pain Symptom Manage.* 2003;25:406–411.

Flor H. Painful memories: can we train chronic pain patients to forget' their pain? *EMBO Rep.* 2002;3(4):288–291.

Gear RW, Miaskowski C, Gordon NC, Paul SM, Heller PH, Levine JD. Kappa-opioids produce significantly greater analgesia in women than in men. *Nat Med.* 1996;2:1248–1250.

Hassett L, Epel E, Clauw DJ, et al. Pain is assaociated with short leukocyte telomere length in women with fibromyalgia. *J Pain.* 2012;13(10):959–969.

Iannetti GD, Mouraux A. From the neuromatrix to the pain matrix (and back). *Exp Brain Res.* 2010;205:1–12.

Jensen MP. Neurophysiological model of pain: research and clinical implications. *J Pain.* 2010;11(1):2–12.

Legrain V, Iannetti GD, Plaghki L, Mouraux A. The pain matrix reloaded: a salience detection system for the body. *Prog Neurobiol.* 2011;93:111–124.

Marquand A, Howard M, Brammer M, et al. Quantitative prediction of subjective pain intensity from whole-brain fMRI data using Gaussian processes. *Neuroimage.* 2010;49:2178–2189.

Melzack R. Evolution of the neuromatrix theory of pain. The Prithvi Raj Lecture: presented at the third World Congress of World Institute of Pain, Barcelona 2004. *Pain Pract,* 2005;5:85–94.

Meunier D, Lambiotte R, Bullmore ET. Modular and hierarchically modular organization of brain networks. *Front Neurosci.* 2012;4 (article 200):1–11.

Mogil, JS. The nature and nurture of pain: The role of genetics and environmental issues in the experience of pain. In Mahajan G, Fishmen SM, eds. *Plenary Proceedings of the 24th Annual Meeting of the American Academy of Pain Medicine, AAPM, Glenview, IL.* 2008:81–94.

Mouraux A, Diukova A, Lee MC, Wise RG, Iannetti GD. A multisensory investigation of the functional significance of the "pain matrix." *Neuroimage.* 2011;54:2237–2249.

Muralidharan A, Smith MT. Pain, analgesia and genetics. *J Pharm Pharmacol.* 2011;63:1387–1400.

Nagi K, Piñeyro G. Regulation of opioid receptor signaling: implications for the development of analgesic tolerance. *Mol Brain.* 2011;4(25):2–9.

Ostrowsky K, Magnin M, Ryvlin P, Isnard J, Guénot M, Mauguière F. Representation of pain and somatic sensation in the human insula: a study of responses to direct electrical cortical stimulation. *Cereb Cortex.* 2002;12(4):376–385.

Petrovic P. Opioid and placebo analgesia share the same network. *Semin Pain Med.* 2005;3:31–36.

Robinson MA, Staud R, Price DD. Pain measurement and brain activity: will neuroimaging replace pain ratings? *J Pain.* 2013;14(4):323–327.

Rodriguez-Raeche R, Niemeier A, Ihler K, Ruether W, May A. Structural brain changes in chronic pain reflect probably neither damage or atrophy. *PLoS ONE.* 2013;8(2):e54475.

Sachy TH. Use of opioids in pain patients with psychiatric disorders. *Pract Pain Manage.* 2010;10(7):17–26.

Schwartz JM, Stapp HP, Beauregard M. Quantum physics in neuroscience and psychology: a neurophysical model of mind–brain interaction. *Philos Trans R Soc Lond B Biol Sci.* 2005;360(1458):1309–1327.

Seifert F, Maihofner C. Functional and structural imaging of pain-induced neuroplasticity. *Curr Opin Anesthesiol.* 2011;24:515–523.

Seo S, Grzenda A, Lomberk G, Ou XM, Cruciani RA, Urrutia R. Epigenetics: a promising paradigm for better undestanding and managing pain. *J Pain.* 2013;14(6):549–557.

Sibille KT, Witek-Janusek L, Mathews HL, Filligim RB. Telomeres and epigenetics: potential relevance to chronic pain. *Pain.* 2012;153:1789–1793.

Song S, Carr DB. Pain and memory. *Pain: Clinical Updates.* 1999;7(1):1–7.

Sporns O. The human connectome project: a complex network. *Ann N Y Acad Sci.* 2011;1224:109–125.

Sporns O, Tononi G, Kötter R. The human connectome: a structural description of the human brain. *PLoS Comput Biol.* 2005;1(4):e42.

Sullivan MD, Cahana A, Derbyshire S, Loeser JD. What does it mean to call chronic pain a brain disease? *J Pain.* 2013;14(4):317–322.

Szyf M, Meaney MJ. Epigenetics, behaviour, and health. *Allergy Asthma Clin Immunol.* 2008;4(1):37–49.

Tinetti ME, Fried T. The end of the disease era. *Am J Med.* 2004;116:179–185.

Todd KH. Clinical versus statistical significance in the assessment of pain relief. *Ann Emerg Med.* 1996;27:439–441.

Tracey I. Can neuroimaging studies identify pain endophenotypes in humans? *Nat Rev Neurol.* 2011;7:173–181.

Turk DC, Wilson HD, Cahana A. Treatment of chronic non-cancer pain. *Lancet.* 2011;377:2226–2235.

Wager TD, Atlas LY, Lindquist MA, Roy M, Woo C, Kross E. An fMRI-based neurologic signature of physical pain. *N Engl J Med.* 2013;368(15):1388–1397.

Wall P. Independent mechanisms converge on pain. *Nat Med.* 1995;1:740–741.

Younger J, McCure R, Mackey S. Pain outcomes: a brief review of instruments and techniques. *Curr Pain Headache Rep.* 2009;13(1):39–43.

Zhang TY, Meaney MJ. Epigenetics and environmental regulation of the genome and its function. *Annu Rev Psychol.* 2010;61:439–466.

Appendix
Introduction to Genetics:
Terms and Definitions

Genes make up segments of DNA (deoxyribonucleic acid) occurring at specific points on the chromosomes by which hereditary characteristics are determined and transmitted. Genes are the basic units of heredity, and most are pleiotropic in that they are involved in the mediation of several traits. Genes are like recipes providing information needed by the organism to build or perform a given function. Human DNA contains about 23,000 of these "recipes" (genes). Genes contain both coding sequences that determine what the gene does, and non-coding sequences that determine when the gene expresses itself. Genes can be expressed in a cell, tissue, or organ. The patchy coloring on a cat, for example, reflects different levels of expression of the pigmentation genes on different areas of the skin.

When active, the coding and non-coding sequences of the gene are copied, resulting in an RNA (ribonucleic acid) copy of the gene's information. This process is called *transcription*. This piece of RNA can now direct the synthesis of proteins through the application of the genetic code. *Gene products* are those molecules resulting from gene expression, whether RNA or protein. These gene products are responsible for the development and functioning of all living things. In the past, it was thought that genetic information only flowed in one direction, that is, DNA to RNA to proteins, which would then determine the genetic trait. However, it is now clear that the information flow is bidirectional, that is, proteins can affect how DNA is read.

Each person has an individual genotype. Humans have two copies (alleles) of each gene. A trait *is* determined by the combination of inherited alleles. If one allele overrides another it is the *dominant* allele and the other, the *recessive* allele. The *genotype* refers to all of the genes or alleles a person inherits. How these genes express themselves is our phenotype. The *phenotype* represents the observable traits or manifest characteristics of an organism including anatomical and psychological, resulting from both heredity and its environment. A person's phenotype may differ from their genotype. Diseases, drugs, environment, and learning can influence gene expression; this is called *epigenetics*.

The term *epigenetics* has been used to describe heritable changes in gene expression that do not involve DNA mutation. For example, a particular male might inherit genes associated with height, but if he comes from an underdeveloped country and does not have adequate nutrition, these genes may not get fully expressed and the man would be shorter than one with a similar genotype but with access to better nutrition. More to the point, one's susceptibility to cancer is reflected in the oncogene. When mutated or expressed at high levels, the oncogene helps to turn a normal cell into a cancer cell. However, its expression is greatly influenced by lifestyle, for example, smoking, diet, and stress. Environmental stresses have been shown to alter genetic expression in the pregnant female which can be passed on to the offspring in the form of increased vulnerability and susceptibility. This is referred to as epigenetic modification of gene expression (EMGEX). These basic examples help to emphasize the importance of examining the interaction between genes and the environment ($G \times E$) and should discourage adoption of a genetic determinism view.

The function of genes is to provide information necessary for the production of protein molecules in cells. Proteins consist of chains of 20 different amino acids and carry out most of the functions required for the cell to live. Proteins (a) form the structural basis for many biological tissues, (b) catalyze chemical actions, (c) transport molecules across lipid barriers, and (d) receive molecular signals. Cells are the smallest functioning units in the human body, which contains about 100 trillion cells. All cells contain the same DNA sequence, or genome. An individual's particular DNA sequence is his or her genotype and unique biological traits. A cell's transcriptome determines how the genes are transcribed into proteins (the cell's proteome). Although biological traits are determined by the genome, the manner in which the organism appears physically, functions, perceives, and processes events is determined by the proteome. Environmental factors are capable of affecting the transcriptome and proteome and thus of influencing the phenotypic expression of the genome.

DNA represents a molecule made up of a chain of four different nucleotides: A (adenine), T (thymidine), G (guanine), and C (cytosine). These nucleotides must match up in a specific fashion and are referred to as *base pairs*. Chromosomes are composed of both proteins and DNA. Chromosomes carry a single long piece of DNA and provide a mechanism for carrying DNA into the cell, conveying hereditary information. The largest human chromosome contains about 247 million base pairs. In essence, genes give instructions and proteins carry them out. A sequence of nucleotides in the gene is translated by the cells producing amino acid chains, which in turn create proteins. Some complex proteins function as enzymes and are capable of serving as a catalyst to stimulate chemical changes in other substances without undergoing any changes themselves. A change in the DNA of a gene can result in changes in the protein's amino acids. This can have a remarkable effect on the organism as a whole. Cells use the DNA to manufacture a matching messenger RNA (mRNA). This process is called *transcription*. mRNA passes through a structure called a *ribosome*, which translates the sequence of nucleotides in the RNA into the correct sequence of amino acids. These amino acid sequences are then joined to make up a complete protein chain. *Translation* is the process of moving the information from the language of the DNA into the language of amino acids.

When the sequence of the DNA in a gene is changed, a mutation is said to have occurred. The genome cannot be altered by the environment but can be by mutated DNA. Mutations create new alleles that have new DNA sequences, resulting in the production of proteins with new properties. For example, animals with a color of fur that makes them easily identified by their natural predators will ultimately have a genetic mutation that changes the color of the fur. If this new color of fur provides better camouflage, this group is more likely to thrive and reproduce, while the other does not, thus resulting in a new strain. This represents an example of natural selection. Genetic engineering occurs when a new piece of DNA is intentionally introduced into the cell to produce a new trait or characteristic.

Single-nucleotide polymorphisms (SNPs) are common genetic variations and the focus of a good deal of research in the area of pain. A *haplotype* represents a block of such SNPs or alleles. Therefore, in place of searching for a specific SNP, the haplotype map (HapMap) emphasizes a pattern of a few SNPs that make up a given haplotype. In essence, the HapMap is a resequencing of the genome with emphasis on cataloging the more common allelic variations. The allelic differences often involve significant portions of the gene's nucleotide base, whereas the SNP represents a minor alteration in the gene's sequence.

GENETICS IN UNDERSTANDING PAIN: RESEARCH METHODOLOGIES

Common laboratory approaches using animals for the study of genetics in relation to pain include inbreeding, transgenic, and knockout models as a means of studying the effect or effects of altering the organism's genetic makeup. *Inbreeding* is the selective mating of organisms that show strong evidence of the characteristic under study, for example, heightened sensitivity to certain experimental stimuli. Transgenic animals are engineered by incorporating an exogenous gene into the animal's genome. Knockout technology involves the deactivation ("knocking out") of a specific gene as a means of studying its effect. Knockout models of pain-related genes are very rare in nature. Given the necessity of pain for survival, it is doubtful that any such alteration would persist. It is estimated that genetic mutations resulting in decreased pain sensitivity probably occur in well under 1% of the population. Undetected diseases and injuries make it unlikely that these individuals would live long enough to pass on their genetic endowment.

There are a number of common genetic variations that occur naturally in humans which can be used to establish a basis for genetic research. For example, some seven million SNPs are said to exist in at least 5% of the population and another four million in 1 to 4% of the population. In addition, certain experimental procedures can indentify pain-sensitive or pain-insensitive persons (phenotypes), allowing for a comparison of their genetic structure. Technological advances have made it possible to scan for and identify any number genes.

There are three main types of genetic analysis: genetic epidemiology, linkage mapping, and association studies. One example of genetic epidemiology is that of twin studies. This methodology is intended to examine the concordance of a trait or characteristic in monozygotic twins (MZ; identical twins formed from the same egg) compared to dizygotic twins (DZ; fraternal twins). Presumably, all other things being equal, which is a critical consideration, the strength or contribution of heritability can be calculated given that MZ twins share all of the genetic alleles, whereas DZ, much like non-twin siblings, only share half of the genetic alleles. In addition to the use of twin studies to determine heritability, multifactorial traits such as pain can also be studied through family analysis, by comparing polymorphism genotypes with allele transmission through families.

After determining the trait, behavior, or phenotype of interest that is inherited, at least to some degree, it then becomes necessary to determine what gene or genes are responsible. Linkage mapping and genetic association studies are employed for this purpose. The genetic linkage methodology is used to examine the coinheritance of a particular trait of interest and some DNA variant or marker in a specific population over a few generations. Genetic linkage is more common among genetic loci that are located physically close to one another on the same chromosome and thus tend to stay together (genetically linked). A linkage map is a genetic map of a particular group or population which shows the position of its known genes or genetic markers.

Genetic association studies focus on the co-occurrence of a trait and a specific DNA variant, single allele, or genotype frequency among different groups. Genetic association studies are based on the principle that genotypes can be compared directly across independent groups of patients. For example, one can examine multiple pain phenotypes involving specific pain conditions such as temporomandibular disorder or low back pain. Although patients in a particular group may have the same diagnosis, the group itself is likely to be quite heterogeneous. Alternatively, one might examine a broader category of clinical pain, such as postoperative pain or neuropathic pain, each of which would inevitably include numerous subcategories.

Association studies sometimes are limited to a few SNPs at specific genes. One type of association study, the case–control study, involves collecting phenotype data and DNA samples from patients and unrelated controls, followed by genotyping of polymorphisms (usually SNPs) of candidate genes. These candidate genes are chosen on the basis of their encoded proteins being involved (or proposed to be involved) in pathways that are logically expected to affect the phenotype expression. Putative pain candidate genes and pathways are specific genes thought to be involved in pain processing. In contrast to exploring candidate genes, genome-wide association studies obtain genotypes from thousands or even millions of SNPs across the genome of hundreds or thousands of subjects, using high-throughput platforms. ("Throughput" refers to the amount of work a computer can do at any given time. High-throughput screening seeks to screen large numbers of compounds rapidly and in parallel. Positive high-throughput screening results are referred to as *hits*.) As one can imagine, massaging the data is a daunting task, to say the least. Furthermore, this methodology is an expensive venture. PHASE technology can be used to generate haplotypes and diplotypes for tightly linked SNPs within a gene. Along with indentifying one or more SNPs, recognizing haplotypes and diplotypes of strongly associated SNPs within a gene can be the source of invaluable information. The presumed effect of an SNP may, indeed, be a consequence of a nearby functional change or associated with an entire haplotype.

Unfortunately, the failure of one researcher to replicate the findings of another when using genetic association methodology is not uncommon (Chanock et al, 2007). This failure to replicate findings may be attributed to sample size, population stratification, differences in phenotype, or the identification of a rare allele or haplotype that is camouflaged in a larger cohort of subjects. Differences in the ancestral background of the cases may affect allele frequencies. It is also feasible that multiple different pathways are involved in a trait, with some having more impact in certain genetic backgrounds. Max and Stewart (2008) have noted that the use of different statistical methods may yield conflicting results. Most often this is due to finding significance with rare alleles and haplotypes, which would disappear with larger cohorts or analysis of other close SNPs, as that may affect allele frequencies.

Ultimately, it is the establishment of a functional relationship between a particular gene or gene variant, not its mere existence, and an observed trait (pain resistant or pain sensitive) that is meaningful. A gene variant can have its effect "directly on a nociceptive pathway, on a physiological pathway affecting disease susceptibility, or on a psychological pathway secondarily affecting the likelihood of experiencing chronic pain....Multiple genes with relatively small effects likely influence vulnerability to pain, and there may be no correspondence between pain phenotypes and individual genotypes" (Kim et al, 2009, p. 683). For example, patients susceptible to diseases such as diabetes and herpes zoster are more likely to develop pain in the form of diabetic peripheral neuropathy or postherpetic neuralgia, respectively. Some genetic variants alter peripheral nociceptive structure and function. Certain genetic variants may be responsible for the suppression of sodium channels expressing Nav1.8. This type of sodium channel is necessary to the experience of mechanical, cold, and inflammatory pain. Finally, genetic alterations can affect the ability of analgesics such as morphine to suppress pain.

REFERENCES

Chanock SJ, Manolio T, Boehnke M, et al. Replicating genotype–phenotype associations. *Nature.* 2007;447:655–660.

Introduction to genetics. Http://en.wikipedia.org/wik/Introduction-to-genetics

Kim H, Clark D, Dionne RA. Genetic contributions to clinical pain and analgesia: avoiding pitfalls in genetic research. *J Pain.* 2009;10:663–693.

Max MB, Stewart WF. The molecular epidemiology of pain: a new discipline for drug discovery. *Nat Rev.* 2008;7:647–658.

Index

Note: Page numbers followed by *f* or *t* indicate a figure or table.